SUBSTANCE USE DISORDERS
in the U.S. Armed Forces

Committee on Prevention, Diagnosis, Treatment and Management of Substance Use Disorders in the U.S. Armed Forces

Board on the Health of Select Populations

Charles P. O'Brien, Maryjo Oster, and Emily Morden, *Editors*

INSTITUTE OF MEDICINE
OF THE NATIONAL ACADEMIES

THE NATIONAL ACADEMIES PRESS
Washington, D.C.
www.nap.edu

THE NATIONAL ACADEMIES PRESS   500 Fifth Street, NW   Washington, DC 20001

NOTICE: The project that is the subject of this report was approved by the Governing Board of the National Research Council, whose members are drawn from the councils of the National Academy of Sciences, the National Academy of Engineering, and the Institute of Medicine. The members of the committee responsible for the report were chosen for their special competences and with regard for appropriate balance.

This study was supported by the U.S. Department of Defense through an interagency agreement with the U.S. Department of Health and Human Services under Contract No. HHSP23337030T. Any opinions, findings, conclusions, or recommendations expressed in this publication are those of the author(s) and do not necessarily reflect the view of the organizations or agencies that provided support for this project.

International Standard Book Number-13: 978-0-309-26055-8
International Standard Book Number-10: 0-309-26055-8

Additional copies of this report are available from the National Academies Press, 500 Fifth Street, NW, Keck 360, Washington, DC 20001; (800) 624-6242 or (202) 334-3313; http://www.nap.edu.

For more information about the Institute of Medicine, visit the IOM home page at: **www.iom.edu.**

Printed in the United States of America

The serpent has been a symbol of long life, healing, and knowledge among almost all cultures and religions since the beginning of recorded history. The serpent adopted as a logotype by the Institute of Medicine is a relief carving from ancient Greece, now held by the Staatliche Museen in Berlin.

Suggested citation: IOM (Institute of Medicine). 2013. *Substance use disorders in the U.S. armed forces*. Washington, DC: The National Academies Press.

"Knowing is not enough; we must apply.
Willing is not enough; we must do."
—Goethe

INSTITUTE OF MEDICINE
OF THE NATIONAL ACADEMIES

Advising the Nation. Improving Health.

THE NATIONAL ACADEMIES

Advisers to the Nation on Science, Engineering, and Medicine

The **National Academy of Sciences** is a private, nonprofit, self-perpetuating society of distinguished scholars engaged in scientific and engineering research, dedicated to the furtherance of science and technology and to their use for the general welfare. Upon the authority of the charter granted to it by the Congress in 1863, the Academy has a mandate that requires it to advise the federal government on scientific and technical matters. Dr. Ralph J. Cicerone is president of the National Academy of Sciences.

The **National Academy of Engineering** was established in 1964, under the charter of the National Academy of Sciences, as a parallel organization of outstanding engineers. It is autonomous in its administration and in the selection of its members, sharing with the National Academy of Sciences the responsibility for advising the federal government. The National Academy of Engineering also sponsors engineering programs aimed at meeting national needs, encourages education and research, and recognizes the superior achievements of engineers. Dr. Charles M. Vest is president of the National Academy of Engineering.

The **Institute of Medicine** was established in 1970 by the National Academy of Sciences to secure the services of eminent members of appropriate professions in the examination of policy matters pertaining to the health of the public. The Institute acts under the responsibility given to the National Academy of Sciences by its congressional charter to be an adviser to the federal government and, upon its own initiative, to identify issues of medical care, research, and education. Dr. Harvey V. Fineberg is president of the Institute of Medicine.

The **National Research Council** was organized by the National Academy of Sciences in 1916 to associate the broad community of science and technology with the Academy's purposes of furthering knowledge and advising the federal government. Functioning in accordance with general policies determined by the Academy, the Council has become the principal operating agency of both the National Academy of Sciences and the National Academy of Engineering in providing services to the government, the public, and the scientific and engineering communities. The Council is administered jointly by both Academies and the Institute of Medicine. Dr. Ralph J. Cicerone and Dr. Charles M. Vest are chair and vice chair, respectively, of the National Research Council.

www.national-academies.org

COMMITTEE ON PREVENTION, DIAGNOSIS, TREATMENT AND MANAGEMENT OF SUBSTANCE USE DISORDERS IN THE U.S. ARMED FORCES

CHARLES P. O'BRIEN (*Chair*), Kenneth E. Appel Professor of Psychiatry and Vice-Chair of Psychiatry, and Director, Center for Studies of Addiction, University of Pennsylvania School of Medicine, Philadelphia

HORTENSIA D. AMARO, Associate Vice Provost for Community Research Initiatives and Dean's Professor of Social Work and Preventive Medicine, University of Southern California, Los Angeles

RHONDA ROBINSON BEALE, Chief Medical Officer, OptumHealth Behavioral Solutions, Glendale, CA

ROBERT M. BRAY, Senior Research Psychologist and Senior Director of the Substance Abuse Epidemiology and Military Behavioral Health Program, RTI International, Research Triangle Park, NC

RAUL CAETANO, Regional Dean and Professor, Dallas Regional Campus of the University of Texas School of Public Health

MATHEA FALCO, President, Drug Strategies, Inc., Washington, DC

JOYCE M. JOHNSON, Vice President of Health Services, Battelle Memorial Institute, Arlington, VA

THOMAS KOSTEN, J.H. Waggoner Chair and Professor of Psychiatry, Pharmacology and Neuroscience, Baylor College of Medicine, Houston, TX

MARY JO LARSON, Senior Scientist, Schneider Institutes for Health Policy, Heller School, Brandeis University, Waltham, MA

DAVID C. LEWIS, Professor Emeritus of Community Health and Medicine, and the Donald G. Millar Distinguished Professor of Alcohol and Addiction Studies, Brown University, Providence, RI

DENNIS McCARTY, Professor of Public Health and Preventive Medicine and Division Head, Health Services Research, Oregon Health and Science University, Portland

MARY ANN PENTZ, Professor of Preventive Medicine and Director, Institute for Health Promotion and Disease Prevention Research, University of Southern California, Los Angeles

TRACY STECKER, Assistant Professor of Community and Family Medicine, Dartmouth Medical School, Lebanon, NH

CONSTANCE WEISNER, Professor of Psychiatry, University of California, and Associate Director for Health Services Research, Kaiser Permanente, Oakland

IOM Staff

MARYJO M. OSTER, Study Director
EMILY C. MORDEN, Research Associate
JON Q. SANDERS, Program Associate
NANCY LESTER, Uniformed Services University of the Health Sciences Intern (Spring 2012)
ANDREA COHEN, Financial Associate
FREDERICK (RICK) ERDTMANN, Director, Board on the Health of Select Populations

Reviewers

This report has been reviewed in draft form by individuals chosen for their diverse perspectives and technical expertise, in accordance with procedures approved by the National Research Council's Report Review Committee. The purpose of this independent review is to provide candid and critical comments that will assist the institution in making its published report as sound as possible and to ensure that the report meets institutional standards for objectivity, evidence, and responsiveness to the study charge. The review comments and draft manuscript remain confidential to protect the integrity of the deliberative process. We wish to thank the following individuals for their review of this report:

Thomas F. Babor, University of Connecticut Health Center
Mady Chalk, Treatment Research Institute
Arthur T. Dean, Community Anti-Drug Coalitions of America
Michael Fitzsimons, Massachusetts General Hospital
Deirdre Hiatt, Managed Health Network
Cristine S. Hunter, U.S. Office of Personnel Management
Kimberly C. Kirby, Treatment Research Institute
Daniel Kivlahan, VA Puget Sound Health Care System
James McKay, Treatment Research Institute
Thomas McLellan, Treatment Research Institute
Roland S. Moore, Pacific Institute for Research and Evaluation
Rumi Kato Price, Washington University School of Medicine
Eve E. Reider, National Institute on Drug Abuse
Stephen N. Xenakis, U.S. Army (Ret.)

Although the reviewers listed above have provided many constructive comments and suggestions, they were not asked to endorse the conclusions or recommendations nor did they see the final draft of the report before its release. The review of this report was overseen by **Richard J. Bonnie,** University of Virginia, and **Susan J. Curry,** The University of Iowa. Appointed by the National Research Council and the Institute of Medicine, they were responsible for making certain that an independent examination of this report was carried out in accordance with institutional procedures and that all review comments were carefully considered. Responsibility for the final content of this report rests entirely with the authoring committee and the institution.

Preface

Substance abuse has long been an issue of concern for the U.S. population and for its military in particular. Dating as far back as the Revolutionary War, Dr. Benjamin Rush detailed the effects of alcohol on the troops. During the Civil War, addiction to opium prescribed for pain became known as the "soldier's disease." Drug problems in both the military and civilian sectors have intensified throughout the 20th century as the types and formulations of substances being used have increased.

Since the 1970s, the Institute of Medicine (IOM) has been called upon numerous times to advise the government on both medical and legal solutions to the problem of substance abuse. Experts from various fields, ranging from mathematics and epidemiology to pharmacology and law, have spent many hours on about a dozen different committees struggling with this thorny problem, which affects our country on societal, economic, personal, and public health levels. While the popular substances of abuse may shift from decade to decade, the overarching problem continues. In the 21st century, prescription opioid abuse has arisen as a major area of concern while problems of alcohol, nicotine, and stimulants have persisted as well. Research has demonstrated that stress and availability are important background factors for causing the initiation and abuse of drugs. As the United States approaches the end of the longest continuous period of war in our history, the stresses faced by our military population are apparent. Our all-volunteer military has endured long periods of deployment and redeployment in highly taxing and demanding environments. Consequently, posttraumatic stress, traumatic brain injury, substance abuse, and suicide are at very high levels.

Press reports of substance abuse among the military stimulated congressional interest and a call for action. The Department of Defense requested that the IOM take a fresh look at the policies and programs of each of the branches of the military and evaluate the adequacy and appropriateness of their prevention, screening, diagnosis, and treatment of substance use disorders. The committee approached this task by holding public meetings to gather information from representatives of each of the military branches and TRICARE (the military's purchased care health plan), as well as from academic researchers and interested members of the public. The committee also conducted visits to military bases and met with a variety of care providers, including those working in substance abuse specialty programs and those in primary care, behavioral health, and pain management.

The committee requested information from each branch of the military and from TRICARE Management Activity regarding program descriptions, access, utilization, and evaluation results. We also requested data on the providers in the substance abuse programs. We extend our appreciation for the exceptional cooperation from all of those who presented at our meetings, hosted our visits to military bases, and assisted with our information gathering efforts.

In addition, the committee wishes to express our appreciation to the study director, Dr. Maryjo Oster, and to the IOM staff, Ms. Emily Morden, Mr. Jon Sanders, and Dr. Rick Erdtmann.

Charles P. O'Brien, *Chair*
Committee on Prevention, Diagnosis, Treatment and Management of Substance Use Disorders in the U.S. Armed Forces

Acknowledgments

The committee thanks the Department of Defense, the individual service branches, and TRICARE Management Activity for the opportunity to review and comment upon the organization and content of their substance used disorders prevention and treatment services. We appreciate their assistance and collaboration in the review.

Many individuals assisted the committee in its work by providing useful data and presenting information at the committee's public meetings and during its site visits. We thank the following people for their contributions: Capt. Robert DeMartino, Alfred Ozanian, Greg Woskow, Frank Lee, and Diana D. Jeffery, TRICARE Management Activity; Les McFarling, Army Center for Substance Abuse Programs; Charles Gould, U.S. Navy Bureau of Medicine and Surgery; Lt. Col. Mark S. Oordt, U.S. Air Force Medical Operations Agency; Keith Humphreys, Stanford University; Don Jansen, Congressional Research Service; Brig. Gen. Margaret Wilmoth, Office of the Assistant Secretary of Defense for Health Affairs; Col. John J. Stasinos, Department of the Army, Office of the Surgeon General; Capt. Mary Rusher, Naval Medical Center San Diego; Vladimir Nacev, Defense Centers of Excellence; Col. Charles Milliken, Walter Reed Army Institute of Research; Wilson Compton and Eve Reider, National Institute on Drug Abuse; John Veneziano, Marine Corps Consolidated Substance Abuse Counseling Center; Ted Jutson and Jerry Sinel, Navy Drug and Alcohol Counselor School; John Sparks, TRICARE Regional Office-West; Andrea Brooks Tucker, TRICARE Regional Office-South; Marie Mentor, TRICARE Regional Office-North; Frank Maguire, TriWest; Debbie Del Rosario and Gary Proctor, ValueOptions; Ian Schaffer and John Wagoner,

Healthnet Federal Services; John M. Morrow, Substance Abuse and Mental Health Services Administration; Abigail Gewirtz, University of Minnesota; Ron Astor, University of Southern California; Barbara Cohoon, National Military Family Association; Lisa Najavits, Harvard University; Anthony Hassan, University of Southern California; Eugene Moore, Cdr. Joseph B. Lawrence, Josh Devine, and Libby Hearin, TRICARE Pharmacy Operations; Isabel Jacobson, Naval Health Research Center; Lt. Gen. David Fridovich, United States Special Operations Command; Lt. Col. Kevin Galloway, Army Pain Management Task Force; Col. Chester Buckenmaier, Walter Reed Army Medical Center; Anthony H. Dekker, Ben Krepps, and Jennifer Weaver, Fort Belvoir Community Hospital; Chideha Ohuoha, Doryan Dixon, Jorge Grandella, and Susan Jessup, Dewitt Army Hospital, Ft. Belvoir; Bob Huebner, National Institute on Alcohol Abuse and Alcoholism; Col. Charles Engel, Department of Defense Deployment Health Clinical Center; Harold Holder, Prevention Research Center of the Pacific Institute for Research & Evaluation; Daniel Kivlahan, Office of Mental Health Services, Veterans Health Administration; 1Lt. Julianna Petrone, SSgt. Cecilia Cardenas, Paul Ahlberg, SrA. Stephanie Tipton, Kim Perez, Eva Shinka, Myron Horn, and Maj. David Cordry, Keesler Air Force Base; Capt. Mary K. Rusher, Joanne Rigoloso, Capt. Warren Peter Klam, Tara Leverett, Valerie Sudduth, Nelson Ferrer, Richard Arriaga, Steven Sovich, and Steven Hanling, Naval Medical Center, San Diego; LTC Sharette Gray, Nicolette Dennis, MAJ Agius, and April Arrington, Carl R. Darnall Army Medical Center, Fort Hood; Dan Harris, CNA; and Caryn Blitz, U.S. Department of Health and Human Services.

Contents

ACRONYMS AND ABBREVIATIONS xxi

SUMMARY 1

1 INTRODUCTION 15
Background, 16
Charge to the Committee, 19
Approach to the Charge, 20
Organization of the Report, 21
References, 22

2 UNDERSTANDING SUBSTANCE USE DISORDERS IN THE MILITARY 25
Understanding Substance Use Disorders, 25
Scope of the Problem, 29
Development of Military Substance Abuse Policy: A Brief Overview, 30
Composition and Sociodemographic Characteristics of the Armed Forces, 32
Prevalence of Substance Use in the Military, 38
Health Care Burden of Substance Use Disorders, 55
Conceptual Approach to Prevention, Intervention, and Treatment of Alcohol Use Problems, 60
Summary, 62
References, 64

3 THE MILITARY HEALTH SYSTEM 69
Eligibility for Care, 70
Direct Care: Military Treatment Facilities, 74
Purchased Care: TRICARE, 78
Care for Substance Use Disorders for Military Service Members and Dependents, 80
Summary, 83
References, 83

4 CHANGING STANDARDS OF CARE FOR SUBSTANCE USE DISORDERS 85
Health Care Reform and Parity Requirements, 85
Office of National Drug Control Policy's National Drug Control Strategy, 89
National Quality Forum's Voluntary Consensus Standards, 91
Practice Improvement Efforts, 91
Clinical Practice Guideline of the Department of Veterans Affairs and DoD, 93
Summary, 94
References, 94

5 BEST PRACTICES IN PREVENTION, SCREENING, DIAGNOSIS, AND TREATMENT OF SUBSTANCE USE DISORDERS 97
Prevention, 97
Screening, Diagnosis, and Treatment, 107
Summary, 124
References, 124

6 POLICIES AND PROGRAMS ON SUBSTANCE USE DISORDERS 137
Department of Defense, 139
Air Force, 148
Army, 153
Navy, 159
Marine Corps, 162
SUD Policies and Programs for Military Dependents in the Direct Care System, 165
Summary of Key Findings, 169
References, 180

7 ACCESS TO CARE FOR SUBSTANCE USE DISORDERS 185
Framework for Access to Care, 186

Care Availability, Access, and Utilization in the Direct Care System, 192
Care Availability, Access, and Utilization in the Veterans Health Administration, 203
Care Availability, Access, and Utilization in the Purchased Care System, 206
Summary of Key Findings, 216
References, 223

8 **SUBSTANCE USE DISORDER WORKFORCE** 227
Air Force Workforce, 228
Army Workforce, 231
Navy Workforce, 232
Marine Corps Workforce, 235
DoD Efforts to Review Staffing Requirements, 237
Summary of Key Findings, 238
References, 244

9 **CONCLUSIONS AND RECOMMENDATIONS** 247
Increasing Emphasis on Efforts to Prevent Substance Use Disorders, 249
Developing Strategies for Identifying, Adopting, Implementing, and Disseminating Evidence-Based Programs and Best Practices for SUD Care, 254
Increasing Access to Care, 260
Strengthening the SUD Workforce, 265
Conclusion, 269
References, 269

APPENDIXES

A Study Activities 271
B S. 459 (111th): SUPPORT for Substance Use Disorders Act 283
C Section 596 of Public Law 111-84, October 28, 2009 297
D Program Reviews 305
E Features of TRICARE and Related Purchased Care Plans 357
F Workforce Standards for Substance Use Disorder (SUD) Care 361
G Access Standards for TRICARE Prime Enrollees 369
H Levels of Care 371
I Summary of Policy-Relevant Strategies for the Prevention of Alcohol-Related Problems 373
J Biosketches of Committee Members and Staff 381

Tables, Figures, and Boxes

TABLES

1-1 Military Policies Addressing Substance Use Disorders as of February 2009, 18
1-2 Military Policies Addressing Substance Use Disorders as of May 2012, 19

2-1 Size of the Military Active Duty and Reserve Components in Fiscal Year 2010, 33
2-2 Sociodemographic Characteristics of Active Duty and Reserve Component Personnel in Fiscal Year 2010, 35
2-3 Sociodemographic Correlates of Past 30-Day Heavy Alcohol Use, Cigarette Use, and Illicit Drug Use, Including Prescription Drug Misuse, 2008, 44
2-4 Alcohol AUDIT Scores of Active Duty and Reserve Component Personnel, 49
2-5 Health Care Burden Attributable to Substance Use Disorder and Three Other Mental Disorders, and Rank Among 139 Diseases and Conditions, Active Duty Component of U.S. Military, 2011, 57

3-1 Reserve Component Health Care Continuum, 75
3-2 Continuum of Care When on Active Duty, 76
3-3 Military Treatment Facilities That Provide Specialty Care for Substance Abuse, by TRICARE Region, 78
3-4 TRICARE Regions and Contractors, 79

5-1 Best-Practice Domains and Recommendations of the National Institutes of Health's Behavior Change Consortium, 115
5-2 A Delivery System Approach Based on the Center for Substance Abuse Treatment's (CSAT's) Treatment Improvement Protocol No. 47, 117

6-1 Military Programs Mentioning Dependents, 166

7-1 Utilization of Alcohol and Drug Abuse Prevention and Treatment (ADAPT) Services by Active Duty Air Force Personnel, 193
7-2 Army Active Duty Initial Referrals to the Army Substance Abuse Program (ASAP), 195
7-3 Utilization of Substance Abuse and Rehabilitation Program (SARP) Treatment by Active Duty Navy and Marine Corps Members, 198
7-4 Numbers of Active Duty Marines Receiving Substance Abuse Counseling Center (SACC) Screening and Completing Treatment, 199
7-5 Numbers of Dependent Beneficiaries Receiving SUD Care in Military Treatment Facilities by TRICARE Region (FY 2010), 200
7-6 Number of Active Duty Service Members (ADSMs) and Active Duty Family Members (ADFMs) Who Accessed Care at Military Treatment Facilities for an SUD Diagnosis by Type of Service (FY 2010), 200
7-7 Substance Use Disorders of Operation Iraqi Freedom (OIF)/ Operation Enduring Freedom (OEF)/Operation New Dawn (OND) Veterans in Department of Veterans Affairs Programs, 2002-2012, 207
7-8 Number of Operation Iraqi Freedom (OIF)/Operation Enduring Freedom (OEF)/Operation New Dawn (OND) Veterans Treated in Department of Veterans Affairs Programs for an SUD Diagnosis, 207
7-9 Average Number of Beneficiaries by TRICARE Region for Fiscal Year 2010, 210
7-10 Number and Rate per 1,000 Beneficiaries Utilizing the Purchased Care Sector for SUD Care, by TRICARE Region (FY 2010), 210
7-11 Medications for Addiction Treatment Given to Active Duty Service Members and Active Duty Family Member Adult Dependent Beneficiaries (aged 18 and over), All Systems of Care (FY 2010), 212
7-12 Number of Beneficiaries Receiving SUD Care by Type of Purchased Care Facility, North Region (FY 2010), 213

7-13 Number of Beneficiaries Receiving SUD Care by Type of Purchased Care Facility, West Region (FY 2010), 214
7-14 Number of Beneficiaries Receiving SUD Care by Type of Purchased Care Facility, South Region (FY 2010), 214
7-15 Number of Beneficiaries with Claims in Purchased Care Settings, by Type of SUD Care (FY 2010), 215

8-1 Alcohol and Drug Abuse Prevention and Treatment (ADAPT) Workforce, 229
8-2 Army Substance Abuse Program (ASAP) Prevention Workforce, 232
8-3 Army Substance Abuse Program (ASAP) Clinical Workforce as of December 2011, 233
8-4 Substance Abuse Rehabilitation Program (SARP) Workforce, 234
8-5 Substance Abuse Counseling Center (SACC) Workforce, 236

I-1 Ratings of Policy-Relevant Strategies and Interventions, 374

FIGURES

2-1a Active duty component members with and without children, 36
2-1b Reserve component members with and without children, 36
2-2a Active duty component family status, 37
2-2b Reserve component family status, 37
2-3 Substance use trends for active duty military personnel, past 30 days, 1980-2008, 39
2-4 Use of selected categories of illicit drugs, past 30 days, DoD branches, 2002, 2005, and 2008, 40
2-5a Standardized comparisons of active duty component personnel and civilians, heavy alcohol use and past 30-day smoking, by age group, 2008, 46
2-5b Standardized comparisons of active duty component personnel and civilians, past 30-day illicit drug use, by age group, 2008, 47
2-6 Prevalence of alcohol-related disorders among the active duty component (rates per 100,000), 51
2-7 Prevalence of drug-related disorders among the active duty component (rates per 100,000), 52
2-8 Prevalence of alcohol- and other drug-related disorders among the reserve component (rates per 100,000), 53
2-9 Prevalence of alcohol- and other drug-related disorders among dependents, 56

2-10 Incidence rates of acute and chronic alcohol-related inpatient and outpatient cases, active duty component, U.S. military, 2001-2010, 59
2-11 Alcohol use problems and interventions, 60

3-1 Defense Enrollment Eligibility Reporting System (DEERS), 71
3-2 TRICARE organization of services, 72
3-3 The uniformed services, 72
3-4 Terminology related to the uniformed services health care system, 73

7-1 Number of Army Substance Abuse Program (ASAP) treatment enrollments by substance of abuse for fiscal year 2010, 195

H-1 Components of health care delivery systems, 371

BOXES

3-1 TRICARE Patient Priority System, 77

4-1 ACO Accreditation Standards, 87
4-2 Dimensions of American Society of Addiction Medicine's (ASAM's) Patient Placement Criteria, 88
4-3 National Quality Forum's Voluntary Consensus Standards for the Treatment of Substance Use Conditions, 92

6-1 Policies and Directives Related to Substance Use Disorders, 138
6-2 Army Substance Abuse Program (ASAP) Prevention and Treatment Capabilities, 154
6-3 Military Studies of the National Institute on Drug Abuse and National Institute on Alcohol Abuse and Alcoholism, 176

7-1 A Soldier's Untreated Substance Abuse, 189
7-2 DoD-Wide Programs to Increase Access to Behavioral Health Care Services and Encourage Help Seeking, 202
7-3 Access Standards of the Veterans Health Administration for SUD Care, 204
7-4 TRICARE Policies Governing Access to SUD Care, 209

8-1 12 Core Functions of Substance Abuse Counselors, 231
8-2 Psychological Health Risk-Adjusted Model for Staffing (PHRAMS) Diagnosis and Risk Groups, 239

Acronyms and Abbreviations

AA	Alcoholics Anonymous
ABAM	American Board of Addiction Medicine
ABC	Alcohol Brief Counseling
ACO	Accountable Care Organization
ACSAP	Army Center for Substance Abuse Programs
ADAMS	Alcohol and Drug Abuse Management Seminar
ADAPT	Alcohol and Drug Abuse Prevention and Treatment
ADC	alcohol and drug counselor
ADCO	alcohol and drug control officers
ADFM	active duty family member
ADMITS	Alcohol and Drug Management Information Tracking System
ADSM	active duty service member
ADT	active duty training
AFI	Air Force Instruction
AFIP	Armed Forces Institute of Pathology
ALARACT	All Army Activities
APA	American Psychiatric Association
AR	Army regulation
ARI	alcohol-related incident
ARM	Alcohol-Related Misconduct
ASAC	Adolescent Substance Abuse Counseling
ASAM	American Society of Addiction Medicine
ASAP	Army Substance Abuse Program

AUD	alcohol use disorder
AUDIT	Alcohol Use Disorders Identification Test
BAM	Brief Addiction Monitor
BASIC	Building Alcohol Skills Intervention Curriculum
BHIVES	Buprenorphine and HIV Care Evaluation and Support
BHOP	Behavioral Health Optimization Program
BUMED	Bureau of Medicine and Surgery
CARF	Commission on Accreditation of Rehabilitation Facilities
CATEP	Confidential Alcohol Treatment and Education Pilot
CBT	cognitive-behavioral therapy
CDC	Centers for Disease Control and Prevention
CD-MART	Controlled Drug Management Analysis and Reporting Tool
CEOA	comprehensive effects of alcohol
CFR	Code of Federal Regulations
CHCBP	Continued Health Care Benefit Program
CM	contingency management
CO	commanding officer
COBRA	Consolidated Omnibus Budget Reconciliation Act
CoRC	Culture of Responsible Choices
CPG	Clinical Practice Guideline
CSAP	Center for Substance Abuse Prevention
CSAT	Center for Substance Abuse Treatment
CSF	Comprehensive Solider Fitness
DAPA	Drug and Alcohol Program Advisor
DCoE	Defense Centers of Excellence
DDCAT	Dual Diagnosis Capability in Addiction Treatment
DEA	Drug Enforcement Agency
DEERS	Defense Enrollment Eligibility Reporting System
DEFY	Drug Education for Youth
DoD	Department of Defense
DODD	Department of Defense Direction
DODI	Department of Defense Instruction
DOJ	Department of Justice
DOT	Department of Transportation
DRI	drug-related incident
DSM	Diagnostic and Statistical Manual
DUI	driving under the influence
DWI	driving while intoxicated

EAP	Employee Assistance Program
EBP	evidence-based practices
ECF	executive cognitive function
EUDL	Enforcing Underage Drinking Laws
FEHBP	Federal Employees Health Benefits Program
FOCUS	Families OverComing Under Stress
FTE	full-time equivalent
FY	fiscal year
GAO	Government Accountability Office
GAT	Global Assessment Tool
GBL	gamma butyrolactone
GHB	gamma-hydroxybutyric acid
HRB	Health Research Board
HRSA	Health Resources and Services Administration
IC&RC	International Certification and Reciprocity Consortium
ICD	International Classification of Diseases
IDS	integrated delivery system
IDT	Inactive Duty Training
IHI	Institute of HealthCare Improvement
IMCOM	Installation Management Command
IntNSA	The International Nurses Society on Addictions
IOM	Institute of Medicine
IOP	intensive outpatient
JCAHO	Joint Commission on Accreditation of Healthcare Organizations
LCSW	Licensed Clinical Social Worker
LIP	Licensed Independent Practitioner
LMFT	Licensed Marriage and Family Counselor
LOD	line of duty
LPC	Licensed Professional Counselor
LSD	lysergic acid diethylamide
MAAC	Marine Alcohol Awareness Course
MCO	Marine Corps Order
MDMA	3,4-methylenedioxy-N-methylamphetamine
MDR	M2 Data Repository

MEDCOM	Medical Command
MET	motivational enhancement therapy
MHAT	Mental Health Advisory Team
MHS	Military Health System
MORE	My Ongoing Recovery Experience
MOU	Memorandum of Understanding
MTF	military treatment facility
NCQA	National Committee for Quality Assurance
NDAAC	Navy Drug and Alcohol Advisory Council
NDACS	Navy Drug and Alcohol Counselor School
NIAAA	National Institute on Alcohol Abuse and Alcoholism
NIDA	National Institute on Drug Abuse
NOAA	National Oceanic and Atmospheric Administration
NORTH STAR	New Orientation to Reduce Threats to Health from Secretive Problems That Affect Readiness
NQF	National Quality Forum
NRC	National Research Council
NREPP	National Registry of Evidence-Based Programs and Practices
OEF	Operation Enduring Freedom
OIF	Operation Iraqi Freedom
OND	Operation New Dawn
ONDCP	Office of National Drug Control Policy
PC	prevention coordinator
PCM	primary care manager
PCP	phencyclidine
PDHA	Post-Deployment Health Assessment
PDHRA	Post-Deployment Health Reassessment
PDMP	Prescription Drug Monitoring Program
PEC	Pharmacoeconomic Center
PFL	Prime for Life
PHA	Periodic Health Assessment
PHRAMS	Psychological Health Risk-Adjusted Model for Staffing
PMART	Prescription Medication Analysis Reporting Tool
POC	Pharmacy Operations Center
POS	point of service
PREVENT	Personal Responsibility and Values Education and Training
PTSD	posttraumatic stress disorder

RE	Resiliency Element
ROSC	recovery-oriented systems of care
RT	resiliency training
RTCQ	Readiness to Change Questionnaire
SACC	Substance Abuse Counseling Center
SACO	Substance Abuse Control Officer
SAIC	Science Applications International Corporation
SAMHSA	Substance Abuse and Mental Health Services Administration
SAODAP	Special Action Office for Drug Abuse Prevention
SAPST	Substance Abuse Prevention Specialist Training
SARP	Substance Abuse Rehabilitation Program
SBIRT	screening, brief intervention, and referral to treatment
SECNAVINST	Secretary of the Navy Instruction
SIP	Short Index of Problems
SM	service member
STD	sexually transmitted disease
SUAT	Substance Use Assessment Tool
SUD	substance use disorder
SUDRF	Substance Use Disorder Rehabilitation Facility
TAMP	Transitional Assistance Management Program
TAP	Technical Assistance Publication
TBI	traumatic brain injury
TDP	TRICARE Dental Plan
TMA	TRICARE Management Activity
TPR	TRICARE Prime Remote
TRS	TRICARE Reserve Select
TSF	twelve-step facilitation
UPL	Unit Prevention Leader
URI	unit risk inventory
USAF	U.S. Air Force
USMC	U.S. Marine Corps
VA	Department of Veterans Affairs
VET	veterans
VHA	Veterans Health Administration
WHO	World Health Organization
WTB	Warrior Transition Brigade
WTU	Warrior Transition Units

Summary

Problems stemming from the misuse and abuse of alcohol and other drugs are by no means a new phenomenon, although the face of the issue has changed in recent years. National trends indicate substantial increases in the abuse of prescription medications. These increases are particularly prominent within the military, a population that also continues to experience long-standing issues with alcohol abuse. The problem of substance abuse within the military has come under new scrutiny in the context of the two concurrent wars in which the United States has been engaged during the past decade—in Afghanistan (Operation Enduring Freedom) and Iraq (Operation Iraqi Freedom and Operation New Dawn). Increasing rates of alcohol and other drug misuse adversely affect military readiness, family readiness, and safety, thereby posing a significant public health problem for the Department of Defense (DoD).

To better understand this problem, DoD requested that the Institute of Medicine (IOM) assess the adequacy of current protocols in place across DoD and the different branches of the military pertaining to the prevention, screening and diagnosis, and treatment of substance use disorders (SUDs). The IOM committee charged with conducting this study was also tasked with assessing access to SUD care for service members, members of the National Guard and Reserves, and military dependents, as well as the education and credentialing of SUD care providers, and with offering specific recommendations to DoD on where and how improvements in these areas could be made.

APPROACH TO THE CHARGE

The charge presented to the committee was substantial and expansive. It involved several distinct topic areas (prevention, diagnosis, treatment, and management) and subpopulations (active duty service members, members of the National Guard and Reserves, and military dependents). Additionally, it entailed an investigation of six sets of policies and programs (DoD, Air Force, Army, Navy, Marine Corps, and TRICARE), some discrete and some overlapping.

This broad charge necessitated a comprehensive approach. The committee engaged in three types of information gathering. First, the committee held four public information gathering meetings that featured presentations by representatives from each of the military branches and TRICARE, as well as academic researchers. Second, the committee conducted five site visits to military bases. During these visits, the committee met with a variety of care providers, including SUD-specific providers as well as those in primary care, behavioral health, and pain management clinics. Third, the committee submitted to each of the military branches and TRICARE Management Activity formal requests for information and numerical data on program reach, service access and utilization, and evaluation results, along with data on the numbers and types of SUD care providers.

The committee compared all of the information thus collected with the best practices and modern standards of care in the scientific literature to assess the adequacy and appropriateness of policies and programs, access to care, and workforce standards. The committee then formulated a set of conclusions and recommendations for improvement in each of these areas, with the aim of helping DoD provide the highest-quality SUD care to military service members and their dependents.

SETTING THE STAGE

The military has a long history of use and abuse of alcohol and other drugs, often exacerbated by deployment and combat exposure. To address these issues, DoD and the individual branches developed a series of policy directives starting in the early 1970s, largely as an outgrowth of concern about substance use during the Vietnam era. Substance abuse has well-known negative health consequences and detrimental effects on military readiness, levels of performance, and discipline. Thus, current DoD policy strongly discourages alcohol abuse (i.e., binge or heavy drinking), illicit drug use, and tobacco use by members of the military. Despite these official policies, however, substance use and abuse remain a concern for the military. Many of the medical conditions that prevail in a heavily deployed force have led to frequent prescriptions for controlled substances, increasing the risk for addiction or misuse. Further, the military's reliance on drug testing limits the identification of misuse to those drugs within the laboratory panel, and does not fully address evolving patterns of drug and alcohol use.

Standards of care and best practices in the prevention, diagnosis, treatment, and management of SUDs have changed considerably over the course of the past decade to reflect developments in the evidence base. Health care reform and federal parity legislation have enhanced access to health insurance and mandated that commercial health plans provide similar coverage for general health, mental health, and alcohol and other drug use disorders. Advocates and policy makers also have called for increased integration of addiction treatment and primary care. Greater integration of prevention and treatment services with primary care could reduce the stigma of alcohol and other drug use disorders and encourage individuals to seek care. The continuum of care for substance misuse in the Military Health System (from prevention through intervention and aftercare) has not been modified to accord with current understanding of factors that motivate individuals to seek help, settings in which care or interventions can be delivered most effectively, training/skills required by key staff, and medications that have proven useful in achieving or maintaining abstinence. These developments set the stage for a comprehensive review and critique of existing SUD policies and programs within DoD and of standards for access to care and SUD care providers.

FINDINGS

The committee's research yielded the findings summarized below regarding the military's policies and programs pertaining to SUDs, access to care for substance misuse and abuse, and the workforce of SUD care providers.

SUD Policies and Programs in the Military

In assessing the SUD policies and programs in place in DoD and each of the branches, the committee arrived at the following findings. First, while DoD and branch policies emphasize screening as a key strategy in combating SUDs, these policies fall short with respect to identifying all service members who have or are at risk of developing these disorders because of a failure to screen for all substances of interest, as well as a lack of confidentiality protections. The committee's review made clear that drug testing also is considered an integral component of DoD's prevention strategy. The committee found very different attitudes toward alcohol and other drugs. These differences are reflected in the screening and drug testing policies, in norms and culture, and in disciplinary actions and repercussions following alcohol-related incidents versus positive urinalyses indicating drug use.

The committee's research further revealed wide variability in SUD-related policies, programs, processes, and instruments across the branches, resulting from the lack of standardization mechanisms in place at the DoD level. The existence of distinct programs in each of the military branches creates the potential for unnecessary duplication and variation from best practices. Further, branch-specific policies that divide program responsibility among the military human resources, legal, installation management, and medical domains create challenges for delivering SUD services. In addition, neither DoD nor the individual branches evaluate their respective programs or initiatives consistently or systematically.

While support for and promotion of evidence-based practices are pervasive in the language of DoD and branch policies and programs, the specifics of which evidence-based practices and programs are utilized and the extent to which they are adopted and implemented are highly variable both across and within the branches. The committee found that current DoD and branch policies and efforts could have much greater efficacy if they were better informed by scientific evidence on the nature of alcohol and other drug use behaviors and made better use of efficacious prevention approaches and modern treatments for the full range of SUDs. While the *VA/DoD Clinical Practice Guideline for Management of Substance Use Disorders* (VA and DoD, 2009) represents an excellent guide for screening, diagnosis, and treatment, the committee found the guideline is not being implemented in a systematic way in DoD settings.

Finally, the committee observed a lack of integration of SUD care with other behavioral health and medical care within the Army and Marine Corps, notably following the Army's shifting of its substance abuse rehabilitation program from its Medical Command to its Personnel Command.

Access to Care

The second major focus of the committee's review was on access to care for SUDs for military members and their dependents. The committee's framework for assessing access is based on its view that alcohol and other drug use behaviors exist on a continuum, and that certain patterns of alcohol and other drug use place some individuals at high risk of developing medical and social problems and possibly abuse or dependence.

Addressing access to brief intervention and treatment for alcohol and other drug use is a complex undertaking. Access includes both the availability of services and the use of appropriate modalities and types of services at the appropriate times. Contemporary substance use treatment systems include frequent screening, brief counseling, brief interventions in primary care settings, a focus on client-centered motivational interviewing, multiple entry points to treatment, pharmacotherapies that reduce cravings and maintain functioning, outpatient counseling, intensive outpatient programs, residential treatment when needed, and continuous contact with counseling professionals after an intense period of treatment. Modalities of care utilize evidence-based environmental, psychosocial, and medication interventions. The standard of practice in modern SUD treatment no longer relies on inpatient hospital services except for the most medically complex patients. Continuity and duration of ambulatory services are more important than the provision of care in residential settings (IOM, 2006).

Available data on the number of military personnel and family members accessing treatment suggest there is unmet need for services in comparison with epidemiological estimates: the committee's review in this area indicated that while services are available through military treatment facilities for active duty service members, the number of patients treated is below epidemiological expectations. Barriers to care apparently inhibit use of these services. These barriers include the structure and location of the services, a reliance on residential care, and stigma that inhibits help-seeking behavior early on. Access is even more problematic in TRICARE's purchased care system, which is utilized by active duty service members and their dependents. The restriction of services to certified Substance Use Disorder Rehabilitation Facilities leads to an expensive reliance on geographically distant hospital-based treatment services, a lack of access to community-based outpatient and intensive outpatient services, and poor transition between inpatient and outpatient services.

The committee found that many policies (e.g., drug testing and Command involvement in treatment planning) may actually inhibit rather than enhance (as intended) access to early SUD treatment and discourage screening and brief intervention in medical settings for alcohol use disorders. For instance, military cultural norms and Command notification requirements, as well as circumstances that diminish confidentiality or attach disciplinary consequences, limit care-seeking behavior. Access to prevention and treatment services that incorporate the latest scientific evidence and are used predominantly in the commercial sector (pharmacotherapy, individual therapy, intensive outpatient programs, and care in individual practitioners' offices as well as outpatient clinics) is limited in the military by an outdated benefit structure, benefit limits, and other policy restrictions. TRICARE regulations that emphasize residential treatment in Substance Use Disorder Rehabilitation Facilities rather than office-based interventions (including integration of SUD treatment into primary care) impact access, especially for family members. Finally, the committee found that members of the National Guard and Reserves, in particular, have limited access to SUD care within the Military Health System when not on active duty.

The SUD Workforce

The third and final component of the committee's charge involved the training/credentialing and staffing requirements for SUD care providers in DoD. The increased prevalence of comorbid behavioral health diagnoses necessitates access to providers with advanced levels of training rather than certified counselors or peer support by individuals in recovery. The results of the committee's review on this topic revealed, first, that credentialing and training vary considerably across the different branches. Second, the committee found that the training manuals for counselors in the Air Force and Navy are dated, do not address the use of evidence-based pharmacological and behavioral therapies, and do not reference the *VA/DoD Clinical Practice Guideline for Management of Substance Use Disorders* (VA and DoD, 2009). Third, physicians who have received SUD-related training in addiction medicine or psychiatry are a rarity in any of the branches. Fourth, the committee observed that the Psychological Health Risk Adjusted Model for Staffing (PHRAMS) includes many of the variables required to calculate the optimal quantitative relationship between need and staffing levels. The databases used for the PHRAMS analysis, however, do not include most encounters for SUD treatment and therefore underestimate staffing needs for SUD care. Finally, the committee identified shortages of SUD counselors across all branches of the military.

RECOMMENDATIONS

The committee recognizes the challenge of managing one of the nation's largest health systems, but notes that the different branches tend to operate their SUD services with minimal direction from and accountability to DoD. Consequently, DoD needs to (1) acknowledge that the current levels of substance use and misuse among military personnel and their dependents constitute a public health crisis; (2) require consistent implementation of prevention, screening, and treatment services; and (3) assume the leadership necessary to achieve this goal. Accordingly, the committee offers the following recommendations for DoD, the service branches, and TRICARE, based on the findings summarized above.

Emphasis on Efforts to Prevent SUDs

Previous IOM reports have differentiated among three levels of prevention: universal, selective, and indicated. Successful universal, population-based environmental prevention strategies that DoD and the service branches should adopt include consistent enforcement of regulations on underage drinking, a reduced number of alcohol outlets, and limited hours of operation of such outlets. Also within this category, DoD and the individual branches should proactively prevent the misuse and abuse of prescription medications by inhibiting access to controlled medications. In the arenas of selective and indicated prevention, the committee advises routine screening and brief intervention in medical settings. Integration of SUD care into primary care may reduce the stigma associated with seeking such care, as well as expand eligibility for such care. The military branches should also coordinate the sharing and implementation of evidence-based programs and models of standardized annual training for program implementers and their supervisors. Finally, the committee advises annual evaluation of prevention programs and encourages DoD to sponsor a study on the cost-effectiveness of the current urinalysis programs in particular. Collectively, these elements make up the committee's first recommendation:

> **Recommendation 1: DoD and the individual branches should implement a comprehensive set of evidence-based prevention programs and policies that include universal, selective, and indicated interventions.**

Evidence-Based and Best Practices for SUD Care

The use of evidence-based practices in SUD care is integral to ensuring that individuals receive effective, high-quality care. While DoD and the individual branches advocate for the adoption and implementation of evidence-based practices throughout their policies and program literature, there is scant detail on the specific practices to be used; consequently, adoption and implementation are highly variable both across and within branches. The lack of standardization, monitoring, and evaluation of SUD policies and programs by DoD and the individual branches contributes to a variety of strategic and quality control problems. Consequently, the committee makes the following recommendation:

> **Recommendation 2: DoD should assume leadership in ensuring the consistency and quality of SUD services. DoD also should require improved data collection on substance use and misuse, as well as the operation of SUD services.**

While DoD and the branches have policies that emphasize screening as a key strategy for combating SUDs in the military, their screening policies and programs fall short of identifying all service members who have or are at risk of developing these disorders. Additionally, these policies reflect very different (and somewhat disconcerting) attitudes toward alcohol and other drugs. Accordingly, the committee makes the following recommendation:

Recommendation 3: DoD should conduct routine screening for unhealthy alcohol use, together with brief alcohol education interventions.

The *VA/DoD Clinical Practice Guideline for Management of Substance Use Disorders* (VA and DoD, 2009) describes procedures for screening, assessment, and management of SUDs in specialty SUD care and in general health care settings, and provides guidance on the use of evidence-based pharmacotherapy and psychosocial interventions. The committee understands that DoD supports implementation of this guideline, but found little evidence of its implementation within the branches. DoD should move forward to promote evidence-based treatment modalities, such as the use of agonist and antagonist medications without restrictions on duration of care and office-based outpatient therapy for the treatment of addiction. Further, DoD and the individual branches should adopt as a consistent practice reviewing the language and content of their policies to ensure that they reflect changes such as those in the definition of SUDs in the forthcoming fifth edition of the *Diagnostic and Statistical Manual of Mental Disorders* (DSM-5), as well as future advances in the field:

Recommendation 4: Policies of DoD and the individual branches should promote evidence-based diagnostic and treatment processes.

The committee's research uncovered a lack of integration of SUD care with other behavioral health and medical care, most notably within the Army and the Marine Corps. Integration of care can occur at two levels: (1) integration of care for mental health disorders and SUDs, and (2) integration of drug and alcohol education with primary care. Primary care is the single greatest missed opportunity in the military for early and confidential identification of and brief education on the misuse of alcohol, and provider credentialing restrictions within the Army also limit service provision of treatment for those with comorbid disorders. Therefore, the committee recommends improvements in integration that will ultimately increase the reach and improve the quality of SUD care:

Recommendation 5: DoD and the individual branches should better integrate care for SUDs with care for other mental health conditions and ongoing medical care.

Finally, the committee observed sufficient access to inpatient beds within the current system, but limited capacity for outpatient and intensive outpatient services. Contemporary systems of care for SUDs rely on outpatient services for continuing disease management. For many individuals, SUDs are relapsing conditions that require ongoing monitoring and periodic stabilization. The elements critical to the high rates of recovery in interventions such as physicians' health programs (for physicians with alcohol and other drug use disorders) appear to be ongoing, continuing care in an outpatient setting, coupled with routine monitoring and clear consequences associated with a return to use. A similar program in military treatment facilities would facilitate retention of trained personnel, noncommissioned leadership, and commissioned leadership while enhancing unit capacity and safety. The individual branches are well positioned to provide these levels of care. Thus the committee makes the following recommendation:

> **Recommendation 6: The Military Health System should reduce its reliance on residential and inpatient care for SUDs in its direct care system and build capacity for outpatient and intensive outpatient SUD treatment using a chronic care model that permits patients to remain connected to counselors and recovery coaches for as long as needed.**

Increased Access to Care

As discussed above, the committee's review revealed substantial unmet need for SUD care, as well as policies and practices that inhibit access to evidence-based SUD treatment in the DoD direct care system and under the TRICARE purchased care system. As noted, best practices for SUD treatment include the use of agonist and antagonist medications and a focus on outpatient rather than residential care. However, the current TRICARE SUD benefit does not permit use of opioid agonist medications for the treatment of addiction and therefore deprives patients access to medications that could help reduce craving and support long-term recovery. Further, the TRICARE SUD benefit does not cover the use of office-based outpatient therapy for SUDs, although such therapy is permitted for other mental disorders. These limitations are inconsistent with both current best practices and requirements for parity. TRICARE benefits for mental health and SUDs should conform to the Mental Health Parity and Substance Abuse Equity Act, and quantitative and nonquantitative limits on behavioral health services should be eliminated. The requirement to use Substance Use Disorder Rehabilitation Facilities should be removed from the TRICARE benefit for the treatment of SUDs, and the benefit should be expanded to include care in outpatient and intensive outpatient treatment settings. Accordingly, the committee makes the following recommendation:

> **Recommendation 7: DoD should update the TRICARE SUD treatment benefit to reflect the practices of contemporary health plans and to be consistent with the range of treatments available under the Patient Protection and Affordable Care Act.**

The committee was impressed by the Army's implementation of the Confidential Alcohol Treatment and Education Pilot (CATEP). CATEP attracted a broader range of patients (including higher-ranking officers) than is routinely seen in the Army Substance Abuse Program (ASAP). CATEP demonstrated that when given an opportunity for confidential treatment, greater numbers of active duty service members will seek care. Such programs should be expanded to all ASAP sites within the Army, as well as to the other branches. Policies should be updated to facilitate Command support for recovery through these confidential programs. The committee understands the need to balance health and discipline. Access to confidential brief counseling, brief treatment, and more intensive treatment promotes good care, reduces stigma, and builds resilience. Delivery of these services without sanctions would promote an effective response to alcohol and other drug use problems as they emerge and foster a system in which individuals seek help rather than hide problems. To promote increased utilization of SUD care, the committee makes the following recommendation:

Recommendation 8: DoD should encourage each service branch to provide options for confidential treatment of alcohol use disorders.

Over the last 10 years, the military has relied heavily on its reserve component (National Guard and Reserve) in the ongoing military operations in Iraq and Afghanistan. These individuals are at high risk for developing SUDs and in many cases lack continuity of care for ongoing mental health services once demobilized. In its review, the committee found a lack of access to SUD care for National Guard and Reserve members in particular and several needs pertaining specifically to this subpopulation. These needs include (1) mounting new programs to reach demobilized and discharged reserve component personnel, (2) making provisions for veterans with other than honorable discharges to receive outreach and continued SUD assessment and services by designated community-based providers, (3) providing options for the receipt of confidential screening and assessment in alternative venues to the Veterans Health Administration (VHA), (4) developing alternative procedures for reserve component demobilized and discharged veterans with elevated postdeployment health reassessment scores to receive a "warm hand-off" to a VHA or community-based provider with specialty training in serving veterans at risk of SUDs and/or suicide, (5) collaborating with the VHA to contract with community providers or existing programs (e.g., Military OneSource) to perform active outreach telephone contacts and facilitated linkage for particularly high-risk or difficult-to-contact reserve component members who are demobilized or discharged, and (6) funding research and evaluation on the most effective technologies and strategies for active engagement of high-risk reserve component members in order to refine future programming. Based on these findings, the committee makes the following recommendation with regard to access to care for reserve component members:

> **Recommendation 9: DoD should establish a joint planning process with the VHA, with highly visible leadership (perhaps recently retired military personnel), to address the SUD needs and issues of access to care of reserve component personnel before and after mobilization.**

Given that DoD and the individual service branches have the added challenge of providing SUD care to service members and their dependents in remote locations and deployment settings, innovative service delivery methods should be explored. Increasing the use of technology in care for SUDs has the potential to substantially reduce counselor workloads and permit more effective and efficient treatment. DoD has an admirable track record in the implementation and adoption of new technology, and should explore the use of technology for prevention, assessment, treatment, and continuing care for SUDs. With the use of Internet technology, for example, patients can participate remotely in prevention courses, treatment groups, counseling sessions, or continuing care, even when deployed. The committee makes the following recommendation with regard to increasing the use of technology:

> **Recommendation 10: DoD and the individual service branches should evaluate the use of technology in the prevention, screening, diagnosis, treatment, and management of SUDs to improve quality, efficiency, and access.**

Changing SUD Workforce Requirements

Since the 1970s, the SUD patient population has become considerably more complex: poly-substance use has become common, the rates and severity of psychiatric and medical comorbidities have increased, and SUD services have increasingly become integrated with behavioral health and primary care services. The committee found high levels of comorbid mental health disorders among active duty service members, reserve component members, and their dependents who seek care for alcohol and other drug use disorders. Accepted standards of care for the treatment of SUDs and other mental health disorders in the civilian sector rely on multidisciplinary teams led by licensed independent practitioners. Licensed independent practitioners complete multidimensional assessments (which include assessments of mental and physical disorders), develop comprehensive treatment plans, and provide integrated SUD and mental health treatment using evidence-based pharmacological and behavioral therapies. With the evolution from residential services to ambulatory treatment systems with continuing care, moreover, a varied workforce is required, and licensed independent practitioners can be integrated into primary care settings as members of medical treatment teams. Such integrated and coordinated care is likely to be more effective and efficient. Furthermore, certified alcohol and drug counselors and individuals in recovery may provide support and continuing care services under the direction of licensed independent practitioners, but they do not have sufficient training to provide SUD treatment independently. Individuals in recovery no longer dominate the workforce; counselors with graduate degrees are prevalent, and health care reforms are likely to demand counselors who are licensed independent practitioners. While individuals certified as alcohol and drug counselors remain a key component of the civilian workforce treating SUDs, their role is increasingly limited and in the near future may disappear.

Rather than continuing to use a 20th century workforce to treat SUDs, DoD is challenged to structure and staff treatment services for alcohol and drug use disorders for the 21st century. The emerging model of care uses multidisciplinary treatment teams to create a varied workforce with carefully articulated roles and training. Individuals in recovery provide peer support instead of serving as primary counselors. Certified counselors work under the supervision of licensed independent practitioners. Treatment plans include evidence-based pharmacological and behavioral therapies and long-term continuing care with peer support. To increase caseloads and enhance productivity, services emphasize outpatient and intensive outpatient modalities, rely on group therapy, and use computer-assisted cognitive-behavioral training. Findings resulting from the committee's comparison of DoD's credentialing and staffing requirements against these standards informed the following recommendation:

Recommendation 11: The individual service branches should restructure their SUD counseling workforces, using physicians and other licensed independent practitioners to lead and supervise multidisciplinary treatment teams providing a full continuum of behavioral and pharmacological therapies to treat SUDs and comorbid mental health disorders.

The statement of task for this study included providing guidance on how to calculate appropriate ratios of physicians and licensed practitioners for the population of DoD beneficiaries to provide sufficient services for alcohol and other drug use disorders. Calculating these ratios is an imprecise process. They vary widely in civilian health plans, reflecting variations in the organization of care, productivity expectations, and the balance of group and individual therapy. Systems that rely on residential and inpatient care require more intensive staffing ratios than those that emphasize ambulatory care. Integration with primary care and behavioral health services requires different ratios than freestanding care. Treatment systems that build automated tools and information technology infrastructure require fewer staff. Population needs and the prevalence of SUDs also affect staffing needs. Finally, continuing care and peer support services require different staffing patterns from those for acute care services.

To determine appropriate staffing ratios, the committee reviewed DoD's PHRAMS, which forecasts psychological health staffing requirements to meet the estimated annual need for care. The committee suggests that the PHRAMS program provides a reasonable starting point for determining the quantitative relationship between need and staffing levels. However, PHRAMS underestimates the need for SUD treatment practitioners because the Military Health System Data Repository (MDR) database used by PHRAMS excludes many SUD encounters and appears to exclude encounters in specialty SUD treatment programs. Despite being careful and logical, PHRAMS estimates are far below the number of existing SUD counselors in DoD. The committee's findings led to the following recommendation with regard to estimating staffing ratios:

> **Recommendation 12: DoD should incorporate complete data on SUD encounters into the MDR database and recalculate the PHRAMS estimates for SUD counselors.**

REFERENCES

IOM (Institute of Medicine). 2006. *Improving the quality of health care for mental and substance-use conditions: Quality chasm series*. Washington, DC: The National Academies Press.

VA (Department of Veterans Affairs) and DoD (Department of Defense). 2009. *VA/DoD clinical practice guideline for management of substance use disorders*. Washington, DC: VA and DoD.

1

Introduction

Problems stemming from the misuse and abuse of alcohol and other drugs are by no means a new phenomenon, although the face of the issue has changed to some extent in recent years. National trends indicate substantial increases in the abuse of prescription medications, specifically pain medications such as opioids. Similar increases have been found within the military, a population that also continues to experience long-standing issues with alcohol abuse (Bray et al., 2009). The problem of substance abuse within the military has come under new scrutiny in the context of the two concurrent wars in which the United States has been engaged during the past decade—in Afghanistan (Operation Enduring Freedom) and Iraq (Operation Iraqi Freedom and Operation New Dawn).

To better understand this problem, the Department of Defense (DoD) requested that the Institute of Medicine (IOM) analyze the current policies and programs in place across the different branches of the military pertaining to the prevention, screening and diagnosis, and treatment of substance use disorders (SUDs) for active duty service members, members of the National Guard and Reserves, and military dependents. The IOM committee charged with conducting this study was also tasked with assessing access to SUD care within each of these subpopulations, as well as the education and credentialing of SUD care providers, and with offering specific recommendations to DoD on where and how improvements in these areas could be made.

BACKGROUND

The impetus for this study began when criminal cases involving the illegal sale and distribution of prescription pain medications, coupled with rising rates of prescription drug abuse, reported staffing shortages in Army SUD treatment programs, concerns about access to care, and allegations of misconduct at Fort Leonard Wood, led Missouri Senator Claire McCaskill to question whether these issues were indicative of more systemic problems across the military.

The Comprehensive Plan

To answer this question, Senator McCaskill's office sponsored the Support for Substance Use Disorders Act (S. 459) in February 2009, "a bill to improve and enhance substance use disorder programs for members of the Armed Forces, and for other purposes."[1] The bill would have directed DoD to conduct a comprehensive review of its programs and activities for the prevention, diagnosis, mitigation, treatment, and management of, as well as research on, SUDs among members of the armed forces, and based on this review, to develop a plan for improving these programs and activities for service members and their dependents. This plan was to include recommendations for SUD prevention, training for health care professionals treating SUDs, SUD services for military dependents, and the dissemination of SUD prevention materials. The bill did not become law, but it did lead to a provision within the National Defense Authorization Act for Fiscal Year 2010.[2] Section 596 of the act authorized the *Comprehensive Plan on Prevention, Diagnosis, and Treatment of Substance Use Disorders and Disposition of Substance Abuse Offenders in the Armed Forces* (*Comprehensive Plan*), which mandates an internal program review on these matters by DoD, as well as an external review conducted by an independent organization such as the IOM. (The full text of S. 459 and Section 596 of Public Law 111-84 can be found in Appendixes B and C, respectively.)

To develop the *Comprehensive Plan*, the Assistant Secretary of Defense for Health Affairs formed an expert workgroup to review and assess (1) the availability of and access to SUD care, (2) DoD oversight of SUD programs, (3) credentialing requirements for providers of SUD care, (4) the epidemiology of SUDs, and (5) disciplinary actions and separations for substance abuse. The resulting *Comprehensive Plan* analyzes policies related to prevention, screening and diagnosis, and treatment of SUDs and

[1] S. 459: Support for Substance Use Disorders Act, 111th Cong., 1st sess. (February 24, 2009).

[2] National Defense Authorization Act for Fiscal Year 2010, Public Law 111-84 (October 28, 2009).

identifies areas for improvement. The report's concise summary notes a lack of standardized tools for screening and diagnosis of SUDs in primary care and other health care settings. Policies related to SUDs, moreover, do not specify common outcome and quality measures, and it is difficult to distinguish more from less effective programs and services. Similarly, the report notes that the *VA/DoD Clinical Practice Guideline for Management of Substance Use Disorders* (VA and DoD, 2009) is implemented inconsistently because policies and standards do not require the use of evidence-based practices. The report indicates that TRICARE has plans to modify its policies prohibiting reimbursement of individual practitioners for treatment of SUDs; placing yearly and lifetime limits on the use of behavioral health care, including treatment for SUDs; and restricting the use of ongoing maintenance drugs for opioid dependence for family member beneficiaries. The Military Health System also is modifying policies requiring licensed mental health practitioners to practice under the supervision of physicians and prohibiting the use of opioid agonist therapy. The *Comprehensive Plan* observes that because of "ongoing, overseas military operations, the Services are facing increasing demand for substance abuse and mental health services" (DoD, 2011, p. 26).

Recent Reports and Research Findings

Senator McCaskill's concern about the pervasiveness of the above issues was not off target. During the latter portion of the past decade, various public health agencies and the popular press documented increases in the prescription of opioid pain medications and subsequent increases in opioid dependence and abuse in both the civilian and military populations. Zoroya (2010) reports that military physicians wrote nearly 3.8 million prescriptions for pain medications in 2009, more than quadruple the number written in 2001. While these increases have been seen in both the civilian and military populations, the latter increases must be understood in the context of the two wars in which the United States has been engaged for the past decade. Multiple deployments, for example, have resulted in increases in combat-related injuries, as well as aches and strains incurred by "carrying heavy packs, body armor, and weapons over rugged and mountainous terrain" (Zoroya, 2010).

While misuse of prescription drugs has been on the rise among both civilians and military personnel and has become a national concern (Bray et al., 2010; DoD, 2009; IOM, 2010; Manchikanti and Singh, 2008; U.S. Army, 2012), Brewin's *Broken Warriors* series documents the unique features of the prescription drug epidemic within the military population, calling prescribing policies and practices into question for this population (Brewin, 2011). Likewise, recent research has shown that alcohol abuse among military personnel returning from Iraq and Afghanistan has increased substantially since the start of the wars (Bray et al., 2009). Although there have been reductions in the use of tobacco and illicit drugs, the stress of multiple deployments has been linked with increases not only in heavy drinking but also in posttraumatic stress disorder, depression, and suicidal ideation and attempts (Blume et al., 2010; Bray et al., 2010; Marshall et al., 2012). In addition, new substances, such as "Spice" and "bath salts," are posing new challenges for public health in both the civilian and military populations (Horgan et al., 2001; Rosenbaum et al., 2012; SAMHSA, 2011; U.S. Air Force Special Operations Command, 2011).

Outdated Policies

Another concern among some members of Congress was the outdated policies on SUD care that DoD and many of the branches continued to implement. Many of these policies had been drafted more than 10 years previously and had not been revised to reflect emerging knowledge on evidence-based practices for the prevention, screening and diagnosis, and treatment of SUDs. Table 1-1 displays the SUD policies in place when Senator McCaskill first introduced S. 459. Since Senator McCaskill and other

TABLE 1-1 Military Policies Addressing Substance Use Disorders as of February 2009

Policy Number	Policy Name	Date of Enactment
DoD Directive 1010.1	Military Personnel Drug Abuse Testing Program	9 December 1994[a]
DoD Directive 1010.4	Drug and Alcohol Abuse by DoD Personnel	3 September 1997[a]
DoD Instruction 1010.6	Rehabilitation and Referral Services for Alcohol and Drug Abusers	13 March 1985
DoD Directive 1010.9	DoD Civilian Employee Drug Abuse Testing Program	23 August 1988[b]
DoD Instruction 6490.03	Deployment Health	11 August 2006
Army Regulation 600-85	The Army Substance Abuse Program	2 February 2009
AFI44-121	Alcohol and Drug Abuse Prevention and Treatment (ADAPT) Program	26 September 2001
SECNAVINST 5300.28D	Military Substance Abuse Prevention and Control	5 December 2005
OPNAVINST 5350.4C	Drug and Alcohol Abuse Prevention and Control	15 October 2003
MCO P1700.24B	Marine Corps Personal Services Manual	27 December 2001

[a] Incorporating Change 1, January 11, 1999.
[b] Incorporating Change 1, January 20, 1992.

members of Congress first raised concern about this issue, several of the branches have updated their policies addressing SUDs. Table 1-2 displays the SUD policies in place as of this writing (May 2012).

CHARGE TO THE COMMITTEE

As required by Public Law 111-84, DoD sponsored this independent review by the IOM. The IOM was awarded the contract through the Department of Health and Human Services' Contracting Office in October 2010 and commenced its search for committee members in December. The committee's composition was finalized in April 2011, and its first information gathering meeting was held in Washington, DC, in March 2011. The committee's review concluded in June 2012.

The committee was charged with addressing the following issues:

- *Protocols for the prevention, diagnosis, treatment, and management of SUDs in members of the armed forces*—The committee's report was to provide an assessment of the adequacy and appropriateness of protocols used by the Military Health System with respect to the prevention, diagnosis, treatment, and management of SUDs in members of the armed forces.
- *Care for SUDs in military medical treatment facilities and under the TRICARE program*—The report was to provide an assessment of the adequacy of the availability of and access to care for SUDs in military medical treatment facilities and under the TRICARE program. It was to address the following areas: the sufficiency of clinical scope (i.e., the range and depth of clinical activities) to meet the needs of the population served by programs and services

TABLE 1-2 Military Policies Addressing Substance Use Disorders as of May 2012

Policy Number	Policy Name	Date of Enactment
Army Regulation 600-85	Rapid Action Revision	2 December 2009
Air Force Instruction 44-121	Alcohol and Drug Abuse Prevention and Treatment Program	11 April 2011
SECNAVINST 5300.28E	Military Substance Abuse Prevention and Control	23 May 2011
OPNAV Instruction 5350.4D	Navy Alcohol and Drug Abuse Prevention and Control	4 June 2009
Marine Corps Order 5300.17	Marine Corps Substance Abuse Program	11 April 2011

in military treatment facilities and the TRICARE program; whether active duty and reserve component personnel and their dependents needing SUD treatment are able to make use of the existing programs and services; what obstacles exist to providing preventive services for individuals (e.g., active duty, Reserve, and National Guard personnel and their dependents); and what obstacles exist to providing substance use treatment for individuals (e.g., active duty, Reserve, and National Guard personnel and their dependents) who need such treatment.

- *Credentials and other requirements for physician and nonphysician health care professionals*—The report was to provide an analysis of the adequacy and appropriateness of current credentials and other requirements for physician and nonphysician health care professionals who treat members of the armed forces with SUDs.
- *Staffing ratio of physician and nonphysician care providers*—The report was to address and offer recommendations on evidence-based methodology(ies) for determining the advisable ratio of physician and nonphysician health care providers of SUD care for members of the armed forces.
- *Availability of and access to care for the active duty and reserve components of the armed forces*—The report was to compare the adequacy of the availability of and access to care for SUDs for members of the active duty and reserve components of the armed forces.
- *Adequacy of SUD programs for dependents of armed forces members*—The report was to assess the adequacy of programs for the prevention, diagnosis, treatment, and management of SUDs for dependents of members of the armed forces, whether such dependents suffer from their own SUD or are affected by the SUD of a member of the armed forces. The following areas were to be addressed: whether such programs and services are sufficient in scope and capacity to meet the needs of dependents, whether dependents with a need for SUD treatment are able to make use of these programs and services, and what obstacles exist to providing preventive services and/or SUD treatment to individuals who need such treatment.

APPROACH TO THE CHARGE

To respond to this broad charge, the IOM assembled a committee with diverse expertise in the areas of SUD prevention, screening and diagnosis, treatment, access, and workforce education and credentialing. Additionally, because the study required examination of three distinct populations (active duty service members, Reserve and National Guard members, and military dependents), the committee's membership needed to be well versed in the specific characteristics and needs of each of these groups. Once assembled, the committee undertook several strategies to gather the necessary information for this report.

First, the committee carried out a thorough review of all DoD, Army, Navy, Air Force, and Marine Corps policies and programs related to the prevention, diagnosis, treatment, and management of SUDs to gain an understanding of how SUDs are addressed in the military. To examine services available outside the direct care system for military members and their dependents, the committee also examined the TRICARE benefit for SUD care and the accessibility and availability of such care. DoD's *Comprehensive Plan* was particularly helpful for these tasks.

To supplement the information thus gathered, the committee held four public information-gathering meetings during the first year of the study. Invited speakers included representatives of the sponsoring agency and other relevant government agencies, as well as experts and researchers in the fields of SUD prevention, diagnosis, and treatment; military families; and pain management. Appendix A provides a list of the speakers who addressed the committee at these public meetings and the topics of their presentations. The committee also made site visits to SUD programs at Camp Pendleton, Fort Belvoir, San Diego Naval Hospital, Keesler Air Force Base, and Fort Hood to speak directly with individuals who provide SUD care to service members in the settings in which this care is provided. Appendix A provides more information on the committee's site visits.

The literature the committee consulted to determine the standards by which it would assess the military policies and programs reviewed and the evidence base upon which it would issue its recommendations consisted primarily of peer-reviewed journal publications. Most of this literature addressed SUD issues among the general public, although some was military-specific. Finally, in addition to researching the etiology, epidemiology, prevention, diagnosis, treatment, and relapse of SUDs, the committee reviewed literature on SUDs and comorbid disorders such as posttraumatic stress disorder (PTSD) and depression. The committee focused its attention on alcohol and other drug use and excluded tobacco use from the purview of its investigation. The IOM (2009) report *Combating Tobacco in Military and Veteran Populations* examines this issue in great detail and offers a variety of recommendations for tobacco use prevention and cessation.

ORGANIZATION OF THE REPORT

This report consists of nine chapters. Following this introduction, Chapter 2 provides more detailed background information on the issue of substance abuse, both among the general population and within the military in particular. Chapter 3 provides a summary of the structure of the Military Health System and describes the avenues for SUD care within this system. Chapter 4 examines the changing standards of care for SUDs, the impact of recent health care reform and drug control strategies, and current standards for addiction treatment. Chapter 5 reviews best practices in prevention, screening and diagnosis, and treatment of SUDs. Chapter 6 summarizes the existing SUD policies and programs in DoD, the Army, the Navy, the Air Force, and the Marine Corps. Chapter 7 tackles the issue of access to care for active duty service members and their dependents, as well as for members of the Reserves and National Guard. Chapter 8 reviews the regulations and instructions governing addiction counselors and licensed practitioners in each branch of the U.S. armed forces to assess current standards. The report concludes with a chapter reviewing all of the committee's major findings and recommendations for improvements to SUD prevention, diagnosis, and treatment for active duty service members, members of the Reserves and National Guard, and military dependents.

REFERENCES

Blume, A. W., K. B. Schmaling, and M. L. Russell. 2010. Stress and alcohol use among soldiers assessed at mobilization and demobilization. *Military Medicine* 175(6):400-404.

Bray, R. M., M. R. Pemberton, L. L. Hourani, M. Witt, K. L. Olmsted, J. M. Brown, B. Weimer, M. E. Lance, M. E. Marsden, and S. Scheffler. 2009. *Department of Defense survey of health related behaviors among active duty military personnel.* Research Triangle Park, NC: RTI International.

Bray, R. M., M. R. Pemberton, M. E. Lane, L. L. Hourani, M. J. Mattiko, and L. A. Babeu. 2010. Substance use and mental health trends among U.S. military active duty personnel: Key findings from the 2008 DoD Health Behavior Survey. *Military Medicine* 175(6):390-399.

Brewin, B. 2011. Military's drug policy threatens troops' health, doctors say. *Nextgov*, http://www.nextgov.com/health/2011/01/militarys-drug-policy-threatens-troops-health-doctors-say/48321/ (accessed June 12, 2012).

DoD (Department of Defense). 2009. *Status of drug use in the Department of Defense personnel.* Falls Church, VA: DoD.

DoD. 2011. *Comprehensive plan on prevention, diagnosis, and treatment of substance use disorders and disposition of substance use offenders in the armed forces.* Washington, DC: Office of the Under Secretary of Defense.

Horgan, C. M., G. Strickler, and K. Skwara. 2001. *Substance abuse: The nation's number one health problem. Key indicators for policy—update.* Waltham, MA: Heller School, Brandeis University.

IOM (Institute of Medicine). 2009. *Combatting tobacco in military and veteran populations.* Washington, DC: The National Academies Press.

IOM. 2010. *Returning home from Iraq and Afghanistan: Preliminary assessment of readjustment needs of veterans, service members, and their families.* Washington, DC: The National Academies Press.

Manchikanti, L., and A. Singh. 2008. Therapeutic opioids: A ten-year perspective on the complexities and complications of the escalating use, abuse, and nonmedical use of opioids. *Pain Physician* 11(Suppl. 2):S63-S88.

Marshall, B. D. L., M. R. Prescott, I. Liberzon, M. B. Tamburrino, J. R. Calabrese, and S. Galea. 2012. Coincident posttraumatic stress disorder and depression predict alcohol abuse during and after deployment among Army National Guard soldiers. *Drug and Alcohol Dependence* [Epub ahead of print].

Office of the Surgeon General. 2004. *2004 Surgeon General's report—the health consequences of smoking*. Atlanta, GA: Office of the Surgeon General.

Rosenbaum, C. D., S. P. Carreiro, and K. M. Babu. 2012. Here today, gone tomorrow. And back again? A review of herbal marijuana alternatives (K2, Spice), synthetic cathinones (bath salts), kratom, salvia divinorum, methoxetamine, and piperazines. *Journal of Medical Toxicology* 8(1):15-32.

SAMHSA (Substance Abuse and Mental Health Services Administration). 2011. *Results from the 2010 National Survey on Drug Use and Health: Summary of national findings*. Rockville, MD: SAMHSA.

U.S. Air Force Special Operations Command. 2011. AFSOC to airmen: Use Spice, may lose career. *Air Force Print News Today*, http://www.afsoc.af.mil/news/story.asp?id=123255852 (accessed June 12, 2012).

U.S. Army. 2012. *Army 2020: Generating health & discipline in the force*. Washington, DC: U.S. Army.

VA (Department of Veterans Affairs) and DoD. 2009. *VA/DoD clinical practice guideline for management of substance use disorders*. Washington, DC: VA and DoD.

Zoroya, G. 2010. Abuse of pain pills by troops concerns Pentagon. *USA Today*, March 17, http://www.usatoday.com/news/military/2010-03-16-military-drugs_N.htm (accessed June 27, 2012).

2

Understanding Substance Use Disorders in the Military

Substance use and abuse has long been a concern for the nation, both in and out of the workplace (IOM, 1994), with consequences that include lost productivity, disease, and premature death. Indeed, it has been estimated that more than one in four deaths in the United States each year can be attributed to the use of alcohol, illicit drugs, or tobacco (Horgan et al., 2001). Thus, it is no surprise that substance abuse is a significant issue for the U.S. military.

This chapter provides essential background information on substance use disorders (SUDs) in the military. It begins with a summary of our current understanding of SUDs, the scope of the problem in the military, and the development of military substance abuse policy. The chapter then details the composition and sociodemographic characteristics of the armed services as context for a discussion of the prevalence of substance use in the military. Next is a review of the health care burden of SUDs in the armed services, followed by the description of a conceptual approach to prevention, intervention, and treatment of alcohol use problems—the substance use concern of greatest significance for the military. The final section presents a summary.

UNDERSTANDING SUBSTANCE USE DISORDERS

The classification system of the current (fourth) edition of the *Diagnostic and Statistical Manual* (DSM-IV) includes two possible diagnoses for SUDs: abuse and dependence. In 2013, however, a fifth edition (DSM-5) will replace this classification to reflect the recent scientific literature. A catch-all diagnosis of "substance use disorder" will replace the "abuse" and "dependence" diagnoses, and its severity will be rated according to the number of symptoms of compulsive drug-seeking behavior. Thus, alcoholism will become "alcohol use disorder," and services based on the diagnosis of "dependence" versus "abuse" will have to be redefined. The symptoms as described in DSM-IV will remain the same except that "legal problems" has been eliminated as a symptom, and "craving" has been added as a symptom (APA, 2011). Several papers have analyzed the proposed criterion changes and demonstrate support for the new classification in DSM-5 (Hasin, 2012). The prevalence of SUDs will not be significantly affected by this change.

The modern approach to SUDs begins with prevention that involves educating the population in the avoidance of risky behaviors and establishing and enforcing policies to discourage such behaviors. One such behavior is binge drinking, defined as five or more standard drinks on a single occasion for a male or four or more for a female (NIAAA, 2005). This is a common behavior among young adults, whether in the military or not, and it increases the likelihood of developing alcohol use disorders. Weekly volume of alcohol consumption also has been used as an early indicator of the risk of developing an alcohol use disorder. For men the danger level is 14 standard drinks per week and for women 7 drinks per week. Early detection of problem drinking should lead to further evaluation and specific intervention according to the needs of the individual. Environmental strategies that have been effective in preventing alcohol problems include such approaches as raising the minimum legal drinking age to 21, enforcing minimum purchase age laws, increasing alcohol taxes and reducing discount drink specials, and holding retailers liable for damage inflicted on others by intoxicated and underage patrons. These strategies are reviewed in greater detail in Chapter 5.

The dimensional approach of DSM-5, in contrast to previous categorical diagnoses, mirrors research findings that SUDs occur along a continuum. While some patients with milder, recent onset may be managed with outpatient therapy, those with more severe disorders may require inpatient care followed by a long period of aftercare. The tradition of 30 days of inpatient or residential care with uncertain follow-up is no longer considered the optimal approach. Clinical research also supports medication-assisted treatment using an array of Food and Drug Administration–approved medications, as discussed later in this report.

The past three decades have seen enormous advances in our understanding of the neurobiology of addiction. Until the 1940s, addiction was regarded as a moral failure that could happen only to people with "bad character." As recently as 1988, the Supreme Court declared that the

Department of Veterans Affairs (VA) did not have to pay benefits to alcoholics because their drinking was due to "willful misconduct."[1]

As a result of the pioneering work of scientists at the Public Health Service Hospital in Lexington, Kentucky (Ludwig et al., 1978) and the discovery of the reward system by psychologists such as Olds (1958), our view of addiction has changed. We now know that addiction, defined as a compulsion to seek and take specific substances, is based on an aberration of normal brain function.

The reward system is a set of circuits and structures that work as a unit in lower animals as well as primates and humans. Previously, animals were thought to be incapable of addiction; now they can serve as models for research relevant to human patients. The reward system developed early in evolution and is present in modern humans in a form that remains essentially unchanged from that of our early ancestors (Maclean, 1955). It is a part of the brain that is essential for survival because it is activated by all types of rewards, including the basic ones such as food, water, and sex. Activation of this system (pleasure) produces reinforcement of specific behaviors that are needed for survival. The reward system also is involved in the formation of memories. The pursuit of pleasure and the avoidance of pain, at a very fundamental level, are completely normal.

Unfortunately, certain plant products, such as opioids and cocaine, are, by coincidence, able to fit perfectly into receptors in the reward circuits where they can directly produce a sensation of reward or euphoria. Other substances, such as alcohol, are able to activate the reward system by stimulating the release of neurotransmitters called endorphins or by other more complex mechanisms. While normal activation of the reward system by constructive behaviors is important for survival, activation of the reward system by the use of drugs can lead to behaviors that are nonproductive or harmful.

Whereas a sense of pleasure normally is earned through constructive behaviors and natural drives, even a small amount of cocaine can directly activate this same pleasure system without the need for the usual work. Cocaine's chemical structure blocks the reuptake mechanism of the neurotransmitter dopamine. Normally, nerve cells release dopamine and take it back up again after their signals are sent; cocaine blocks the reuptake process, causing continued high stimulation of the reward system. Dopamine accumulates in the space between nerve cells where signaling occurs (the synapses), and the cocaine effect takes over or "hijacks" the reward system (Ritz et al., 1987). Other addictive drugs, such as alcohol, nicotine, marijuana, and opioids, also directly activate the reward system; although

[1] Traynor v. Turnage, 485 U.S. 535 (1988).

they do so through different mechanisms, the net result is a similar hijacking (Koob and Bloom, 1988).

When the reward system is hijacked in this way, the human or animal begins to choose the rapid drug activation over natural rewards such as food, water, and sex. Activation through drugs becomes repeatedly reinforced, establishing strong memories that are difficult to change. Theoretically, any human or animal can develop these strong, fixed memories that underlie addiction; however, hereditary factors influence the ease with which these memories develop. Genetic influences on addiction have been studied in both humans and animals. Large population studies have shown that many humans try drugs and do not particularly like the experience, while others experience pleasure and repeat the drug taking and, within a period of time that depends on genetic variables, become compulsive users (Anthony et al., 1994). Most addictions show substantial evidence of heritability (Goldman et al., 2005), suggesting that many alleles contribute to each type of addiction, but only in a few instances have the alleles been identified. Examples include alleles for ethanol metabolizing enzymes in alcoholism and alpha 5 nicotinic receptor subunit alleles in nicotine addiction. The net result is that only a few of those who initiate drug use go on to become addicts. The variables that influence the risk of progressing from a user to an addict are both genetic and environmental, but the influence of the genetic variables is similar to the strength of the genetic risk for other chronic diseases, such as diabetes or hypertension. Vulnerability to addiction thus depends largely on the luck of the genetic sorting at conception. Good people, smart people—anyone is at risk of developing an addiction given the presence of the right variable.

Using animal models, researchers can predict whether a drug will be abused by humans because of the similarity between the reward system in lower animals and humans (Brady and Griffiths, 1983). In cases where animals demonstrate liking a drug by working to obtain it, we can surmise that humans will be highly likely to like it as well. By developing addiction in animals, we can test different treatments to see which ones will reduce the animal's drug taking with high predictive value. These advancements with animal models have served a great advantage in the development of new medications for addiction and substantially increased our understanding of addiction mechanisms (IOM, 1996; IOM and NRC, 2004; O'Brien, 2012).

Addiction tends to be a chronic disorder with remissions and relapses. Short-term treatments usually are followed by relapses. Expensive residential programs lasting 30 days or more are not successful unless followed by long-term (months or years) outpatient care and supported by 12-step programs (O'Brien and McLellan, 1996). Medications have been developed that reduce the craving for drugs and increase the probability of remaining abstinent. Other medications that are pharmacologically similar to drugs of abuse, such as methadone or buprenorphine for opioid addiction, can be used for maintenance to help stabilize the patient and permit normal functioning. Chapter 5 reviews these and other effective treatments for SUDs.

SCOPE OF THE PROBLEM

Historically, the use of alcohol, illicit drugs, and tobacco has been common in the military. Heavy drinking is an accepted custom (Ames and Cunradi, 2004; Ames et al., 2009; Bryant, 1979; Schuckit, 1977) that has become part of the military work culture and has been used for recreation, as well as to reward hard work, to ease interpersonal tensions, and to promote unit cohesion and camaraderie (Ames and Cunradi, 2004; Ames et al., 2009; Ingraham and Manning, 1984). Alcoholic beverages have long been available to service members at reduced prices at military installations, including during "happy hours" (Bryant, 1974; Wertsch, 1991). Studies of the conflicts of the past decade in Iraq and Afghanistan have shown that military deployments and combat exposure are associated with increases in alcohol consumption, binge and heavy drinking, and alcohol-related problems (Bray et al., 2009; Jacobson et al., 2008; Lande et al., 2008; Santiago et al., 2010; Spera, 2011). These increases in alcohol use may be associated with the challenges of war, the alcohol being used in part as an aid in coping with stressful or traumatic events and as self-medication for mental health problems (Jacobson et al., 2008; Thomas et al., 2010). The availability of and easy access to alcohol on military installations, due in part to reduced prices, may also play a role in its increased use.

Service members have engaged in illicit drug use (i.e., the use of illegal drugs such as cocaine, heroin, and marijuana and the nonmedical use of prescription drugs) since discovering that they reduced pain, lessened fatigue, or helped in coping with boredom or panic that accompany battle. In the modern U.S. military, drug use surfaced as a problem during the Vietnam War in the late 1960s and early 1970s. Heroin and opium were widely used by service members in Vietnam, partly to help them tolerate the challenges of the war environment (Robins et al., 1975). It was estimated that almost 43 percent of those who served in Vietnam used these drugs at least once, and half of those who used were thought to be dependent on them at some time (Robins, 1974). In the active duty component of the military, marijuana has been the most widely used illicit drug since the early 1980s (Bray et al., 2009).

More recently, increasing misuse of prescription drugs among both civilians and military personnel has become a national concern (Bray et al., 2012; Manchikanti, 2007; Manchikanti and Singh, 2008). Unfortunately, misuse of these drugs has risen more rapidly in military than civilian populations, making this a substantial issue for military leaders (Bray et al., 2009, 2010a, 2012). Misuse of prescription drugs in the military is associated with increases in the number of prescriptions for these medications that have been written to alleviate chronic pain among service members who have sustained injuries during a decade of continuous war. Indeed, Bray and colleagues (2012) found that the key driver of prescription drug misuse in the military is misuse of pain medications. Holders of prescriptions for pain medications were found to be nearly three times more likely to misuse prescription pain relievers than those who did not have a prescription.

Although opioid misuse has been increasing, little is known about the demographic, psychiatric, clinical, deployment, or medication regimen characteristics that may be related to such misuse. Nonphysician medics and corpsmen represent one source of prescription opioids for military personnel in the field. While opioids are an important tool in first aid on the battlefield, the increasing prevalence of opioid abuse in the military services suggests that both nonphysician and physician providers need more training in the use of opioids in the management and treatment of pain and the risks of opioid medication. During the conflicts in Iraq and Afghanistan, the military has increased its use of prescription medications for the treatment of pain and other health conditions (U.S. Army, 2012). This increase has raised awareness that greater availability of prescription medications may lead to greater potential for abuse. To begin addressing this concern, the Army has taken a positive step by curtailing the length of time for which a prescription is valid, but additional efforts will be needed to mount a comprehensive response to this complex issue.

Tobacco use also has long been common in the military, particularly after it was sanctioned in connection with World War I (Brandt, 2007), a stance that continued during World War II (Conway, 1998). Cigarettes became readily accessible to service members, partly because the War Department began issuing tobacco rations. Cigarettes were included in K-rations and C-rations and sometimes became more valuable for trading or selling than the food items in the rations (Conway, 1998). The harmful effects of tobacco have been well established (Office of the Surgeon General, 1967, 1979, 2004). Tobacco use has a negative effect on military performance and readiness and results in enormous costs (an estimated cost of $564 million to the Military Health System in 2006) (IOM, 2009).

DEVELOPMENT OF MILITARY SUBSTANCE ABUSE POLICY: A BRIEF OVERVIEW

The Department of Defense's (DoD's) series of policy directives aimed at decreasing and possibly preventing alcohol and other drug abuse originated in the early 1970s (DoD, 1970, 1972; The Controlled Substances Act of

1970[2]), whereas policies directed toward smoking prevention were developed in the 1980s and 1990s (DoD, 1986a,b, 1987, 1994). DoD convened a task force in 1967 to investigate alcohol and other drug abuse in the military, and the resulting recommendations led to a policy directive in 1970 that guided military efforts targeting alcohol and other drug abuse during the 1970s (DoD, 1970). This policy emphasized the prevention of alcohol and other drug abuse through education and law enforcement procedures focused on detection and early intervention. Treatment was provided for problem users, with the goal of returning them to service. A urinalysis testing program was established to help deter illicit drug use, but the program was challenged in the courts[3] and was discontinued from 1976 until the early 1980s.

In 1980, DoD updated its policy on alcohol and other drug abuse in a new directive (DoD, 1980) that focused on prevention and emphasized the goal of being free from the negative effects of such abuse. The policy emphasized the incompatibility of alcohol and other drug abuse with military performance standards and readiness. It continued to emphasize education and training, but gave less emphasis to treatment. This policy shift to prevention resulted from the view that many drug users were not addicted and thus were not in need of treatment (Allen and Mazzuchi, 1985). In 1981, however, drug use was one factor implicated in the crash of a jet on an aircraft carrier, resulting in further attention to the military's drug problem. A new program to stop drug abuse was introduced, based largely on increased drug testing and the discharge of repeat offenders. Improvements in chemical testing procedures led to the decision that drug test results could be used as evidence if the procedures were strict enough to ensure that service members' urine samples could not be misidentified. In 1981, the Navy introduced its "War on Drugs," which initiated DoD's emphasis on zero tolerance of illicit drug use. The other military branches soon followed the Navy's lead and developed related programs, with drug testing playing a central role.

Beginning in 1986, policies on alcohol and other drug abuse were placed in the broader context of a health promotion policy directive. This directive, which focused on activities designed to support and influence individuals in managing their health through lifestyle decisions and self-care (DoD, 1986a), included prevention and cessation of smoking and prevention of alcohol and other drug abuse. In a related effort, DoD launched an antismoking campaign in 1986 that emphasized the negative health impacts of smoking. Subsequent efforts to curtail tobacco use resulted in further restrictions on smoking behavior, such as permitting smoking on base only

---

[2]The Controlled Substances Act of 1970, Public Law 91-513, 91st Cong. (October 27, 1970).

[3]U.S. v. Ruiz, Court Martial Reports 48:797 (23 U.S. Court of Military Appeals 181) (1974).

in designated smoking areas and offering smoking cessation programs to encourage smokers to quit (DoD, 1994; Kroutil et al., 1994). A 2009 Institute of Medicine committee that reviewed tobacco use in the armed services and the VA urged the military to become smoke-free, although many challenges to making this a reality remain (IOM, 2009).

Current DoD policy strongly discourages alcohol abuse (i.e., binge or heavy drinking), illicit drug use, and tobacco use by members of the military forces because of their negative effects both on health and on military readiness and the maintenance of high standards of performance and discipline (DoD, 1997). The U.S. military defines alcohol abuse as alcohol use that has adverse effects on the user's health or behavior, family, or community or on DoD, or that leads to unacceptable behavior. Alcohol use is considered illegal for individuals under the age of 21 in the United States. Drug abuse is defined as the wrongful use, possession, distribution, or introduction onto a military installation of a controlled substance (e.g., marijuana, heroin, cocaine), prescription medication, over-the-counter medication, or intoxicating substance (other than alcohol) (DoD, 1997). Tobacco use is defined as use of cigarettes, cigars, pipes, snuff, or chewing tobacco and is discouraged because of its negative effects on performance and association with disease.

COMPOSITION AND SOCIODEMOGRAPHIC CHARACTERISTICS OF THE ARMED FORCES

To better understand factors that influence substance use in the military, it is important to know the characteristics of the military population. The DoD services have an active duty component, comprising those who serve on active duty, and a reserve component, comprising those who serve in the Reserves and National Guard. The active duty component includes personnel from the Army, Navy, Marine Corps, and Air Force; the reserve component includes personnel from the Army National Guard, Army Reserve, Navy Reserve, Marine Corps Reserve, Air Force National Guard, and Air Force Reserve. All Reserve and Guard members are assigned to one of three groups: the Ready Reserve, the Standby Reserve, or the Retired Reserve. The Ready Reserve is further divided into the Selected Reserve, the Individual Ready Reserve, and the Inactive National Guard. Because Selected Reserve members train throughout the year and participate annually in active duty training exercises, they are the Reserve group of greatest interest and can be thought of as Traditional Reservists.

Table 2-1 provides data on the size of the active duty and reserve components. As shown, the active duty component consists of slightly more than 1.4 million service members. The Army is the largest branch, representing nearly 40 percent of the active duty component, followed by

TABLE 2-1 Size of the Military Active Duty and Reserve Components in Fiscal Year 2010

	Enlisted		Officers		Total	
	Number	Percent	Number	Percent	Number	Percent of Component
Active Duty Component						
Army	467,537	83.2	94,442	16.8	561,979	39.6
Navy	270,460	83.7	52,679	16.3	323,139	22.8
Marines	181,221	89.4	21,391	10.6	202,612	14.3
Air Force	263,439	79.9	66,201	20.1	329,640	23.3
Total Active	1,182,657	83.4	234,713	16.6	1,417,370	62.5
Reserve Component						
Army National Guard	319,846	88.3	42,169	11.7	362,015	42.6
Army Reserve	168,717	82.2	36,564	17.8	205,281	24.2
Navy Reserve	50,718	78.0	14,288	22.0	65,006	7.6
Marine Corps Reserve	35,423	90.3	3,799	9.7	39,222	4.6
Air National Guard	93,287	86.6	14,389	13.4	107,676	12.7
Air Force Reserve	55,559	79.2	14,560	20.8	70,119	8.3
Total Reserve	723,550	85.2	125,769	14.8	849,319	37.5
Total Active and Reserve	1,906,207	84.1	360,482	15.9	2,267,349	100.0

NOTE: Reserve component refers to the Selected Reserve, which comprises traditional drilling Reservists.
SOURCE: DoD, 2011a.

the Air Force and Navy, which are similar in size, and then the Marine Corps, which is the smallest. The reserve component (Selected Reserve) is much smaller than the active duty component, consisting of nearly 850,000 members. The Army National Guard is the largest branch of the reserve component (42.6 percent), followed by the Army Reserve, Air National Guard, Air Force Reserve, Navy Reserve, and Marine Corps Reserve. The Army National Guard and Army Reserve account for about two-thirds of the Selected Reserve. Together, the active duty and reserve components have just over 1.9 million members—62.5 percent in the active duty component and 37.5 percent in the reserve component.

Table 2-2 presents sociodemographic characteristics of active duty and reserve component personnel based on 2010 personnel counts reported by the Defense Manpower Data Center (DoD, 2011a). As shown, the groups are similar with regard to the distributions of gender and race/ethnicity. For example, the majority of both components are male (85.6 percent active duty, 82.1 percent reserve) and white (70.0 percent active duty, 75.9 percent reserve). Likewise, the two components have fairly similar levels of education and similar rank distribution. For example, the majority of personnel in both components are in the lower and mid-level enlisted pay grades, E1-E6.

In contrast to these similarities, there are two notable differences in the demographic composition of active duty and reserve component personnel. The first is that members of the active duty component are younger on average than those in the reserve component. For example, 65.3 percent of the active duty component is aged 30 or younger, compared with 51.9 percent of the reserve component. The second notable difference is that active duty component personnel are somewhat more likely to be married (56.4 percent) than reserve component personnel (48.2 percent), a fact that is somewhat surprising given the overall older ages of reserve component personnel.

Figures 2-1 to 2-2 provide additional information on the family status of active duty and reserve component service members. As noted in Figures 2-1a and 2-1b, although the majority of active duty and reserve component personnel do not have children, more than 40 percent of members of both the active duty component (44 percent) and the reserve component (43 percent) do have children. Figures 2-2a and 2-2b provide a further breakdown of the various family configurations. As shown, the family distributions of the active duty and reserve components are highly similar. The largest groups are those who are single with no children (38 percent active duty, 43 percent reserve) and those who are married to civilians and have children (36 percent active duty, 33 percent reserve). The next-largest groups are those who are married to civilians and do not have children (14 percent active duty, 13 percent reserve) and those who are single and have children (5 percent active duty, 9 percent reserve).

TABLE 2-2 Sociodemographic Characteristics of Active Duty and Reserve Component Personnel in Fiscal Year 2010

Sociodemographic Characteristic	Reserve Component (N = 849,319) (%)	Active Duty Component (N = 1,417,370) (%)
Service Branch		
Army	24.2	38.5
Army National Guard	42.6	
Navy	7.6	22.1
Marine Corps	4.6	13.9
Air Force	8.3	22.6
Air National Guard	12.7	
Gender		
Male	82.1	85.6
Female	17.9	14.4
Race		
White	75.9	70.0
African American	14.9	17.0
Asian	2.8	3.7
American Indian or Alaska Native	0.9	1.7
Native Hawaiian or Other Pacific Islander[a]	0.6	0.6
Multiracial[a]	0.7	2.1
Ethnicity		
Hispanic	9.5	10.8
Education		
No high school diploma	2.9	0.5
Less than a bachelor's degree[b]	76.7	79.5
Bachelor's degree	14.0	11.0
Advanced degree	5.4	6.7
Age		
25 or younger	33.3	44.2
26-30	18.6	21.1
31-35	12.2	13.8
36-40	12.1	11.1
41 or older	23.8	8.8
Marital Status		
Not married	51.8	43.6
Married	48.2	56.4
Pay Grade		
E1-E3	19.5	24.6
E4-E6	53.9	49.3
E7-E9	11.8	9.5
W1-W5	1.4	1.4
O1-O3	6.3	9.0
O4-O10	7.1	6.2

NOTE: Reserve component refers to the Selected Reserve of DoD, which comprises traditional drilling Reservists and excludes Department of Homeland Security's Coast Guard Reserve.
[a] The Army does not report "Native Hawaiian or Other Pacific Islander" or "Multiracial."
[b] Includes individuals with at least a high school diploma and possibly additional education less than a bachelor's degree (e.g., associate's degree).
SOURCE: DoD, 2011a.

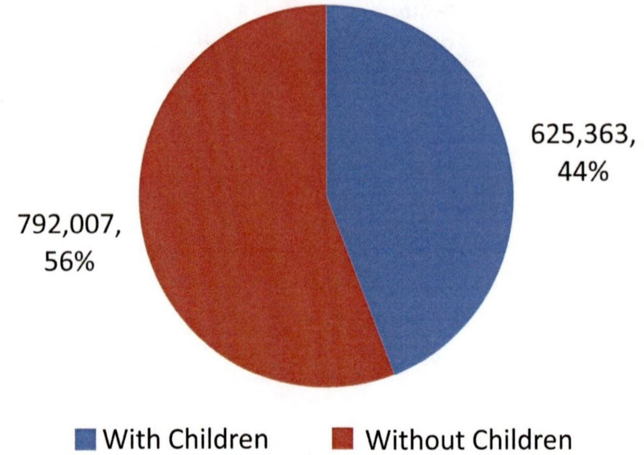

FIGURE 2-1a Active duty component members with and without children.
NOTE: Children include minor dependents aged 20 or younger and dependents aged 22 and younger enrolled as full-time students.
SOURCE: DoD, 2011a, p. 52.

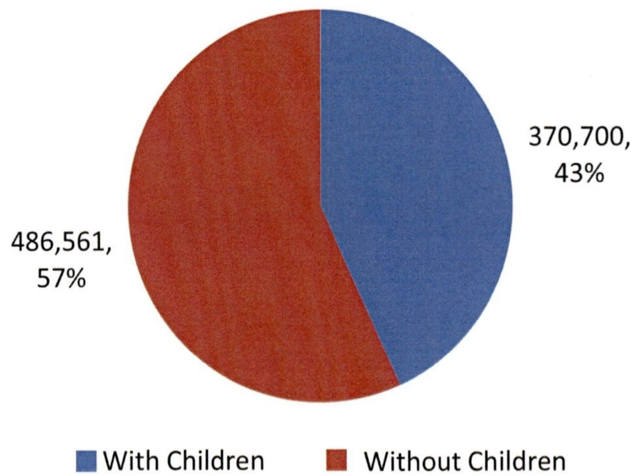

FIGURE 2-1b Reserve component members with and without children.
NOTE: Children include minor dependents aged 20 or younger and dependents aged 22 and younger enrolled as full-time students. Totals here include Department of Homeland Security's Coast Guard Reserve.
SOURCE: DoD, 2011a, p. 116.

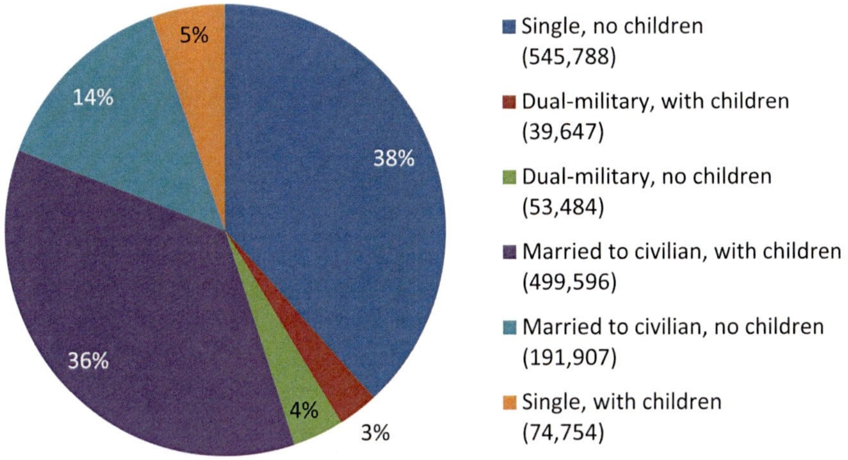

FIGURE 2-2a Active duty component family status.
NOTE: Single includes annulled, divorced, and widowed. Children include minor dependents aged 20 or younger and dependents aged 22 and younger enrolled as full-time students.
SOURCE: DoD, 2011a.

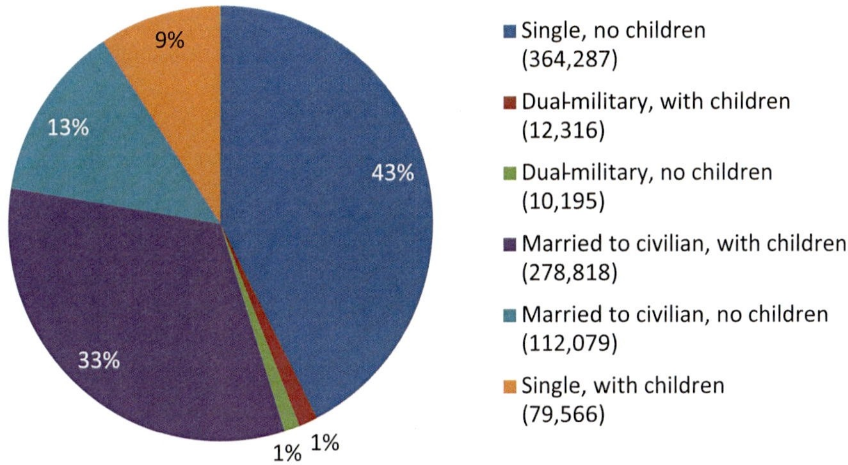

FIGURE 2-2b Reserve component family status.
NOTE: Single includes annulled, divorced, and widowed. Children include minor dependents aged 20 or younger and dependents aged 22 and younger enrolled as full-time students. Totals here include Department of Homeland Security's Coast Guard Reserve.
SOURCE: DoD, 2011a.

PREVALENCE OF SUBSTANCE USE IN THE MILITARY

As background for understanding SUDs in the military, it is useful to know the prevalence of substance use in the military. A much more substantial body of data is available to answer this question for the active duty than for the reserve component. Some data are also available on the prevalence of alcohol use disorders in particular for both components.

Substance Use in the Active Duty Component

The most comprehensive data on substance use in the active duty component come from the 10 DoD Surveys of Health Related Behaviors among Military Personnel (HRB Surveys), conducted from 1980 to 2008 (Bray et al., 2009, 2010a). These cross-sectional studies are particularly valuable in that they are population-based surveys with large sample sizes designed to represent the active duty component population. To encourage honest reporting on sensitive questions, respondents were asked to answer all questions anonymously.

Figure 2-3 presents trends in past-month substance use (cigarettes, heavy alcohol, illicit drugs) for the active duty component from the HRB Surveys (Bray et al., 2009, 2010a). As shown, the prevalence of past-month cigarette smoking decreased significantly from 51 percent in 1980 to 30 percent in 1998, increased significantly from 1998 (30 percent) to 2002 (34 percent), and gradually declined in 2005 (32 percent) and in 2008 (31 percent) such that it was back to the rate reported in 1998.

Heavy alcohol use (defined as five or more drinks/occasion at least once per week) decreased significantly from 1980 (21 percent) to 1988 (17 percent), remained relatively stable with some fluctuations between 1988 and 1998 (15 percent), showed a significant increase from 1998 to 2002 (18 percent), and continued to increase gradually in 2005 (19 percent) and 2008 (20 percent). Rates from 1998 (15 percent) to 2008 (20 percent) show a significant 5 percentage point increase. It is also notable that the heavy drinking rate for 2008 (20 percent) was about the same as the rate when the survey series began in 1980 (21 percent).

Paralleling the increase in heavy drinking from 1998 to 2008, the HRB Surveys showed an increase in binge drinking (five or more drinks/occasion for men, four or more for women, at least once in the past month). Binge drinking increased from 35 percent in 1998 to 47 percent in 2008 (Bray et al., 2009), a 12 percentage point increase in a decade.

The prevalence of any reported illicit drug use (including prescription drug misuse) during the past 30 days declined sharply from 28 percent in 1980 to 3 percent in 2002. In 2005 the rate of illicit drug use was 5 percent, and in 2008 it was 12 percent. Improved question wording in 2005 and

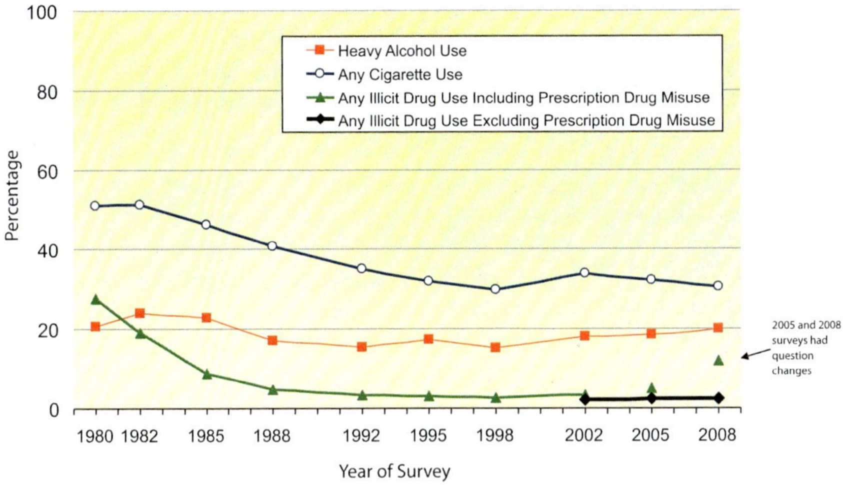

FIGURE 2-3 Substance use trends for active duty military personnel, past 30 days, 1980-2008.
NOTES: Heavy alcohol use = 5 or more drinks on the same occasion at least once a week in the past 30 days. Any illicit drug use including prescription drug misuse = use of marijuana, cocaine (including crack), hallucinogens (PCP/LSD/MDMA), heroin, methamphetamine, inhalants, or GHB/GBL or nonmedical use of prescription-type amphetamines/stimulants, tranquilizers/muscle relaxers, barbiturates/sedatives, or pain relievers. Any illicit drug use excluding prescription drug misuse = use of marijuana, cocaine (including crack), hallucinogens (PCP/LSD/MDMA), heroin, inhalants, or GHB/GBL.
SOURCE: Bray et al., 2009.

2008 may account in part for the higher observed rates. Because of these wording changes, data from 2005 and 2008 are not directly comparable to data from prior surveys and are not included in the trend line. An additional line from 2002 to 2008 shows estimates of illicit drug use excluding prescription drug misuse. As shown, those rates were very low (2 percent in 2008) and did not change across these three iterations of the survey.

To better illustrate the relationship between overall illicit drug use and prescription drug misuse, Figure 2-4 presents three summary measures of illicit drug use in the past 30 days from 2002 to 2008: use of any illicit drug including prescription drug misuse, use of any illicit drug excluding prescription drug misuse, and any prescription drug misuse. As shown, past 30-day any illicit drug use excluding prescription drug misuse for active duty DoD service members remained stable from 2002 to 2008 at 2 percent. However, any illicit drug use including prescription drug misuse and any prescription drug misuse during the past 30 days increased signifi-

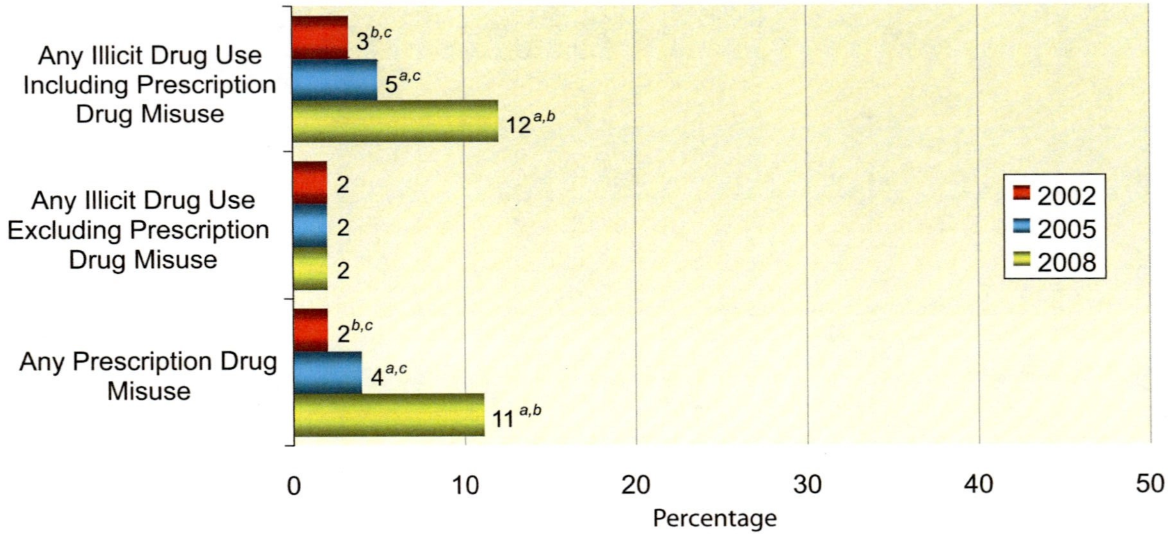

FIGURE 2-4 Use of selected categories of illicit drugs, past 30 days, DoD branches, 2002, 2005, and 2008.
NOTE: Any illicit drug use including prescription drug misuse = use of marijuana, cocaine (including crack), hallucinogens (PCP, LSD, MDMA, and other hallucinogens), heroin, methamphetamine, inhalants, or GHB/GBL or nonmedical use of prescription-type amphetamines/stimulants, tranquilizers/muscle relaxers, barbiturates/sedatives, or pain relievers. Any illicit drug use excluding prescription drug misuse = use of marijuana, cocaine (including crack), hallucinogens (PCP, LSD, MDMA, and other hallucinogens), heroin, inhalants, or GHB/GBL. Any prescription drug misuse = nonmedical use of prescription-type amphetamines/stimulants (including any use of methamphetamine), tranquilizers/muscle relaxers, barbiturates/sedatives, or pain relievers.
[a] Estimate is significantly different from the 2002 estimate at the .05 level.
[b] Estimate is significantly different from the 2005 estimate at the .05 level.
[c] Estimate is significantly different from the 2008 estimate at the .05 level.
SOURCE: Bray et al., 2009.

cantly. Any illicit drug use including prescription drug misuse among DoD personnel increased slightly from 3 percent in 2002 to 5 percent in 2005, but more than doubled from 2005 to 2008, from 5 percent to 12 percent. Any prescription drug misuse doubled from 2 percent in 2002 to 4 percent in 2005 and almost tripled from 2005 to 2008, from 4 percent to 11 percent. Other data from the 2008 HRB Survey not shown in Figure 2-4 indicate that the large majority of prescription drug misuse was attributable to the use of pain medications (10 percent in 2008) (Bray et al., 2009, 2012). Other, more recent data corroborate the military's concern about the problem of prescription drug misuse (U.S. Army, 2012). Because of the punitive measures that result from illicit drug use in the military, there is likely to be some underreporting of drug use on surveys, so these numbers should be viewed as conservative estimates.

Analyses of the military prescription database by the Defense Health Board (2011) support the HRB Survey data in showing increases in drug prescriptions, particularly for narcotic pain killers, from 2001 to 2010. The increasing availability and use of prescription drugs opens up the possibility of higher rates of abuse, as noted by the Army (U.S. Army, 2012).

Other valuable information on illicit drug use comes from DoD statistics on positive drug screens from urinalysis testing (DoD, 2009). Among the active duty component, test results from fiscal year (FY) 2008 indicated a positive rate of 1.07 percent. This figure can be compared with a rate of 2.3 percent illicit drug use (excluding prescription drug misuse) during the past 30 days from the 2008 HRB Survey (Bray et al., 2009). Although these rates are not strictly comparable since they encompass different drugs and time frames, they both point to relatively low rates of illicit drug use.

Two new types of drugs—Spice and bath salts—have recently been gaining in popularity among civilians, partly because they are advertised as safe and legal, but the extent of their use among service members is not well documented. There is some evidence, however, that Spice abuse is beginning to occur among military personnel. The KLEAN Treatment Center reported that the military began conducting urine tests for Spice in March 2011, and that more than half of personnel tested were positive for its use (KLEAN Treatment Center, 2012). Spice is a synthetic cannabinoid that since 2008 has been detected in herbal smoking mixtures and when smoked produces effects similar to THC, the active ingredient in marijuana. Intoxication, withdrawal, psychosis, and death have been reported after consumption. Because it is easy to modify the chemical composition of the compounds (e.g., more than 140 different variations of Spice have been identified), it is also easy to avoid legal efforts to ban these substances (Fattore and Fratta, 2011; Vandrey et al., 2012; Wells and Ott, 2011).

Bath salts, known by such street names as "Ivory Wave," "Purple Wave," "Vanilla Sky," and "Bliss," are new drugs in the form of synthetic powder that can be used to get high and are usually taken orally, inhaled, or injected. Bath salts, which can be obtained legally in mini-marts, smoke shops, or over the Internet, contain various amphetamine-like chemicals that can trigger intense cravings and pose a high risk for overdose (Winder et al., 2012). Referred to by some as a cocaine substitute, bath salts can result in chest pains, increased blood pressure, increased heart rate, agitation, hallucinations, extreme paranoia, and delusions and have been responsible for thousands of calls to poison centers (Kasick et al., 2012; Volkow, 2011). There are no published data at present on the use of bath salts in the military.

Characteristics of Active Duty Substance Users

Table 2-3 shows the characteristics of the heavy alcohol, cigarette, and illicit drug users from the 2008 HRB Survey (Bray et al., 2009, 2010b). It presents prevalence estimates and odds ratios adjusted for all of the other characteristics in the table. As shown, the overall prevalence of heavy drinking was 20 percent. The highest rates of heavy alcohol use occurred among those who were serving in the Marine Corps or Army, were men, were white or Hispanic, had less than a college degree, were single or married but unaccompanied by their spouse, and were in any pay grade except senior officers (O4-O10).

The prevalence of cigarette use was 30.7 percent. Smokers were more likely to be serving in the Army, Navy, or Marine Corps relative to the Air Force, and were more likely to be men, to be white non-Hispanic, to have less than a college degree, to be single, to be enlisted (especially pay grades E1-E6), and to be stationed outside the continental United States. The demographic profile shown in Table 2-3 is highly similar for heavy alcohol users and cigarette users.

The overall prevalence of illicit drug use (including prescription drug misuse) was 12 percent. Drug users were most likely to be serving in the Army, Navy, or Marine Corps relative to the Air Force; they were more likely to be women, to be Hispanic or "other" race/ethnicity, to be married but unaccompanied by their spouse, and to be enlisted.

Comparison of Active Duty Component and Civilian Substance Use Rates

To provide some perspective on whether the levels of substance use in the military are higher or lower than might be expected, it is valuable to compare them against a benchmark such as rates of use in the civilian population. To this end, Bray and colleagues (2009) compared military data from the 2008 HRB Survey for active duty component personnel with civilian data from the 2007 National Survey on Drug Use and Health, a nationwide survey of substance use. The two data sets were equated for age and geographic location of respondents, and civilian demographics were adjusted (reweighted) to reflect the demographic distribution of the military. Substance use rates then were recalculated for civilians assuming those demographics. Heavy alcohol use, cigarette smoking, and illicit drug use were compared for four age groups—18-25, 26-35, 36-45, and 46-64.

Figures 2-5a and 2-5b present the findings from these comparisons, which varied by type of substance and by age group. As shown in Figure 2-5a, active duty component military personnel aged 18-25 or 26-35 were significantly more likely than their civilian counterparts to have engaged in heavy drinking. There was no difference in rates for those aged 36-45, and the military rate was lower for those aged 46-64. Rates of past month cigarette use were lower for military personnel aged 36-45 or 46-64 than for comparable civilians; there was no significant difference in smoking rates between military personnel and civilians aged 18-25 or 26-35.

As shown in Figure 2-5b, service members aged 18-25 were less likely than civilians of similar age to use illicit drugs. This pattern was reversed for service members aged 36-45 or 46-64. Note that the higher prevalence of illicit drug use among these older age groups was due to the misuse of prescription drugs. If one looks just at illicit drug use excluding prescription drugs, the rates were lower for service members than for civilians in each age group.

As observed, substance use patterns in the military often differ from those among comparable-aged civilians. The higher rates of heavy drinking among younger military personnel compared with their civilian counterparts suggest that norms and expectations of military life may encourage heavy drinking or that military policy and prevention programs directed at reducing these rates have not been as effective as similar efforts among civilians. The comparable or lower rates of smoking in the military relative to civilians suggest that military efforts (e.g., restricted smoking areas, smoke-free buildings, antismoking campaigns) and/or secular trends in the civilian population played a role in reducing rates of smoking. The lower rates of drug use (excluding prescription drugs) among military personnel compared with civilians suggest either that military policies and practices deter drug use or that military personnel hold attitudes and values that discourage this behavior. However, the military is facing increasing challenges in managing drug abuse, as indicated by the apparent rise in prescription drug misuse. Given the military's stringent policy prohibiting drug use and the strong deterrence of the urinalysis testing program, it appears likely that the difference in prevalence of drug use between military personnel and civilians is the result of military policies and practices.

TABLE 2-3 Sociodemographic Correlates of Past 30-Day Heavy Alcohol Use, Cigarette Use, and Illicit Drug Use, Including Prescription Drug Misuse, 2008

	Heavy Alcohol Use			
	Adjusted Prevalence		Odds Ratio[a]	
Sociodemographic Characteristics			Adjusted[b]	95% CI[c]
Service				
Army	21.6	(2.3)	1.49*	(1.11, 1.99)
Navy	17.9	(0.7)	1.16	(0.99, 1.35)
Marine Corps	25.2	(1.1)	1.84*	(1.53, 2.22)
Air Force	15.9	(0.9)	1.00	
Gender				
Male	21.8	(1.2)	2.97*	(2.49, 3.56)
Female	8.9	(0.8)	1.00	
Race/Ethnicity				
White, non-Hispanic	21.6	(1.1)	1.00	
African American, non-Hispanic	14.3	(1.2)	0.59*	(0.52, 0.67)
Hispanic	20.7	(1.6)	0.94	(0.83, 1.08)
Other	17.4	(1.3)	0.75*	(0.63, 0.88)
Education				
High school or less	23.4	(1.4)	1.98*	(1.57, 2.49)
Some college	19.6	(1.0)	1.56*	(1.22, 1.98)
College graduate or higher	13.8	(1.3)	1.00	
Family Status				
Not married	24.3	(1.4)	1.83*	(1.63, 2.06)
Married, spouse not present	20.9	(1.5)	1.50*	(1.27, 1.77)
Married, spouse present	15.3	(0.9)	1.00	
Pay Grade				
E1-E3	18.8	(1.5)	2.27*	(1.47, 3.51)
E4-E6	22.6	(1.1)	2.92*	(1.96, 4.33)
E7-E9	16.2	(1.0)	1.88*	(1.26, 2.80)
W1-W5	17.3	(1.5)	2.05*	(1.36, 3.10)
O1-O3	16.7	(1.6)	1.95*	(1.36, 2.81)
O4-O10	9.5	(1.6)	1.00	
Region				
CONUS[d]	19.4	(1.6)	0.89	(0.73, 1.08)
OCONUS[e]	21.2	(0.7)	1.00	
Total	20.0	(1.1)		

NOTE: Prevalence estimates are percentages among military personnel in each sociodemographic group that were classified as heavy alcohol users, cigarette users, or illicit drug users in the past 30 days. The standard error of each estimate is presented in parentheses. These estimates were adjusted to obtain a model-based, standardized estimate. Heavy alcohol use is defined as consumption of 5 or more drinks on the same occasion at least once a week in the past 30 days. Any illicit drug use, including prescription drug misuse, is defined as the use of marijuana, cocaine (including crack), hallucinogens (PCP, LSD, MDMA, and other hallucinogens), heroin, methamphetamine, GHB/GBL, or inhalants or the nonmedical use of prescription-type amphetamines/stimulants, tranquilizers/muscle relaxers, barbiturates/sedatives, or pain relievers.

Cigarette Use				Illicit Drug Use			
Adjusted Prevalence		Odds Ratio[a]		Adjusted Prevalence		Odds Ratio[a]	
		Adjusted[b]	95% CT[c]			Adjusted[b]	95% CI[c]
33.5	(2.2)	1.62*	(1.30, 2.02)	15.8	(0.7)	2.21*	(1.92, 2.54)
31.2	(1.3)	1.44*	(1.24, 1.68)	10.0	(0.6)	1.31*	(1.11, 1.54)
32.3	(1.6)	1.53*	(1.27, 1.83)	11.5	(0.8)	1.53*	(1.28, 1.82)
24.5	(1.1)	1.00		7.9	(0.3)	1.00	
31.9	(1.2)	1.61*	(1.41, 1.84)	11.7	(0.4)	0.85*	(0.76, 0.94)
23.3	(1.5)	1.00		13.5	(0.6)	1.00	
35.3	(1.4)	1.00		11.0	(0.5)	1.00	
19.6	(1.1)	0.42*	(0.38, 0.46)	14.5	(0.8)	1.38*	(1.16, 1.63)
23.4	(1.1)	0.53*	(0.48, 0.59)	12.9	(0.9)	1.20	(0.98, 1.47)
29.4	(1.6)	0.74*	(0.63, 0.88)	13.0	(0.8)	1.21*	(1.05, 1.40)
36.5	(1.4)	2.60*	(2.10, 3.22)	12.9	(0.6)	1.14	(0.88, 1.47)
29.9	(1.2)	1.89*	(1.58, 2.25)	11.5	(0.3)	1.00	(0.79, 1.26)
19.0	(1.4)	1.00		11.5	(1.2)	1.00	
31.7	(1.3)	1.14*	(1.06, 1.22)	12.4	(0.6)	1.11	(0.99, 1.24)
32.2	(1.6)	1.16	(0.98, 1.39)	13.2	(0.9)	1.20*	(1.02, 1.41)
29.3	(1.3)	1.00		11.3	(0.3)	1.00	
33.6	(2.8)	5.02*	(2.94, 8.56)	13.6	(0.8)	1.86*	(1.21, 2.87)
34.7	(0.8)	5.28*	(3.30, 8.45)	13.0	(0.6)	1.77*	(1.21, 2.60)
23.6	(1.4)	2.97*	(1.80, 4.90)	11.8	(1.0)	1.59*	(1.13, 2.22)
14.5	(1.6)	1.59	(0.82, 3.07)	5.6	(2.2)	0.69	(0.25, 1.92)
16.5	(1.5)	1.86*	(1.16, 3.00)	5.7	(0.7)	0.70	(0.44, 1.11)
9.8	(2.0)	1.00		7.8	(1.3)	1.00	
29.6	(1.6)	0.85*	(0.73, 0.98)	12.4	(0.5)	1.13	(0.98, 1.31)
32.8	(1.1)	1.00		11.2	(0.5)	1.00	
30.7	(1.2)			12.0	(0.4)		

[a] Odds ratios were adjusted for branch, gender, race/ethnicity, education, family status, pay grade, and region.

[b] An asterisk beside an estimate indicates that it is significantly different from the reference group.

[c] 95% CI = 95% confidence interval of the odds ratio.

[d] Refers to personnel who were stationed within the 48 contiguous states in the continental United States.

[e] Refers to personnel who were stationed outside the continental United States or aboard afloat ships.

SOURCE: Bray et al., 2010b.

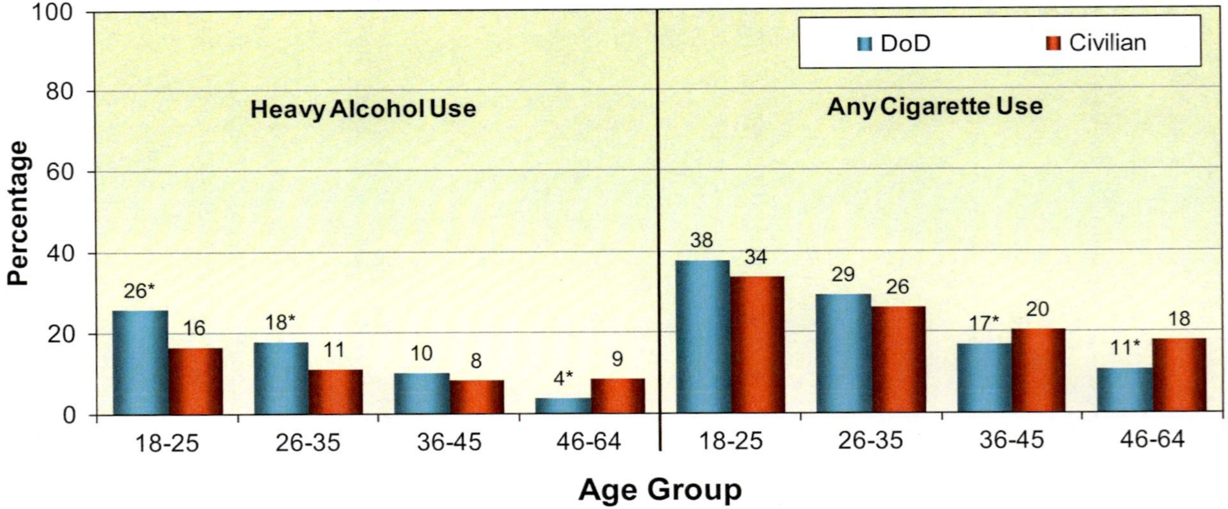

FIGURE 2-5a Standardized comparisons of active duty component personnel and civilians, heavy alcohol use and past 30-day smoking, by age group, 2008.
NOTE: Heavy alcohol use = 5 or more drinks per occasion at least once a week in past 30 days for DoD, 5 or more drinks per occasion 5 or more times in past 30 days for civilians.
*Statistically significant from the civilian rate at the .05 level. Civilian data are from the 2007 National Survey on Drug Use and Health (SAMHSA, 2008) and were standardized to the U.S.-based 2008 military data by gender, age, education, race/ethnicity, and marital status.
SOURCE: Bray et al., 2009.

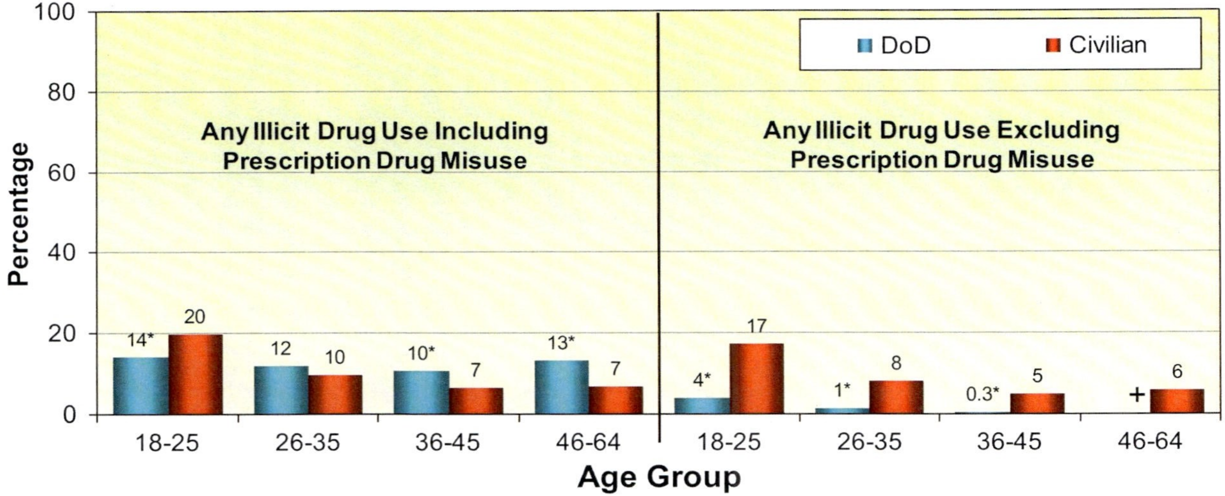

FIGURE 2-5b Standardized comparisons of active duty component personnel and civilians, past 30-day illicit drug use, by age group, 2008.
*Statistically significant from the civilian rate at the .05 level. Civilian data are from the 2007 National Survey on Drug Use and Health (SAMHSA, 2008) and were standardized to the U.S.-based 2008 military data by gender, age, education, race/ethnicity, and marital status.
+ Data not reported; low precision.
SOURCE: Bray et al., 2009.

Substance Use in the Reserve Component

Systematic data on substance use among the reserve component are limited as few surveys have been conducted on this population. The first large-scale population-based survey of the reserve component was conducted in 2006 (Hourani et al., 2007). A more recent follow-on survey of the reserve component was conducted in 2010-2011, but data from that survey were not available as of this writing. Analyses of the 2006 survey found that 6.6 percent of the Selected Reserves had engaged in illicit drug use (including prescription drug misuse) in the past 30 days and 12.0 percent in the last year. The past year estimate did not differ significantly from the past year rate of 10.9 percent for the active duty component from the 2005 HRB Survey. Additionally, 16.7 percent of reserve component personnel (Selected Reserves) reported past month heavy drinking, 40.4 percent reported binge drinking, and 23.7 percent reported cigarette smoking. Analyses that adjusted for demographic differences between the active duty and reserve components found that the rates for the reserve component were significantly lower than those for the active duty component on all three measures (Hourani et al., 2007).

DoD statistics on positive drug screens from urinalysis testing also provide information on members of the reserve component who are not serving on active duty (DoD, 2009). Among the reserve component, urinalysis test results from FY 2006 indicate a positive rate of 1.36 percent for Reservists and 2.26 percent for National Guardsmen. These rates are for a selected panel of drugs that does not include prescription medications and are not directly comparable to the survey data discussed above.

Alcohol Use Disorders Identification Test Findings: Active Duty and Reserve Components

Excessive alcohol use has been shown to result in similar negative outcomes for military personnel and civilians. Mattiko and colleagues (2011) showed that negative outcomes had a curvilinear dose-response relationship with alcohol drinking levels. Higher levels of drinking were associated with higher rates of alcohol-related problems, which were substantially higher for heavy drinkers. Heavy alcohol users reported nearly three times the rate of serious consequences and more than twice the rate of productivity loss relative to the next-lowest level of moderate/heavy drinkers. These findings suggest that a qualitative shift in drinking problems may occur with increasing levels of consumption.

The Alcohol Use Disorders Identification Test (AUDIT), developed by the World Health Organization as a simple method of screening for excessive drinking and assisting in brief assessment, is also useful for characterizing the risk associated with drinking (Babor, 2001; Saunders et al., 1993). It consists of 10 questions scored 0-4 that are summed to yield a total score ranging from 0 to 40. The questions are primarily about consequences of drinking, signs and symptoms of problematic drinking, and quantity and frequency of drinking. Three levels of alcohol use risk can be identified: hazardous alcohol use, harmful alcohol use, and alcohol dependence. Hazardous use is a pattern of alcohol consumption that increases the risk of harmful consequences for the user or others; harmful use refers to alcohol consumption that results in consequences for physical and mental health; and alcohol dependence is a cluster of behavioral, cognitive, and physiological phenomena that may develop after repeated alcohol use (Babor, 2001). As defined by Babor and colleagues, AUDIT scores of 8-15 are indicative of hazardous drinking, scores of 16-19 suggest harmful drinking, and scores of 20 and above suggest possible alcohol dependence.

Table 2-4 presents AUDIT scores for the three risk levels for active duty and reserve component personnel using data from the 2008 HRB Survey for the former and the 2006 HRB Survey for the latter. As shown, 24.6 percent of active duty component service members had scores in the hazardous category of 8-15, 4.2 percent had scores in the harmful category of 16-19, and 4.5 percent had scores of 20 or higher suggestive of possible alcohol dependence. Across all three categories, about one-third (33.2 percent) of active duty component personnel had a score of 8 or higher, indicative of being at risk for some level of alcohol problems or consequences. The rates for reserve component personnel showed a similar pattern but were lower. About one-fifth of reserve component personnel (20.1 percent) had a score of 8 or higher, compared with one-third of active duty component personnel.

These data are informative in several important ways. First, in combination with other data presented above, they indicate that alcohol is a much larger substance use problem in the military than illicit drug use or

TABLE 2-4 Alcohol AUDIT Scores of Active Duty and Reserve Component Personnel

Drinking Level	Active Duty Component (N = 24,640) (%)	Reserve Component (N = 15,212) (%)
AUDIT Score of 8-15 (Hazardous Drinking)	24.6	14.3
AUDIT Score of 16-19 (Harmful Drinking)	4.2	2.7
AUDIT Score of 20+ (Possible Dependence)	4.5	3.1
AUDIT Score of 8+	**33.2**	**20.1**

SOURCES: For active duty component, Bray et al. (2009); for reserve component, Hourani et al. (2007).

prescription drug misuse. Second, they indicate that substantial percentages of military personnel in both the active duty and reserve components are drinking alcohol at rates that place them at risk for alcohol problems, even though they do not meet the current criteria for alcohol dependence. Third, the data suggest that many problem drinkers would benefit from some type of alcohol intervention or treatment before reaching the most severe problem levels. This point is reinforced by an analysis reported by Mattiko and colleagues (2011). The authors compared drinking levels and AUDIT scores and found that more than 75 percent of heavy drinkers had an AUDIT score of 8 or higher, the level at which some type of intervention is recommended. The question then arises of whether personnel in need of treatment or other early intervention are receiving these needed services. The potential unmet need for treatment is examined in Chapter 7 of this report.

Alcohol- and Other Drug-Related Disorders: Active Duty and Reserve Components

To gain insight into the trends in alcohol and other drug use disorders, the military conducted analyses of record data from the Military Health System Data Repository (MDR) and reported these analyses in the Comprehensive Plan. Counts of International Classification of Diseases (ICD)-9 codes indicative of alcohol and other drug use disorders were used to estimate the prevalence of substance abuse disorders among the active and reserve components (DoD, 2011b). Personnel included in the estimates had one or more diagnoses from a health care provider that had been entered into a clinical record. Ratings for alcohol were based on four codes indicative of alcoholic psychoses, dependence, intoxication, and abuse. Ratings for other drugs were based on 20 codes indicative of abuse and dependence for various drugs and drug combinations. Figure 2-6 shows the prevalence of alcohol-related disorders from FY 2000 to FY 2009 for the active duty component. As shown, there were initial increases in alcohol use disorder diagnoses, followed by decreases from 2000 to 2004 for the Army and Marine Corps, but substantial increases from 2005 to 2009. In contrast, the prevalence of these disorders for the Air Force and Navy remained relatively stable.

Figure 2-7 presents results for members of the active duty component who received a drug abuse diagnosis. As shown, there was an increase over the years for all branches, especially from 2004 to 2009. As with alcohol use disorders, the Army showed substantially higher rates of drug-related diagnoses than the other branches throughout the period. For the reserve component, data on alcohol and other drug use disorders were aggregated in the analyses from FY 2004 through FY 2009. Thus these data cannot be compared directly with the data in Figures 2-6 and 2-7. Figure 2-8 shows

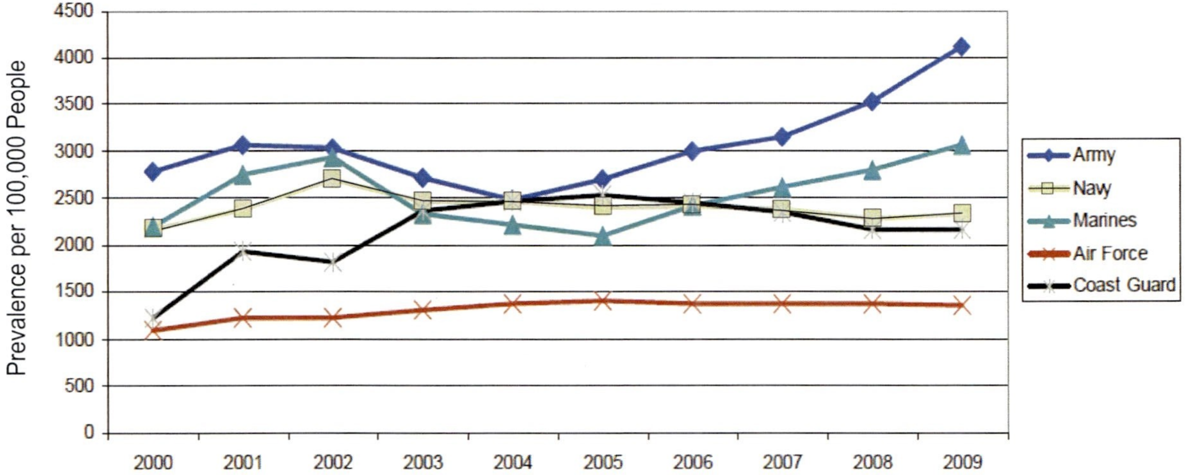

FIGURE 2-6 Prevalence of alcohol-related disorders among the active duty component (rates per 100,000).
SOURCE: DoD, 2011b.

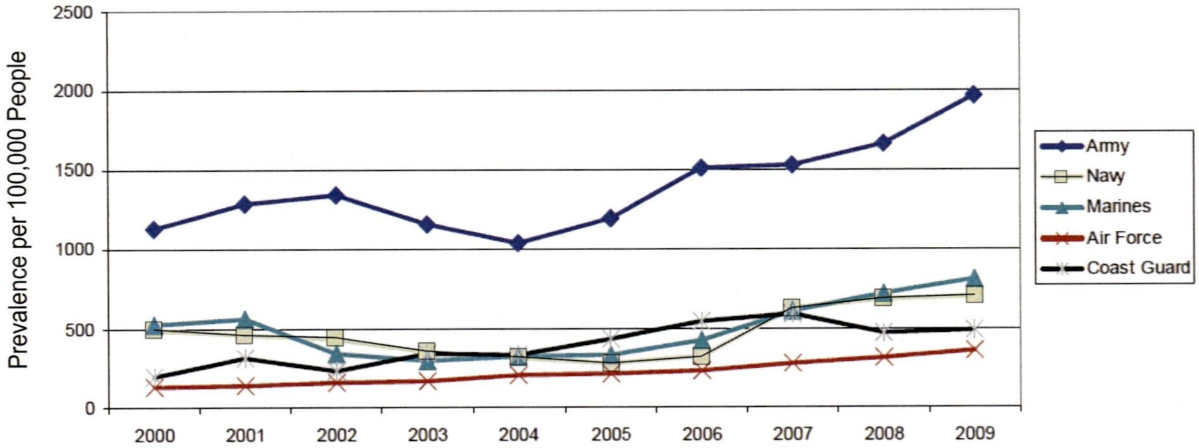

FIGURE 2-7 Prevalence of drug-related disorders among the active duty component (rates per 100,000).
SOURCE: DoD, 2011b.

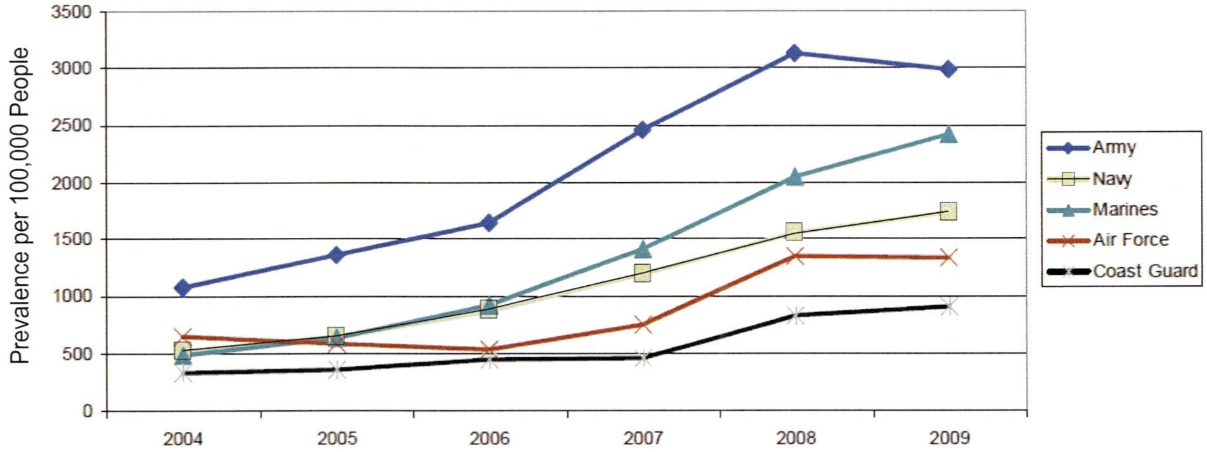

FIGURE 2-8 Prevalence of alcohol- and other drug-related disorders among the reserve component (rates per 100,000).
SOURCE: DoD, 2011b.

this combined trend and, as with the active duty component, shows increasing rates over time, with the Army and Marine Corps having the highest combined rates.

Substance Use and Substance Use Disorders Among Military Dependents

The considerable information available on substance use among service members is in stark contrast to the limited empirical data on substance use among military spouses and children. One small study of military female spouses whose husbands were deployed (Padden et al., 2011) found that 3.9 percent reported illicit drug use, 12.4 percent reported binge drinking, and 27 percent reported tobacco use. Unfortunately, this was a small convenience sample of 105 spouses from a family readiness group, so the results are of limited generalizability.

Studies of military family members have tended to focus on the stress and mental health challenges they face. Indeed, the conflicts in Iraq and Afghanistan over the past decade have placed considerable strain on military families, who have had to cope with frequent and often lengthy separations due to the deployment of their service members. Not surprisingly, some of these deployment stressors, including fear for the safety of loved ones, single parent responsibilities, and marital strain, have had negative impacts on the spouses of military personnel (Schumm et al., 2000). Deployments have been associated with increased mental health diagnoses for spouses (Mansfield and Engel, 2011), with a higher likelihood of child maltreatment in military families (Gibbs et al., 2007), with poorer dietary behaviors, and with poorer stress management and rest (Padden et al., 2011). Eaton and colleagues (2008) found that rates of mental health problems among military spouses were similar to those among service members. However, spouses were more likely to seek mental health care and had less concern about the stigma of receiving that care relative to service members. Spouses also were an important influence on National Guard members who served in the Iraq and Afghanistan wars seeking care for their alcohol or mental health problems (Burnett-Zeigler et al., 2011).

Ahmadi and Green (2011) suggest that the stressors of military life, coupled with the fact that military personnel marry and have children earlier than their civilian counterparts, place service members at increased risk for substance abuse and for the development of adverse coping mechanisms. While this suggestion may have merit, the committee could identify no large-scale published studies examining substance use among military spouses and children. Mansfield and Engel (2011) suggest that this dearth of data with which to assess relationships between deployment stress and substance use points to the need for well-designed epidemiological studies to fill this information gap. The Millennium Cohort Study, an ongoing prospective health analysis in the military, will soon be reporting survey data for military spouses (DoD, 2012). These data may serve as a first step toward providing some of this important information.

Data on trends in combined alcohol and drug use disorders for military dependents (spouses and children up to age 18) were included in the analyses of record data from the MDR database discussed above for active duty and reserve component personnel based on counts of ICD-9 codes (DoD, 2011b). Figure 2-9 displays the trends from FY 2004 to FY 2009. Similar to the patterns for the active duty and reserve components, rates of SUDs show gradual increases over the years for dependents in the Marine Corps, Navy, and Air Force. Dependents in the Army show the highest rates and a gradual increase from 2004 to 2006, but a sharp increase from 2006 to 2008 and a decline in 2009. It is of interest that the pattern for dependents is similar to that for the active duty and reserve components, suggesting that there may be family patterns of alcohol and drug use leading to SUD diagnoses.

HEALTH CARE BURDEN OF SUBSTANCE USE DISORDERS

DoD recently published analyses of the absolute and relative morbidity burden among the armed services in 2011, grouping all medical encounters into 139 diseases and conditions (Armed Forces Health Surveillance Center, 2012a) based on ICD-9 codes. The morbidity burden attributable to a condition had four measures: (1) total number of medical encounters, (2) total number of service members affected (i.e., had one medical encounter for the condition), (3) total bed days during hospitalization, and (4) total number of lost duty days associated with seeking medical care for the condition. Table 2-5 shows the absolute numbers and ranks for the morbidity burden associated with substance abuse disorder and three selected mental disorders on three of these measures. As shown, the burden of substance abuse disorder for medical encounters ranked seventh among 139 conditions and for hospital bed days ranked first, even though it ranked only thirty-sixth for individuals affected. Substance abuse disorder and mood disorders accounted for nearly one-quarter (24 percent) of all hospital days. Together, the four mental disorders shown in the table (substance abuse, mood, anxiety, and adjustment) and two pregnancy- and delivery-related conditions accounted for one-half (50.3 percent) of all hospital bed days. Four conditions—upper respiratory infections, substance abuse disorder, mood disorders, and back problems—accounted for 24 percent of all lost duty days (Armed Forces Health Surveillance Center, 2012a).

These data suggest that DoD should place high priority on the development of new policies and programs to reduce the morbidity burden associated with substance abuse. Given that substance abuse imposes

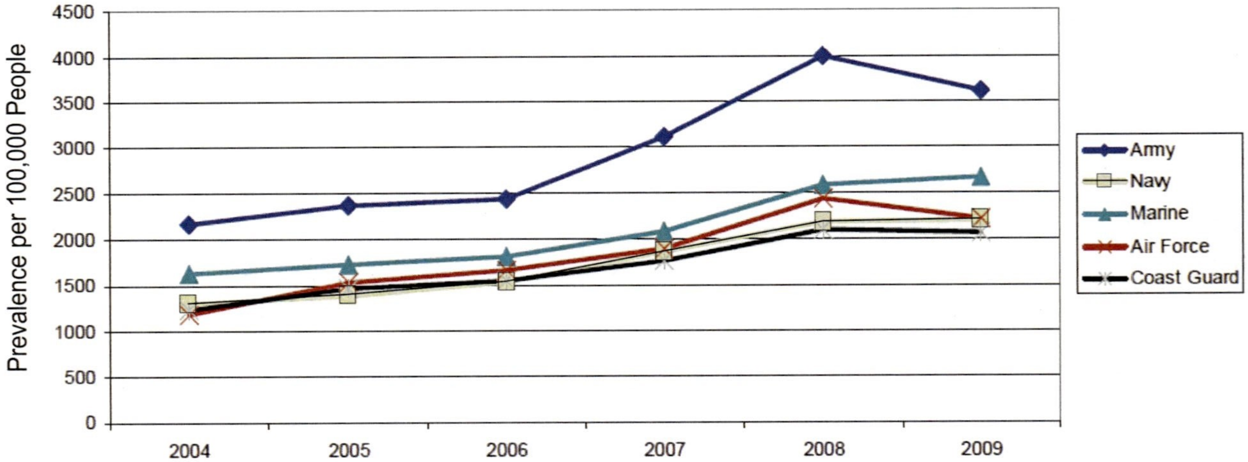

FIGURE 2-9 Prevalence of alcohol- and other drug-related disorders among dependents (rates per 100,0000).
SOURCE: DoD, 2011b.

TABLE 2-5 Health Care Burden Attributable to Substance Use Disorder and Three Other Mental Disorders, and Rank Among 139 Diseases and Conditions, Active Duty Component of U.S. Military, 2011

Major Category/ Condition[a]	Medical Encounters[b]		Individuals Affected[c]		Bed Days[d]	
	No.	Rank	No.	Rank	No.	Rank
Anxiety disorder	475,546	6	68,672	20	28,738	4
Substance abuse disorder	395,021	7	36,276	36	53,589	1
Adjustment disorder	385,122	8	89,563	15	26,456	5
Mood disorder	377,334	9	61,996	23	51,694	2

NOTES: The surveillance period was January 1 to December 31, 2011. The surveillance population included all individuals who served in the active duty component of the U.S. Army, Navy, Air Force, Marine Corps, or Coast Guard at any time during the surveillance period.
[a] Major categories and conditions modified from the Global Burden of Disease study. Rank is rank among 139 major categories and conditions.
[b] Medical encounters = total hospitalizations and ambulatory visits for the condition (with no more than one encounter per individual per day per condition).
[c] Individuals with at least one hospitalization or ambulatory visit for the condition.
[d] Total bed days for hospitalization and lost duty days due to the condition, measured as days confined to quarters and one-half day for a visit for the condition.
SOURCE: Adapted from Armed Forces Health Surveillance Center, 2012a, Table 1.

disproportionately large morbidity and health care burdens relative to the number of service members affected, a further implication is that high priority should be given to focusing prevention resources and research on determining what effective universal, selective, and indicated prevention interventions could be introduced or expanded.

Substance Use and Comorbid Conditions

Substance use disorder prevention, diagnosis, and treatment must take into account the comorbid conditions that often result from the effects of war on service members. A recent Institute of Medicine (IOM) report notes that "the trauma of combat, high-stress environments, or simply being deployed to a theater of war can have immediate and long-term disruptive physical, psychological, and other consequences in those who are deployed to foreign soil and to their family members" (IOM, 2010, p. 39).

Studies have suggested that multiple deployments and the high levels of stress associated with combat exposure and injury may increase the likelihood of behavioral and mental health issues among service members, including drug and alcohol abuse, posttraumatic stress disorder (PTSD), and depression (Shen et al., 2012; U.S. Army, 2012). PTSD has been associated with other comorbid mental disorders (Brady et al., 2000; Keane and Wolfe, 1990). For example, approximately 80 percent of individuals with PTSD have a comorbid psychiatric disorder at some time in their lives (Foa, 2009). Studies of psychiatric inpatients have found that more than 75 percent of PTSD patients have other psychiatric or medical diagnoses, including depression, suicidal ideation and attempts, alcohol and other drug abuse, anxiety, conduct disorder, chronic pain, and metabolic syndrome (Campbell et al., 2007; Floen and Elklit, 2007; Jakovljevic et al., 2006). A study of service members previously deployed to Iraq and Afghanistan (Tanielian et al., 2008) found that 14 percent screened positive for probable PTSD; 14 percent screened positive for probable major depression; 19 percent reported symptoms of probable traumatic brain injury (TBI) during deployment; and about one-third met criteria for PTSD, major depression, or TBI, with 5 percent meeting criteria for all three. Adams et al. (2012) found an association between TBI and past month reported binge drinking by military personnel after controlling for PTSD and combat exposure.

Comparing veterans of the Vietnam era with those of the Iraq and Afghanistan wars, Fontana and Rosenheck (2008) found that, because of the emphasis on PTSD, the latter veterans were less often diagnosed and treated for substance abuse disorders. Regarding this finding, the Army notes that "current treatment of Iraq and Afghanistan veterans should take into consideration the potential for manifestations of substance abuse and violent behavior as well as the potential for recurrence or late onset of PTSD" (U.S. Army, 2012, p. 23).

Alcohol-Related Diagnoses

The Armed Forces Health Surveillance Center (2011, 2012b) examined trends and demographic characteristics for acute, chronic, and "recurrent" alcohol-related diagnoses over a 10-year period from January 1, 2001, through December 31, 2010, for the active duty component of the military. Records of health care encounters, including hospitalizations and ambulatory care, in the Defense Medical Surveillance System were searched to identify those encounters that were associated with ICD-9 diagnostic codes encompassing both alcohol abuse and dependence indicators and were classified as acute or chronic cases. Acute cases were defined by four codes: (1) alcohol abuse/drunk, (2) toxic effect of alcohol, (3) excessive blood alcohol content, and (4) alcohol poisoning. Chronic cases were defined by eight codes: (1) acute intoxication in the presence of alcohol dependence, (2) alcohol-induced mental disorders, (3) other and unspecified alcohol dependence (chronic alcoholism), (4) alcoholic liver disease, (5) alcoholic cardiomyopathy, (6) alcoholic gastritis, (7) alcoholic polyneuropathy, and (8) personal history of alcoholism.

Figure 2-10 presents findings on the acute and chronic inpatient and outpatient cases from 2001 to 2010. As shown, there was a gradual increase in rates of acute and chronic incident (new) alcohol diagnoses during the latter part of the decade. Numbers of hospital bed days for acute alcohol diagnoses increased more than threefold. Incidence rates of acute and chronic alcohol-related diagnoses were highest in men aged 21-24 in the Army; for women, rates were highest among those under 21. In addition, there were sharp increases in alcohol-related medical encounters, especially from 2007 to 2010.

Initial analysis also indicated that approximately 21 percent of acute alcohol-related encounters were classified as "recurrent" diagnoses, meaning that during the 10-year period, personnel had a 12-month period that included three or more acute encounters. Following this initial report, some concern was expressed that individuals receiving treatment may have been misclassified as recurrent cases. A subsequent reanalysis using a revised algorithm found that 79 percent of cases originally classified as recurrent were likely treatment related, and further suggested that with this correction, approximately 4 percent of the initial cases would be considered recurrent (Armed Forces Health Surveillance Center, 2012b).

The results of this study indicate the increasing medical burden imposed on the Military Health System by excessive alcohol use and are especially

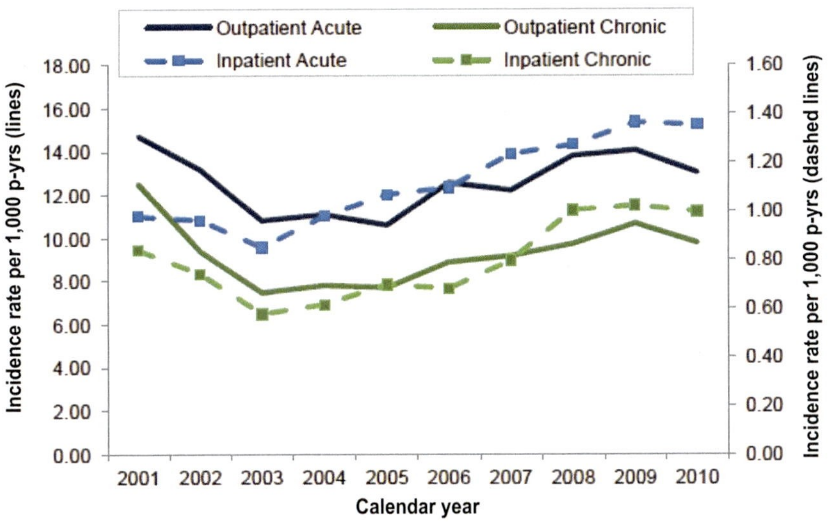

FIGURE 2-10 Incidence rates of acute and chronic alcohol-related inpatient and outpatient cases, active duty component, U.S. military, 2001-2010.
NOTE: p-yrs = person-years.
SOURCE: Armed Forces Health Surveillance Center, 2011.

noteworthy with respect to personnel with chronic alcohol-related diagnoses. The number of bed days attributable to chronic alcohol abuse diagnoses roughly quadrupled over the 10-year period. This finding highlights the need for continued emphasis on the prevention, early identification, and treatment of alcohol-related disorders. (It should be noted that recent increases in incident alcohol-related diagnoses may reflect increasing scrutiny of alcohol use among military members and a concomitant focus on referrals for evaluation of alcohol misuse.)

CONCEPTUAL APPROACH TO PREVENTION, INTERVENTION, AND TREATMENT OF ALCOHOL USE PROBLEMS

As suggested throughout this report, alcohol use is viewed as the key substance use problem in need of intervention and/or treatment among military personnel. Using health care as an example, Figure 2-11 presents a useful approach for conceptualizing alcohol use and likely associated problems in the military as they can be found in primary care, as well as intervention responses in that setting (IOM, 1990). The distribution of alcohol use (and associated problems) includes individuals drinking at nonharmful levels,

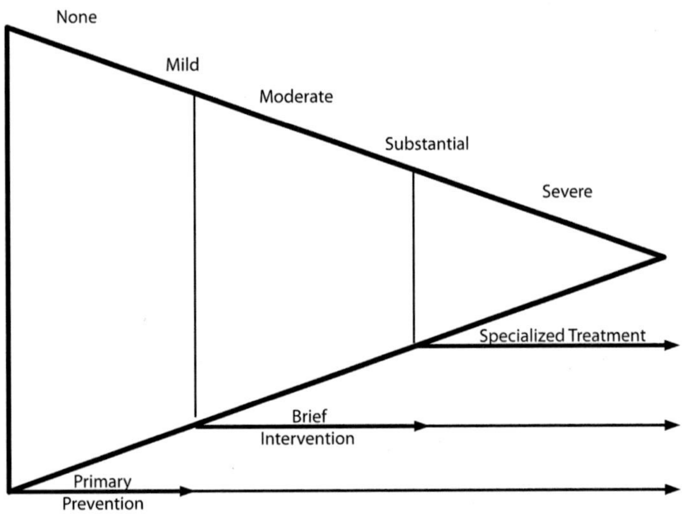

FIGURE 2-11 Alcohol use problems and interventions.
NOTE: The term "primary prevention" in this figure is used in the 1990 IOM report, but subsequent reports (including this one) use the term "universal prevention" instead.
SOURCE: IOM, 1990, p. 212.

those with unhealthy alcohol use who may be at risk for developing severe problems, and those with severe problems. The figure includes the spectrum of services the committee recommends to address alcohol use problems.

The bottom of this horizontal pyramid includes the largest portion of military personnel—those who do not use alcohol or who drink at levels causing no health, social, or public safety problems. (For drinkers in this category NIAAA specifies fewer than 5 drinks in a day and not more than 14 drinks in a week for men and fewer than 4 drinks in a day and not more than 7 drinks in a week for women.) Universal prevention targets this group. In line with evidence-based practice, the committee would suggest implementing programs consistent with the resiliency focus in the armed services—that is, including SUDs in the current teaching of resilience—as well as adding other evidence-based practices and policies that are implemented primarily in the community. The military is ideally structured for base commanders to institute environmental prevention strategies, including enforcement of existing underage drinking policies, removal of tax breaks for alcohol in exchanges (as is now being attempted with tobacco), and elimination of drink specials on premises.

The next-largest group of alcohol users in the pyramid includes those who may have a higher likelihood of developing unhealthy drinking habits as a result of particular risk factors, such as younger age or diagnosis of another mental health condition. These individuals would benefit from a targeted or selective prevention effort.

A third group of individuals includes those who are engaging in risky drinking but have not yet developed problems associated with their drinking. Individuals in this group can be identified through screening in primary care or other appropriate settings, such as the armed services' substance abuse programs, or possibly by military buddies or noncommissioned officers in their units. The majority of these individuals are best served through motivational interviewing and brief advice. Educational interventions should be confidential—within the clinical practice. This approach is classified as indicated prevention and is consistent with DoD and VA guidelines. A subset of this group who have moderate problems often come into contact with Command through law enforcement or other disciplinary mechanisms as a result of being involved in an alcohol-related incident (e.g., driving under the influence); these individuals typically are sent to the substance abuse program of their particular service branch.

At the top of the pyramid is the smallest proportion of individuals—those with substantial or severe problems. This may also be the group most likely to have comorbid PTSD or other mental health problems. These individuals require specialized treatment. Approaches to addressing SUDs need to consider the full spectrum of problems faced by service members.

SUMMARY

The military has a long history of use and abuse of alcohol and other drugs, and substance use often is exacerbated by deployment and combat exposure. To address these issues, DoD and the armed services developed and implemented a series of policy directives beginning in the early 1970s, largely as an outgrowth of concern about substance use during the Vietnam era. Current policy strongly discourages alcohol abuse (i.e., binge or heavy drinking), illicit drug use and prescription drug misuse, and tobacco use among members of the military forces because of the negative effects of these behaviors on health and on military readiness and the maintenance of high standards of performance and military discipline (DoD, 1997). Despite these official policies, however, substance use and abuse remain a concern for the armed services. Studies of substance use in the military show the following:

- Heavy alcohol use in the active duty component declined from 21 percent in 1980 to 17 percent in 1988, remained relatively stable with some fluctuations between 1988 and 1998 (15 percent), showed a significant increase in 2002 (18 percent), and continued to increase gradually in 2005 (19 percent) and 2008 (20 percent). It is also notable that the heavy drinking rate for 2008 (20 percent) was about the same as that when the HRB Survey series began in 1980 (21 percent).
- Binge drinking in the active duty component increased from 35 percent in 1998 to 47 percent in 2008.
- Illicit drug use in the past 30 days among the active duty component declined sharply from 28 percent in 1980 to about 3 percent in 2008.
- Prescription drug misuse among the active duty component doubled from 2 percent in 2002 to 4 percent in 2005 and almost tripled from 2005 to 2008, from 4 percent to 11 percent.
- Two new types of drugs—Spice and bath salts—have recently been gaining in popularity among civilians, partly because they are advertised as safe and legal, but the extent of their use among service members is not well documented.
- Compared with their civilian counterparts, active duty component military personnel were found to be more likely to engage in heavy drinking (a finding driven by personnel aged 18-35); less likely to use illicit drugs (excluding prescription drug misuse) among all age groups; and less likely to use illicit drugs (including prescription drugs) among younger personnel aged 18-25, but more likely to use these drugs among those aged 36 or older (a finding driven by prescription drug misuse).

- Rates of heavy drinking and illicit drug use were significantly lower for the reserve component than for the active duty component.
- Collectively, the data indicate that excessive alcohol use is a much greater substance use problem than illicit drug use or prescription drug misuse.
- Examination of alcohol risk based on AUDIT indicates that substantial percentages of military personnel (among both the active duty and reserve components) are drinking alcohol at rates that place them at risk for alcohol-related problems, even though they do not meet the current criteria for alcohol dependence; many problem drinkers would benefit from some type of alcohol intervention or treatment before reaching the most severe problem levels.
- Analyses of record data by the military indicate that alcohol and other drug use disorders have been increasing in recent years for the active duty component, the reserve component, and military dependents.
- Rates of acute and chronic incident alcohol diagnoses increased from 2001 through 2010, especially during the latter part of the decade for the active duty component. The results indicate the increasing medical burden imposed on the Military Health System by excessive alcohol use and are especially noteworthy for personnel with chronic alcohol abuse diagnoses. The number of bed days attributable to chronic alcohol abuse diagnoses roughly quadrupled over the 10-year period.
- DoD analyses of the morbidity burden for the active duty component in 2011 found that the SUD burden from medical encounters ranked seventh among 139 conditions and from hospital bed days ranked first, even though the number of service members with any medical encounter for SUD ranked only thirty-sixth. SUDs and mood disorders accounted for nearly one-quarter (24 percent) of all hospital bed days.
- Empirical data on substance use among military spouses and children are highly limited. Most studies of families have examined the strain placed by deployments on military families, the mental health problems that often result, and the increased risk for substance use problems. Well-designed studies are needed to understand substance use issues among military dependents.
- Substance use disorder prevention, diagnosis, and treatment must take into account the comorbid conditions that often result from the effects of war on service members. SUDs commonly co-occur with depression, PTSD, and other psychiatric or medical diagnoses.

REFERENCES

Adams, R. S., M. J. Larson, J. Corrigan, C. Horgan, and T. Williams. 2012. Frequent binge drinking after combat-acquired traumatic brain injury among active duty military personnel with a past year combat deployment. *Journal of Head Trauma and Rehabilitation* 27(5):349-360.

Ahmadi, H., and S. L. Green. 2011. Screening, brief intervention, and referral to treatment for military spouses experiencing alcohol and substance use disorders: A literature review. *Journal of Clinical Psychology in Medical Settings* 18(2):129-136.

Allen, J., and J. Mazzuchi. 1985. Alcohol and drug abuse among American military personnel: Prevalence and policy implications. *Military Medicine* 150(5):250-255.

Ames, G. M., and C. Cunradi. 2004. Alcohol use and preventing alcohol-related problems among young adults in the military. *Alcohol Research & Health* 28(4):252-257.

Ames, G. M., M. R. Duke, R. S. Moore, and C. B. Cunradi. 2009. The impact of occupational culture on drinking behavior of young adults in the U.S. Navy. *Journal of Mixed Methods Research* 3(2):129-150.

Anthony, J. C., L. A. Warner, and R. C. Kessler. 1994. Comparative epidemiology of dependence on tobacco, alcohol, controlled substances, and inhalants: Basic findings from the National Comorbidity Survey. *Experimental and Clinical Psychopharmacology* 2(3):244-268.

APA (American Psychiatric Association). 2011. *DSM-5 development.* http://www.dsm5.org/ProposedRevisions/Pages/proposedrevision.aspx?rid=431 (accessed August 10, 2011).

Armed Forces Health Surveillance Center. 2011. Alcohol-related diagnoses, active component, U.S. Armed Forces, 2001-2010. *Medical Surveillance Monthly Report* 18(10):9-13.

Armed Forces Health Surveillance Center. 2012a. Absolute and relative morbidity burdens attributable to various illnesses and injuries, U.S. Armed Forces, 2011. *Medical Surveillance Monthly Report* 19(4):4-9.

Armed Forces Health Surveillance Center. 2012b. Surveillance snapshot: Recurrent medical encounters associated with alcohol abuse-related diagnostic codes, active component, U.S. Armed Forces, 2001-2010. *Medical Surveillance Monthly Report* 19(2):23.

Babor, T. 2001. *AUDIT, the alcohol use disorders identification test: Guidelines for use in primary care* (2nd ed.). Geneva, Switzerland: World Health Organization, Department of Mental Health and Substance Dependence.

Brady, J. V., and R. R. Griffiths. 1983. Testing drugs for abuse liability and behavioral toxicity: Progress report from the laboratories at the Johns Hopkins University School of Medicine. *NIDA Research Monograph* 43:99-124.

Brady, K. T., T. K. Killeen, T. Brewerton, and S. Lucerini. 2000. Comorbidity of psychiatric disorders and posttraumatic stress disorder. *Journal of Clinical Psychiatry* 61(Suppl. 7):22-32.

Brandt, A. M. 2007. *The cigarette century: The rise, fall, and deadly persistence of the product that defined America.* New York: Basic Books. http://site.ebrary.com/lib/alltitles/docDetail.action?docID=10263798 (accessed June 12, 2012).

Bray, R. M., M. R. Pemberton, L. L. Hourani, M. Witt, K. L. Olmsted, J. M. Brown, B. Weimer, M. E. Lance, M. E. Marsden, and S. Scheffler. 2009. *Department of Defense Survey of Health Related Behaviors among Active Duty Military Personnel.* Research Triangle Park, NC: RTI International. http://www.tricare.mil/2008HealthBehaviors.pdf (accessed June 11, 2012).

Bray, R. M., M. R. Pemberton, M. E. Lane, L. L. Hourani, M. J. Mattiko, and L. A. Babeu. 2010a. Substance use and mental health trends among U.S. military active duty personnel: Key findings from the 2008 DoD Health Behavior Survey. *Military Medicine* 175(6):390-399.

Bray, R. M., J. L. Spira, K. R. Olmsted, and J. J. Hout. 2010b. Behavioral and occupational fitness. *Military Medicine* 175(Suppl. 1):39-56.

Bray, R. M., K. L. Rae Olmsted, and J. Williams. 2012. Misuse of prescription pain medications in U.S. active-duty service members: From recruitment to returning troops. In *Pain syndromes—from recruitment to returning troops*, edited by B. K. Wiederhold, Vol. 91. Amsterdam: IOS Press.

Bryant, C. D. 1974. Olive-drab drunks and GI junkies: Alcohol and narcotic addiction in the U.S. military. In *Deviant behavior: Occupational and organizational bases*, edited by C. D. Bryant. Chicago, IL: Rand McNally.

Bryant, C. D. 1979. *Khaki-collar crime: Deviant behavior in the military context*. New York: Free Press.

Burnett-Zeigler, I., M. Ilgen, M. Valenstein, K. Zivin, L. Gorman, A. Blow, S. Duffy, and S. Chermack. 2011. Prevalence and correlates of alcohol misuse among returning Afghanistan and Iraq veterans. *Addictive Behaviors* 36(8):801-806.

Campbell, D. G., B. L. Felker, C. F. Liu, E. M. Yano, J. E. Kirchner, D. Chan, L. V. Rubenstein, and E. F. Chaney. 2007. Prevalence of depression-PTSD comorbidity: Implications for clinical practice guidelines and primary care-based interventions. *Journal of General Internal Medicine* 22(6):711-718.

Conway, T. L. 1998. Tobacco use and the United States military: A longstanding problem. *Tobacco Control* 7(3):219-221.

Defense Health Board. 2011. *Psychotropic medication prescription practices and use and complementary and alternative medicine use*. Falls Church, VA: Defense Health Board.

DoD (Department of Defense). 1970. *Directive 1300.11: Illegal or improper use of drugs by members of the Department of Defense*. Washington, DC: DoD.

DoD. 1972. *Directive 1010.2: Alcohol abuse by personnel of the Department of Defense*. Washington, DC: DoD.

DoD. 1980. *Directive 1010.4: Alcohol and drug abuse by DoD personnel*. Washington, DC: DoD.

DoD. 1986a. *Directive 1010.10: Health promotion*. Washington, DC: DoD.

DoD. 1986b. *Smoking and health in the military*. Washington, DC: DoD.

DoD. 1987. *Department of Defense updated report on smoking and health in the military*. Washington, DC: DoD.

DoD. 1994. *Instruction 1010.15: Smoke-free DoD facilities*. Washington, DC: DoD.

DoD. 1997. *Directive 1010.4: Drug and alcohol abuse by DoD personnel*. Washington, DC: DoD.

DoD. 2009. *Status of drug use in the Department of Defense personnel*. Falls Church, VA: DoD.

DoD. 2011a. *Demographics 2010: Profile of the military community*. Arlington, VA: DoD.

DoD. 2011b. *Comprehensive plan on prevention, diagnosis, and treatment of substance use disorders and disposition of substance use offenders in the armed forces*. Washington, DC: Office of the Under Secretary of Defense.

DoD. 2012. *The Millennium Cohort Study*. http://www.millenniumcohort.org/index.php (accessed July 23, 2012).

Eaton, K. M., C. W. Hoge, S. C. Messer, A. A. Whitt, O. A. Cabrera, D. McGurk, A. Cox, and C. A. Castro. 2008. Prevalence of mental health problems, treatment need, and barriers to care among primary care-seeking spouses of military service members involved in Iraq and Afghanistan deployments. *Military Medicine* 173(11):1051-1056.

Fattore, L., and W. Fratta. 2011. Beyond THC: The new generation of cannabinoid designer drugs. *Frontiers in Behavioral Neuroscience* 5:60.

Floen, S. K., and A. Elklit. 2007. Psychiatric diagnoses, trauma, and suicidiality. *Annals of General Psychiatry* 6(12).

Foa, E. B. 2009. *Effective treatments for PTSD: Practice guidelines from the International Society for Traumatic Stress Studies*. New York: Guilford Press.

Fontana, A., and R. Rosenheck. 2008. Treatment-seeking veterans of Iraq and Afghanistan: Comparison with veterans of previous wars. *Journal of Nervous and Mental Disease* 196(7):513-521.

Gibbs, D. A., S. L. Martin, L. L. Kupper, and R. E. Johnson. 2007. Child maltreatment in enlisted soldiers' families during combat-related deployments. *Journal of the American Medical Association* 298(5):528-535.

Goldman, D., G. Oroszi, and F. Ducci. 2005. The genetics of addictions: Uncovering the genes. *Nature Reviews Genetics* 6(7):521-532.

Hasin, D. S. 2012. Introduction to DSM-5 criteria linked papers in drug and alcohol dependence. *Drug and Alcohol Dependence* 122(1-2):20-21.

Horgan, C. M., G. Strickler, and K. Skwara. 2001. *Substance abuse: The nation's number one health problem—key indicators for policy—update*. Schneider Insitute for Health Policy. Waltham, MA: Heller School, Brandeis University.

Hourani, L. L., R. M. Bray, M. E. Marsden, M. Witt, R. Vandermaas-Peeler, S. Scheffler, K. Rae Olmsted, B. Weimer, J. M. Brown, M. R. Pemberton, S. J. Nielsen, B. Lane, K. Aspinwall, S. Jones, and L. Strange. 2007. *Department of Defense survey of health related behaviors among the Guard and Reserve Force*. Research Triangle Park, NC: RTI International. http://www.tricare.mil/hpae/_docs/RC_2006%20Reserve%20Component_FR_9-07.pdf (accessed May 24, 2012).

Ingraham, L. H., and F. J. Manning. 1984. *The boys in the barracks: Observations on American military life*. Philadelphia, PA: Institute for the Study of Human Issues.

IOM (Institute of Medicine). 1990. *Broadening the base of treatment for alcohol problems*. Washington, DC: National Academy Press.

IOM. 1994. *Under the influence?: Drugs and the American work force. Summary: Conclusion and recommendations*. Washington, DC: National Academy Press.

IOM. 1996. *Pathways of addiction: Opportunities in drug abuse research*. Washington, DC: National Academy Press.

IOM. 2009. *Combating tobacco use in military and veteran populations*. Washington, DC: The National Academies Press.

IOM. 2010. *Returning home from Iraq and Afghanistan: Preliminary assessment of readjustment needs of veterans, service members, and their families*. Washington, DC: The National Academies Press.

IOM and NRC (National Research Council). 2004. *New treatments for addiction: Behavioral, ethical, legal, and social questions*. Washington, DC: The National Academies Press.

Jacobson, I. G., M. A. K. Ryan, T. I. Hooper, T. C. Smith, P. J. Amoroso, E. J. Boyko, G. D. Gackstetter, T. S. Wells, and N. S. Bell. 2008. Alcohol use and alcohol-related problems before and after military combat deployment. *Journal of the American Medical Association* 300(6):663-675.

Jakovljevic, M., M. Saric, S. Nad, R. Topic, and B. Vuksan-Cusa. 2006. Metabolic syndrome, somatic and psychiatric comorbidity in war veterans with post-traumatic stress disorder: Preliminary findings. *Psychiatria Danubina* 18(3-4):169-176.

Kasick, D. P., C. A. McKnight, and E. Klisovic. 2012. "Bath salt" ingestion leading to severe intoxication delirium: Two cases and a brief review of the emergence of mephedrone use. *American Journal of Drug and Alcohol Abuse* 38(2):176-180.

Keane, T. M., and J. Wolfe. 1990. Comorbidity in post-traumatic stress disorder an analysis of community and clinical studies. *Journal of Applied Social Psychology* 20(21):1776-1788.

KLEAN Treatment Center. 2012. *Spice: Military adopts no tolerance policy*. www.kleantreatmentcenter.com/spice-military-adopts-no-tolerance-policy (accessed May 24, 2012).

Koob, G. F., and F. E. Bloom. 1988. Cellular and molecular mechanisms of drug dependence. *Science* 242(4879):715-723.

Kroutil, L. A., R. M. Bray, and M. E. Marsden. 1994. Cigarette smoking in the U.S. military: Findings from the 1992 Worldwide Survey. *Preventive Medicine* 23(4):521-528.

Lande, R. G., B. A. Marin, A. S. Chang, and G. R. Lande. 2008. Survey of alcohol use in the U.S. Army. *Journal of Addictive Diseases* 27(3):115-121.

Ludwig, A. M., F. Bendfeldt, A. Wikler, and R. B. Cain. 1978. "Loss of control" in alcoholics. *Archives of General Psychiatry* 35(3):370-373.

Maclean, P. D. 1955. The limbic system (visceral brain) in relation to central gray and reticulum of the brain stem; evidence of interdependence in emotional processes. *Psychosomatic Medicine* 17(5):355-366.

Manchikanti, L. 2007. National drug control policy and prescription drug abuse: Facts and fallacies. *Pain Physician* 10(3):399-424.

Manchikanti, L., and A. Singh. 2008. Therapeutic opioids: A ten-year perspective on the complexities and complications of the escalating use, abuse, and nonmedical use of opioids. *Pain Physician* 11(Suppl. 2):S63-S88.

Mansfield, A. J., and C. C. Engel. 2011. Understanding substance use in military spouses. *Journal of Clinical Psychology in Medical Settings* 18(2):198-199.

Mattiko, M. J., K. L. R. Olmsted, J. M. Brown, and R. M. Bray. 2011. Alcohol use and negative consequences among active duty military personnel. *Addictive Behaviors* 36(6):608-614.

NIAAA (National Institute on Alcohol Abuse and Alcoholism). 2005. *Helping patients who drink too much: A clinician's guide.* Bethesda, MD: NIAAA.

O'Brien, C. P. 2012. *If addictions can be treated, why aren't they?* http://www.dana.org/news/features/detail_rop.aspx?id=39154 (accessed August 28, 2012).

O'Brien, C. P., and A. T. McLellan. 1996. Myths about the treatment of addiction. *Lancet* 347(8996):237-240.

Office of the Surgeon General. 1967. *The health consequences of smoking: A public health service review.* Atlanta, GA: National Clearinghouse for Smoking and Health.

Office of the Surgeon General. 1979. *Smoking and health: A report of the Surgeon General.* http://profiles.nlm.nih.gov/ps/access/NNBCMD.pdf (accessed June 27, 2012).

Office of the Surgeon General. 2004. *2004 Surgeon General's report—the health consequences of smoking.* Atlanta, GA: U.S. Public Health Service, Office on Smoking and Health.

Olds, J. 1958. Self-stimulation of the brain: Its use to study local effects of hunger, sex, and drugs. *Science* 127(3294):315-324.

Padden, D. L., R. A. Connors, and J. G. Agazio. 2011. Determinants of health-promoting behaviors in military spouses during deployment separation. *Military Medicine* 176(1): 26-34.

Ritz, M. C., R. J. Lamb, S. R. Goldberg, and M. J. Kuhar. 1987. Cocaine receptors on dopamine transporters are related to self-administration of cocaine. *Science* 237(4819):1219-1223.

Robins, L. N. 1974. *The Vietnam drug user returns. Final report.* Washington, DC: Special Action Office for Drug Abuse Prevention.

Robins, L. N., J. E. Helzer, and D. H. Davis. 1975. Narcotic use in southeast Asia and afterward. An interview study of 898 Vietnam returnees. *Archives of General Psychiatry* 32(8):955-961.

SAMHSA (Substance Abuse and Mental Health Services Administration). 2008. *Results from the 2007 National Survey on Drug Use and Health: National Findings.* Rockville, MD: Office of Applied Studies, Substance Abuse and Mental Health Services Administration.

Santiago, P. N., J. E. Wilk, C. S. Milliken, C. A. Castro, C. C. Engel, and C. W. Hoge. 2010. Screening for alcohol misuse and alcohol-related behaviors among combat veterans. *Psychiatric Services* 61(6):575-581.

Saunders, J. B., O. G. Aasland, T. F. Babor, J. R. De La Fuente, and M. Grant. 1993. Development of the Alcohol Use Disorders Identification Test (AUDIT): WHO collaborative project on early detection of persons with harmful alcohol consumption—II. *Addiction* 88(6):791-804.

Schuckit, M. A. 1977. Alcohol problems in the United States armed forces. *Military Chaplain's Review: Alcohol Abuse* (Winter):9-19.

Schumm, W. R., D. B. Bell, and P. A. Gade. 2000. Effects of a military overseas peacekeeping deployment on marital quality, satisfaction, and stability. *Psychological Reports* 87(3, Part 1):815-821.

Shen, Y.-C., J. Arkes, and T. V. Williams. 2012. Effects of Iraq/Afghanistan Deployments on Major Depression and Substance Use Disorder: Analysis of Active Duty Personnel in the US Military. *American Journal of Public Health* 102(S1):S80-S87.

Spera, C. 2011. Relationship of military deployment recency, frequency, duration, and combat exposure to alcohol use in the Air Force. *Journal of Studies on Alcohol and Drugs* 72(1):5-14.

Tanielian, T. L., L. Jaycox, T. L. Schell, G. N. Marshall, M. A. Burnam, C. Eibner, B. R. Karney, L. S. Meredith, J. S. Ringel, and M. E. Vaiana. 2008. *Invisible wounds of war: Summary and recommendations for addressing psychological and cognitive injuries.* Santa Monica, CA: RAND Corporation, Center for Military Health Policy Research.

Thomas, J. L., J. E. Wilk, L. A. Riviere, D. McGurk, C. A. Castro, and C. W. Hoge. 2010. Prevalence of mental health problems and functional impairment among active component and National Guard soldiers 3 and 12 months following combat in Iraq. *Archives of General Psychiatry* 67(6):614-623.

U.S. Army. 2012. *Army 2020: Generating health & discipline in the force.* Washington, DC: Department of the Army.

Vandrey, R., K. E. Dunn, J. A. Fry, and E. R. Girling. 2012. A survey study to characterize use of Spice products (synthetic cannabinoids). *Drug and Alcohol Dependence* 120(1-3):238-241.

Volkow, N. D. 2011. *"Bath salts": Emerging and dangerous products. Messages from the director,* http://www.drugabuse.gov/about-nida/directors-page/messages-director/2011/02/bath-salts-emerging-dangerous-product (accessed June 13, 2012).

Wells, D. L., and C. A. Ott. 2011. The "new" marijuana. *Annals of Pharmacotherapy* 45(3):414-417.

Wertsch, M. E. 1991. *Military brats: Legacies of childhood inside the fortress* (1st ed.). New York: Harmony Books.

Winder, G. S., N. Stern, and A. Hosanagar. 2012. Are "bath salts" the next generation of stimulant abuse? *Journal of Substance Abuse Treatment* [Epub ahead of print].

3

The Military Health System

The Military Health System (MHS) provides care to specific military-connected beneficiaries in military health care facilities and certain civilian facilities where care is purchased. In reality, the MHS is not a single system and is fairly complex. Its beneficiaries are a diverse group, and include active duty service members (ADSMs), members of the National Guard and Reserves, retirees, and family members. The total beneficiary population is about 9.7 million.

Operational oversight of the Defense Health Program, both the direct and purchased care systems, resides in the Office of the Under Secretary of Defense for Personnel and Readiness, through the Office of the Assistant Secretary of Defense for Health Affairs. The Army, Navy, and Air Force each have a designated surgeon general who has management responsibility for the branch-specific services. Since the Marine Corps does not have a Medical Command, any physicians serving with the Marines are Navy officers, and as such, come under the authority of the Navy surgeon general. Increasingly, facilities are being managed jointly by more than one branch. In the National Capital Region, for example, the services provided by the former Army Walter Reed Hospital and the National Naval Medical Center have been integrated into the new Walter Reed National Medical Center on the grounds of the former National Naval Medical Center. This consolidated site is staffed by providers from both the Army and Navy and provides care for service members from different branches of the military.

The general focus of the MHS is on ADSMs, fitness for duty, readiness, and care of the war fighter. In this context, substance use disorders (SUDs) generally are viewed as a condition that interferes with fitness for duty and service members' ability to carry out their job duties, including deployments, particularly since positive identification of an SUD may lead to separation from uniformed service. Thus, SUDs are sometimes viewed as personnel issues and at other times as medical conditions. As a result, both the Personnel and Medical Commands are involved in the identification and management of SUDs. Although the focus of military treatment facilities is operational readiness, the Department of Defense (DoD) for many years has expressed a commitment to providing substance abuse treatment to eligible beneficiaries.

This chapter provides an overview of the MHS. It describes the eligible beneficiaries, the direct care military treatment facilities, and the purchased care system. It also explains how service members and their dependents access SUD care and concludes with a summary.

ELIGIBILITY FOR CARE

To be eligible for health care services in the MHS, including those for substance abuse, one must be either a "sponsor" (generally the person who has served or is serving in the uniformed services) or the sponsor's family member (spouse; dependent child under age 21 or under age 23 if a full-time student, or up to age 26 at additional cost[1]; or adult disabled child if disabled before age 21). Eligibility is determined by enrollment in the Defense Enrollment Eligibility Reporting System (DEERS), a computerized database of all beneficiaries eligible for health care and other uniformed services benefits (see Figure 3-1).

Military treatment facilities and the MHS in general are designed to ensure the operational readiness of the members of the uniformed services. *Readiness* is the ability of the uniformed services to be prepared for operational duties at all times. Readiness requires medical, dental, and mental health. DoD, in conjunction with the Department of Health and Human Services (for Public Health Service officers) and the National Oceanic and Atmospheric Administration (for NOAA officers), has a statutory responsibility to provide health care to identified beneficiaries. This care is provided through the direct care system at military treatment facilities and through the purchased care system by reimbursement to authorized providers via the TRICARE insurance plans (see Figure 3-2).

Members of each of the seven uniformed services (see Figure 3-3) have the same overall health care benefits under the TRICARE plans, which include coverage of behavioral health benefits such as substance abuse services. Further, members of the same beneficiary category (i.e., active duty, Guard/Reserve, retiree, family member) also have similar benefits across the different branches of the military, with the same TRICARE plans from which to choose.

---

[1] TRICARE Young Adult, a provision of the 2010 Patient Protection and Affordable Care Act.

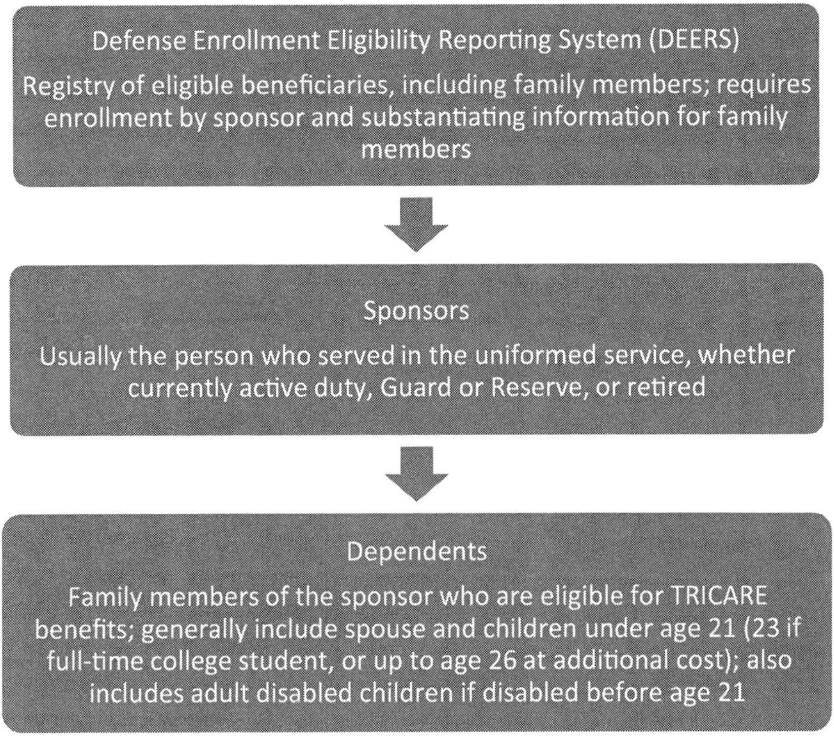

FIGURE 3-1 Defense Enrollment Eligibility Reporting System (DEERS).

Although active duty readiness is a major focus of the MHS, ADSMs and their dependents are becoming an increasingly smaller percentage of the total beneficiary population. In 1999, ADSMs and their dependents represented 57 percent of the beneficiary population, and retirees and their dependents 43 percent. By 2010, the active duty population had shrunk to 43 percent, while the retiree population had grown to 57 percent. By 2015, estimates are that only 35 percent of beneficiaries will be ADSMs and their dependents, while 65 percent will be retirees and their dependents. Because older beneficiaries tend to utilize health care services more than do younger persons, this changing demographic is contributing to the ever-growing costs of military health care (Jansen, 2009). Figure 3-4 provides definitions of terms related to TRICARE and the uniformed services health care system.

Active Duty Service Members and Their Dependents

ADSMs generally receive medical care at military treatment facilities or field health stations. ADSMs are automatically enrolled in TRICARE Prime

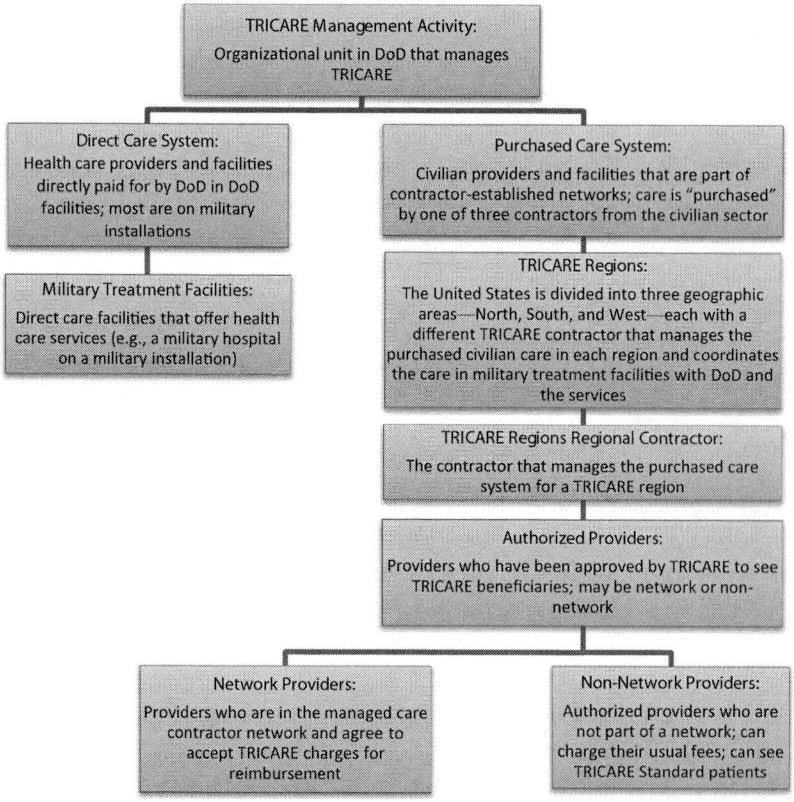

FIGURE 3-2 TRICARE organization of services.

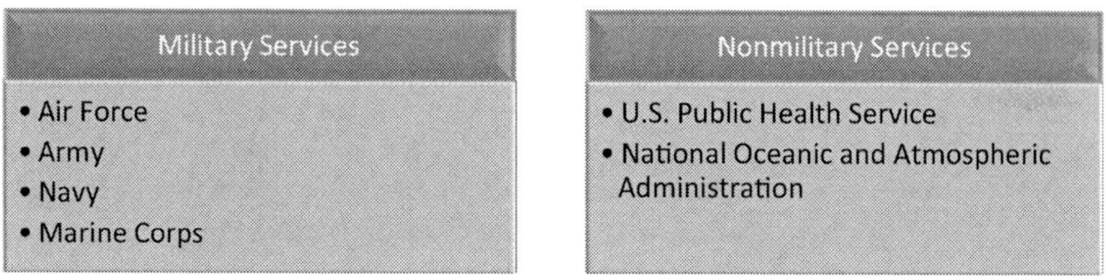
Military Services
• Air Force
• Army
• Navy
• Marine Corps
Nonmilitary Services
• U.S. Public Health Service
• National Oceanic and Atmospheric Administration

FIGURE 3-3 The uniformed services.

and are required to utilize military treatment facilities when those facilities are available. If ADSMs want to utilize a civilian provider outside of the TRICARE system, they must obtain specific permission to do so, even if they have private health insurance (such as from a working spouse) or are willing to pay the costs out of pocket. It is viewed as a readiness issue, and also relates to the Command's "need to know."

Military Health System

- Military and civilian health care providers and facilities that provide care to uniformed services–connected beneficiaries through Department of Defense funding

TRICARE

- The health care program serving uniformed service members and retirees and their families worldwide

National Guard and Reserve

- Refers to members of the Army National Guard, Army Reserve, Navy Reserve, Marine Corps Reserve, Air National Guard, Air Force Reserve, and Coast Guard Reserve

FIGURE 3-4 Terminology related to the uniformed services health care system.

If readiness is to be maintained, the families of ADSMs also must receive the medical care they need. The stress of deployment would only be magnified if an ADSM were concerned about the health care available to his/her family members.

Active Duty Retirees and Their Dependents

Retirees and their dependents have earned their health care benefits through their years of active service. Until age 65, retirees and their family members have the option of participating in various TRICARE options, some with enrollment fees and copayments. When a retiree or family member reaches age 65 or is otherwise eligible for Medicare, TRICARE for Life becomes applicable. TRICARE for Life generally requires participation in Medicare Parts A and B and acts as a secondary payer. Beneficiaries usually bear no out-of-pocket costs for specific medical services received. TRICARE for Life also provides an enhanced benefit package over Medicare. Most TRICARE for Life benefits are provided by civilian TRICARE contractors; however, military treatment facilities provide care to these beneficiaries on a space-available basis as well.

National Guard and Reserve Members and Their Dependents

Members of the National Guard and Reserves and their dependents make up yet another beneficiary group. The specifics of coverage for this group are complex, depending on the particulars of the sponsor's military duty. With the increased support provided by the Guard and Reserves for the wars in Iraq and Afghanistan, greater numbers of Guard members and Reservists have been called to extended active duty. Accordingly, their health care benefit options have increased somewhat over time.

In general, if members of the National Guard or Reserves are on military duty for 30 days or less, such as for drilling, they qualify for care in the line of duty. Also, sponsors and family members are usually eligible for TRICARE Reserve Select, a premium-based program. When sponsors are activated or called to duty for more than 30 days, they and family members become eligible for essentially the same TRICARE benefits as other ADSMs. When Guard and Reserve members transition off active duty service, they are then eligible for the Continued Health Care Benefit Program (CHCBP), which the military offers to be in compliance with the Consolidated Omnibus Budget Reconciliation Act (COBRA). This program allows service members and their eligible dependents to maintain health insurance coverage for 18-36 months by paying the full premium. Additional details are presented in Tables 3-1 and 3-2. Note that since many Guard and Reserve members have private health insurance as part of their civilian jobs, they and their families have a lower TRICARE participation rate than other ADSMs.

Other Beneficiaries

In addition to ADSMs, Guard members and Reservists, retirees, and their family members, the direct care system provides care for a fixed fee to certain government officials on occasion, including the President and members of Congress. However, these populations represent a small fraction of the care given and are not considered further in this report.

DIRECT CARE: MILITARY TREATMENT FACILITIES

The direct care system includes the providers and facilities that are directly managed by the military services. They are organized by service (i.e., Army, Navy, Air Force) and are managed by each service's surgeon general. Thus, there is variation among the branches in the policies and the specific ways in which those policies are implemented to meet overall statutory mandates and DoD directives. However, greater uniformity is expected to develop over time for substance abuse treatment as well as other medical care as the different branches of the military increasingly share resources and facilities to treat service members regardless of their branch. DoD recently was tasked to conduct an evaluation of the proposed shift toward a Unified Medical Command that would oversee the medical services of all

TABLE 3-1 Reserve Component Health Care Continuum

Inactive Duty for Training/ Selected Reserve	Active Duty Service	Predeployment	Deployment	Postdeployment	Transition Off Activity Duty
TRICARE Reserve Select (TRS)	TRICARE for Active Duty	Early Eligibility	TRICARE for Active Duty	Transitional Assistance Management Program (TAMP)	Continued Health Care Benefit Program (CHCBP)
TRICARE Standard	TRICARE Standard/ Extra Prime/TRICARE Prime Remote (TPR)	TRICARE Standard/ Extra Prime/TPR	TRICARE Standard/ Extra Prime/TPR	TRICARE Standard/ Extra Prime	TRICARE Standard/ Extra Prime
Participating Selected Reserve Monthly Premiums (Not eligible if eligible for Federal Employees Health Benefits [FEHB] Program	Inactive duty training (IDT)/active duty training (ADT) orders Coverage begins: • Member—day 1 • Family—day 1 (any order ≥31 days)	Delayed effective date orders Coverage begins: • Up to 180 days prior to deployment • Member and family covered	Active duty orders Coverage begins: • Member—day 1 • Family—day 1 (any order ≥31 days)	Contingency orders ≥31 days Coverage begins: • At release from active duty • Covered for 180 days • Must re-enroll in Prime • TPR not available	• Consolidated Omnibus Budget Reconciliation Act (COBRA)-like benefit • Must enroll within 60 days after separation from active duty or loss of eligibility for military health care • Quarterly premiums • 18-36 months of coverage

SOURCE: Powerpoint presentation by Brigadier General Margaret Wilmoth, Assistant for Mobilization and Reserve Affairs, U.S. Department of Defense, Office of Force Health Protection and Readiness, May 3, 2011, Washington, DC.

TABLE 3-2 Continuum of Care When on Active Duty

	Military Duty (30 days or less)	Preactivation* (90 days early eligibility)	Activation	Deactivation (upon leaving active duty)	Continued Coverage
Medical—Guard/ Reserve Member	Treatment for line of duty (LOD) conditions, TRICARE Reserve Select (TRS)	Full TRICARE coverage as active duty service members	Full TRICARE coverage as active duty service members	Transition Assistance Management Program (TAMP) coverage*	TRS or Continued Health Care Benefits Program (CHCBP)
Medical—Family Members	TRS	Full TRICARE coverage as active duty family members	Full TRICARE coverage as active duty family members	TAMP	TRS or CHCBP
Dental—Guard Reserve Member	Treatment for LOD conditions only	Full TRICARE coverage as active duty service members	Full TRICARE coverage as active duty service memebrs	TRICARE Dental Program (TDP)	TDP
Dental—Family Members	TDP (Reserve Component family member rates)	TDP (active duty family member rates)	TDP (active duty family member rates)	TDP (Reserve Component family member rates)	TDP (Reserve Component family member rates)

*If active duty is in support of a contingency operation.
SOURCE: Powerpoint presentation by Brigadier General Margaret Wilmoth, Assistant for Mobilization and Reserve Affairs, U.S. Department of Defense, Office of Force Health Protection and Readiness, May 3, 2011, Washington, DC.

BOX 3-1
TRICARE Patient Priority System

Priority 1	Active duty service members
Priority 2	Active duty family members enrolled in TRICARE Prime
Priority 3	Retirees, their family members, and survivors enrolled in TRICARE Prime
Priority 4	Active duty family members not enrolled in TRICARE Prime
Priority 5	All other eligible persons

branches.[2] It remains to be seen whether the military will move forward with such a large reorganization of its health services.

DoD is required to provide care to ADSMs at military treatment facilities and also to their dependents on a space-available basis.[3,4] While many categories of beneficiaries have some level of access to military treatment facilities, TRICARE Prime beneficiaries identify a facility where they will receive their primary care, and a specific primary care manager is then assigned. This provider manages their overall care and most referrals, including those for substance abuse treatment. Because of capacity limitations, military treatment facilities are unable to provide care to all eligible beneficiaries. TRICARE Prime beneficiaries generally receive care at their identified facility. Because of space limitations, however, a patient priority system has been developed for all beneficiaries (see Box 3-1). When military treatment facilities lack the capacity or capabilities needed by their primary beneficiaries, these beneficiaries generally can be seen by contracted civilian providers.

The direct care system includes 59 inpatient hospitals and medical centers and 363 ambulatory care clinics, staffed by roughly 85,000 ADSMs and 53,000 civilians. Substance abuse services are provided in only a fraction of these facilities (TMA, 2011a). Table 3-3 details how the 108 (as of July 2012) military treatment facilities that provide specialty care for substance abuse are distributed by TRICARE region and by state or foreign country.

[2] National Defense Authorization Act for Fiscal Year 2012, Public Law 112-81, 112th Cong. (December 31, 2011).

[3] Scope and Duration of Federal Loan Insurance Program, 20 U.S.C. § 1074 (2012).

[4] Medical and Dental Care for Dependents: General Rule, 10 U.S.C. § 1076 (2012).

TABLE 3-3 Military Treatment Facilities That Provide Specialty Care for Substance Abuse, by TRICARE Region

TRICARE Region	State/Country	Total
U.S.-Based		**91**
North Region	Connecticut (1), Delaware (1), District of Columbia (1), Illinois (2), Kentucky (1), Maryland (6), New York (2), North Carolina (3), Ohio (1), Pennsylvania (1), Rhode Island (1), Virginia (3)	23
South Region	Alabama (3), Florida (8), Georgia (5), Kentucky (2) Louisiana (2), Mississippi (2), Oklahoma (3), South Carolina (2), Tennessee (1), Texas (5)	33
West Region	Alaska (2), Arizona (3), California (5), Colorado (3), Hawaii (4), Idaho (1), Kansas (3), Missouri (2), Montana (1), Nebraska (1), Nevada (2), New Mexico (2), North Dakota (1), Utah (1), Washington (4)	35
Overseas		**17**
Overseas Pacific	Japan (5), South Korea (2)	7
Eurasia-Africa	Germany (5), Italy (2), Portugal (1), Turkey (1), United Kingdom (1)	10
Latin America		0
TOTAL		**108**

SOURCE: http://www.tricare.mil/mtf.

PURCHASED CARE: TRICARE

As noted, to augment care provided by military treatment facilities, health care services are purchased from civilian providers. Overall, there are nearly 400,000 network individual providers for primary care, behavioral health, and specialty care. There are also more than 3,100 TRICARE network acute hospitals nationwide (TMA, 2011a). Most of the care is purchased through one of three large TRICARE contractors, one per TRICARE region. Each of these contractors maintains a network of civilian providers that provide a full range of services, including substance abuse services (GAO, 2011). The specific providers vary over time. Table 3-4 shows the states that make up the various TRICARE regions and the contractor responsible for each region.

Care through both the direct and purchased care systems is provided through a cluster of 12 TRICARE plans. The details of the specific plans affect the substance abuse treatment providers accessible to beneficiaries, as well as the co-payments. The 12 plans are based on four general models: (1) Prime, (2) Extra, (3) Standard, and (4) TRICARE for Life. (See Appendix E for a summary of these four models.)

TRICARE Prime options are essentially health maintenance organizations (HMOs). As noted earlier, beneficiaries have assigned primary care

TABLE 3-4 TRICARE Regions and Contractors

TRICARE Region	States	Contractor
U.S.-Based		
North Region	Connecticut, Delaware, District of Columbia, Illinois, Indiana, Iowa, Kentucky, Maine, Maryland, Massachusetts, Michigan, Missouri (St. Louis), New Hampshire, New Jersey, New York, North Carolina, Ohio, Pennsylvania, Rhode Island, Tennessee (Ft. Campbell), Vermont, Virginia, West Virginia, Wisconsin	Health Net
South Region	Alabama, Arkansas, Florida, Georgia, Louisiana, Mississippi, Oklahoma, South Carolina, Tennessee (excluding Ft. Campbell), Texas (excluding El Paso)	Humana
West Region	Arizona, Arkansas, California, Hawaii, Idaho, Iowa (except Rock Island Arsenal), Kansas, Minnesota, Missouri (except St. Louis), Montana, Nebraska, New Mexico, North Dakota, Oregon, South Dakota, Texas (southwest corner), Utah, Washington, Wyoming	TriWEST*
Overseas		International SOS
Overseas Pacific		
Eurasia-Africa		
Latin America		

*TriWEST lost the bid to renew its contract as the provider for the Western Region on March 16, 2012. It appealed this decision on May 3, 2012. The U.S. Government Accountability Office denied the appeal on July 2, 2012.

managers who make referrals for specialty care. The Prime options require pre-enrollment and use of network providers. ADSMs are automatically enrolled in TRICARE Prime.

TRICARE Extra options utilize preferred provider organizations, which domestically are typically networks managed by one of the three national TRICARE contractors. Providers participating in Extra options are authorized providers who agree to accept TRICARE reimbursement, which in most cases is based on Medicare reimbursement schedules. The Extra plans do not require pre-enrollment and have no annual enrollment costs. Although referrals for specialty care are not necessary, preauthorization is required for many services, including substance abuse treatment (TMA, 2012c).

TRICARE Standard is essentially a fee-for-service option utilizing authorized providers. Authorization involves a credential review and approval by TRICARE. Providers charge their usual rates, no pre-enrollment is required, and referrals are not necessary for specialty care. However, preauthorization is required for many services, including substance abuse treatment (TMA, 2012c).

TRICARE for Life is the Medicare "wrap-around." As discussed earlier, TRICARE beneficiaries aged 65 and older who participate in Parts A and B of Medicare are eligible for this plan. They must pay the Medicare enrollment fees but no additional annual TRICARE enrollment fees. Medicare is the first payer; the TRICARE for Life plan generally pays all out-of-pocket Medicare costs and also provides some additional medical benefits (TMA, 2012a).

TRICARE Prime now has a Point of Service option, which allows TRICARE Prime beneficiaries to participate as well in features of TRICARE Standard and TRICARE Extra. Essentially, this option gives beneficiaries a greater choice of providers, although the providers must still be TRICARE authorized. Out-of-pocket expenses also increase. TRICARE Prime provides the most comprehensive benefit, although the choice of providers is more limited than is the case under TRICARE Extra and TRICARE Standard (TMA, 2011b).

TRICARE also has a pharmacy benefit with four options, each of which is available to all TRICARE beneficiaries. Prescriptions can be filled at a pharmacy at a military treatment facility at no cost. Prescriptions can also be filled through a mail order pharmacy program that is managed by a single contracted worldwide pharmacy home delivery vendor. This service is used most often for routine prescriptions taken for chronic conditions. The third option is a retail pharmacy, which includes almost 64,000 contracted network retail pharmacies. The retail pharmacies can dispense a maximum 30-day medication supply. Finally, non-network pharmacies can be used if the other options are not available. The mail order and retail pharmacy programs have some co-payments, which vary with beneficiaries' duty status and whether the prescription is for generic or brand name products. Waivers are possible for nonformulary pharmaceuticals (TMA, 2012b).

CARE FOR SUBSTANCE USE DISORDERS FOR MILITARY SERVICE MEMBERS AND DEPENDENTS

The preceding sections describe how ADSMs, members of the National Guard and Reserves, and their dependents access health care through the direct and purchased care systems. This section explains how each of these groups accesses SUD care in particular.

SUD Care Provided Through the Direct Care System

The SUD care available in the direct care system for service members and their dependents varies by service branch and location. The way each branch approaches prevention, screening, diagnosis, treatment, and management for SUDs is guided by overarching policies laid out by DoD, as well as by branch-specific policies. These policies set forth clear guidelines for zero tolerance of drug and alcohol abuse, as well as the legal and administrative consequences of such abuse (DoD, 1997). The requirement to provide education focused on preventing drug and alcohol abuse, to conduct drug use testing, and to offer rehabilitation for substance use offenders also is laid out in DoD policies and instructions (DoD, 1985, 1994, 1997). Each branch is then responsible for developing its own branch-level policies to guide programs and activities that address SUDs. The branch policies set forth the specifics of how drug prevention, testing, and rehabilitation programs will operate. Some of the branch-level policies are more detailed than others and also address the responsibilities of personnel at different levels, as well as training and credentialing requirements for providers. Chapter 6 of this report provides a thorough review of all DoD and branch-level policies and programs addressing SUDs, while Chapter 8 details the requirements for credentialing and training for providers in these programs.

The branches vary widely in how SUD care is delivered in the direct care system. In the Army, for instance, all SUD prevention activities and nearly all SUD treatment are provided under the authority of the Installation Management Command, which is responsible for all personnel issues. In contrast, the Navy houses all of its SUD treatment services under the Navy Bureau of Medicine and Surgery, its Medical Command, while prevention activities and services are delivered under the Personnel Command. This "ownership" by either the Medical or Personnel Command has implications for how care and services are delivered. Chapter 6 details the various types of SUD services and care that are provided within each branch of the military and the authority under which they operate.

SUD Care Provided Through the TRICARE Network

TRICARE is required to provide care for SUDs under the authority of 32 *Code of Federal Regulations* (CFR) 199.4.[5] This care may include detoxification, rehabilitation, and outpatient group and family therapy. TRICARE provides a lifetime limit of three SUD treatment benefit periods (each benefit period is 365 days from the first visit), although this limit can be waived by the managed care support contractor that oversees the TRICARE plans for the region. Emergency and inpatient hospital services for detoxification and stabilization and for treatment of medical complications from an SUD do not start a benefit period for treatment. Emergency and inpatient hospital services are deemed medically necessary when the personnel and facilities of a hospital are required to manage the patient's

[5] Basic Program Benefits, 32 CFR § 199.4 (2004).

condition. All purchased treatment for SUDs requires prior authorization from the regional TRICARE contractor (TMA, 2008).

Chemical detoxification is covered for up to 7 days, although more days can be covered if medically or psychologically necessary. These 7 days count toward the 30- or 45-day limit for acute inpatient psychiatric care per fiscal year. If an inpatient general hospital setting is not needed, however, up to 7 days of chemical detoxification is covered in addition to any further rehabilitative care. Rehabilitation for SUDs may occur in an inpatient or partial hospitalization setting. Coverage encompasses 21 days (or one inpatient stay per benefit period) in a TRICARE-authorized facility. These 21 days also count toward the 30- or 45-day limit for acute inpatient psychiatric care (TMA, 2008).

Outpatient group therapy for SUDs must be provided by an approved Substance Use Disorder Rehabilitation Facility (SUDRF) (for more information on these facilities, refer to Chapter 7). The benefit includes 60 group therapy sessions in a benefit period. These sessions are in addition to the 15 sessions of outpatient family therapy covered by TRICARE. Family therapy is covered upon the completion of rehabilitative care (TMA, 2010). Note that individual outpatient therapy is not covered for SUDs unless it is provided through a SUDRF. As a TRICARE benefit, access to SUD services through contracted TRICARE providers requires preapproval through the contractor. Each of the contractors has a phone number that begins the preapproval process. SUD services can also be accessed through a provider-based toll-free number that is not limited to TRICARE beneficiaries; TRICARE specialists return all calls to this number and assist with referrals. Chapter 7 of this report describes the availability of and access to SUD care through the TRICARE benefit.

Other Avenues for SUD Care

In addition to the direct care and purchase care systems described above, members of the military and their families have several other avenues for SUD care. Like nearly all employers in the United States, the military has access to employee assistance programs; the specific contract provisions vary somewhat among the branches. An additional avenue is Military OneSource, which includes a website and nonclinical counseling that offer referral information on a wide range of topics, including substance abuse. Service members and their families may also receive care through Warrior Transition Units, the Soldier 360 Program, the Veterans Health Administration, and community programs such as Give an Hour. Some of these programs are reviewed in Chapter 6 and Appendix D of this report.

SUMMARY

Through the direct care system and the TRICARE insurance benefit, the MHS provides comprehensive health care to military service members and their dependents. A multitude of insurance plans are available to eligible beneficiaries, along with a provider network that spans the globe. For the treatment of SUDs, service members and their dependents can access care both in military treatment facilities and through TRICARE network providers. The TRICARE SUD benefit notably does not reimburse for office-based outpatient treatment. The implication of this benefit limitation is discussed further in Chapter 7.

REFERENCES

DoD (Department of Defense). 1985. *Instruction 1010.6: Rehabilitation and referral services for alcohol and drug abusers*. Washington, DC: DoD.

DoD. 1994. *Directive 1010.1: Drug abuse testing program*. Washington, DC: DoD.

DoD. 1997. *Directive 1010.4: Drug and alcohol abuse by DoD personnel*. Washington, DC: DoD.

GAO (U.S. Government Accountability Office). 2011. *Defense health care: Access to civilian providers under TRICARE standard and extra*. Washington, DC: GAO.

Jansen, D. 2009. *Military medical care: Questions and answers*. Washington, DC: Congressional Research Service.

TMA (TRICARE Management Activity). 2008. *TRICARE policy manual 6010.57-M*. Falls Church, VA: TMA.

TMA. 2010. *Treatment for substance use disorders*. http://tricare.mil/substanceusedisorders (accessed May 24, 2012).

TMA. 2011a. *Evaluation of the TRICARE program: FY 2011 report to Congress*. http://www.tricare.mil/tma/downloads/TRICARE2011_02_28_11v8.pdf (accessed June 27, 2012).

TMA. 2011b. *TRICARE prime and TRICARE remote handbook*. Falls Church, VA: TMA.

TMA. 2012a. *TRICARE for life*. http://www.tricare.mil/mybenefit/home/overview/LearnAboutPlansAndCosts/TRICAREForLife (accessed June 14, 2012).

TMA. 2012b. *TRICARE pharmacy program*. http://www.tricare.mil/mybenefit/home/Prescriptions/PharmacyProgram (accessed June 14, 2012).

TMA. 2012c. *TRICARE standard and extra*. http://www.tricare.mil/standardextra (accessed June 14, 2012).

4

Changing Standards of Care for Substance Use Disorders

The committee's review of the Department of Defense's (DoD's) policies and programs for prevention, diagnosis, treatment, and management of substance use disorders (SUDs) included the strongest and most up-to-date evidence in the scientific and industry literature. This chapter reflects on the standards and expectations for SUD care and how they are evolving in a rapidly changing health care environment. Although DoD may be exempt from facets of health care reform, a contemporary set of prevention and treatment services for the U.S. military will embrace the state of the art, encourage evidence-based practices, and reflect emerging standards of care. In addition to health care reform, emerging expectations from the Office of National Drug Control Policy and the National Quality Forum will affect alcohol and other drug prevention and treatment services.

HEALTH CARE REFORM AND PARITY REQUIREMENTS

The Patient Protection and Affordable Care Act of 2010 (hereafter referred to as the Affordable Care Act) aims to better control health care expenses, enhance the quality of health care, and reduce the proportion of individuals who are uninsured. The act is likely to add many millions of individuals to state Medicaid plans (Sommers et al., 2011), and a number of these new enrollees are likely to have alcohol and other drug use disorders (Barry and Huskamp, 2011; Buck, 2011; Garfield et al., 2011). Requirements that state exchanges must cover treatment of alcohol, other drug, and mental health disorders as essential benefits promote access to treatment services for SUDs (Barry and Huskamp, 2011; Buck, 2011).

Under the Affordable Care Act, Medicaid and other health plans will become primary payers for most addiction treatment services. The current system of direct grants and contracts will dissipate as treatment providers' reimbursement from Medicaid and commercial health plans increases. State and federal appropriations designated for addiction prevention and treatment are likely to decline as Medicaid health plans become major payers (Buck, 2011). The substance abuse counseling workforce is likely to change because health plans are typically selective in their purchase of service contracts and screen for evidence of quality care. Practitioners that provide evidence of quality care are likely to have competitive advantages. Medicaid and commercial health plans are likely to limit reimbursement to practitioners with graduate degrees and professional licensure (McCarty et al., 2010). The workforce impact may be substantial because only about 50 percent of counselors in most addiction treatment centers have graduate degrees (i.e., 42 percent of total counselors, 58 percent of outpatient counselors) (McCarty et al., 2007a). With the increasing medicalization of substance abuse treatment services (Buck, 2011), freestanding addiction treatment centers that rely on experientially trained counselors and/or counselors with alcohol and drug certification (but not clinical licensure) may struggle to survive (McCarty et al., 2010). The training of the addiction treatment workforce will also need to evolve to meet new requirements.

Accountable Care Organizations and Integrated Care

The Affordable Care Act generally promotes the integration of mental health and SUD treatment with primary care services and makes integrated care a priority for community-based accountable care organizations (ACOs).[1] ACOs reflect emerging standards and expectations for integrated, patient-centered care provided within a medical home that is financially responsible for coordinating a patient's health care, including care for mental health disorders and SUDs. The National Committee for Quality Assurance (NCQA) met with consumer advocates, purchasers of care, and health plans and released accreditation standards for ACOs in November 2011. The ACO accreditation standards encourage coordination of mental health and SUD services with the development of primary care medical homes and address seven dimensions of care (see Box 4-1).

ACOs will support the integration of behavioral health and primary care. Recognition is increasing that general medicine practitioners "should become the first line 'experts' for substance abuse" (O'Connor and Samet, 2002, p. 398). Alcohol and other drug use is prevalent among patients

[1] Patient Protection and Affordable Care Act, Public Law 111-148, 111th Cong. (March 23, 2010).

BOX 4-1
ACO Accreditation Standards

1. ACO Structure and Operations
2. Access to Needed Providers
3. Patient-Centered Primary Care
4. Care Management
5. Care Coordination and Transitions
6. Patient Rights and Responsibilities
7. Performance Reporting and Quality Improvement

SOURCE: NCQA, 2012.

treated in primary care (Manwell et al., 1998). Habitual alcohol and/or other drug use increases the likelihood of developing or exacerbating disorders of the heart, liver, and gastrointestinal system and conditions such as diabetes and hypertension (Gourevitch and Arnsten, 2005). Despite consensus among medical leadership on the need for a more integrated system (APA, 1994), progress has been slow. Reforms in the health system under the provisions of the Affordable Care Act could eliminate the long-standing separation of training and treatment for SUDs from routine medical care (IOM, 2006).

There are many approaches to integrated care. Most attempt to (1) create a medical home; (2) use health care teams; (3) titrate care based on level of need and capacity for self-care; and (4) differentiate the severity of behavioral health and primary care needs into four quadrants—low primary care and low behavioral health need, low primary care and high behavioral health need, high primary care and low behavioral health need, and high primary care and behavioral health need—with patients with higher needs being referred to specialty services (Collins, 2010). The need for integrated primary care, mental health, and SUD services is further illustrated by increases in prescribed opioids for pain in primary care settings. Analyses by Kaiser Permanente Northern California and Group Health of Seattle suggest significantly higher opioid use for pain in patients with SUDs (Weisner et al., 2009).

The Buprenorphine and HIV Care Evaluation and Support demonstration (sponsored by the HIV/AIDS Bureau of the Health Resources and Services Administration) is a recent example of the value of integrated care. In this study, 10 HIV clinics provided integrated medication-assisted opioid treatment. Study data documented reductions in opioid use (Fiellin et al.,

2011), increased engagement in HIV care (Altice et al., 2011), improved quality of life (Korthuis et al., 2011b), and improved quality of HIV care (Korthuis et al., 2011a). Participating patients voiced strong preferences for buprenorphine integrated into HIV care over referral to an opioid treatment program (Korthuis et al., 2010). This demonstration showed that the advantages of integrated care innovations can extend to patients in HIV primary care and supports the extension of this approach to primary care for patients without HIV infection.

Patient Placement and Levels of Care

Many health care systems use the American Society of Addiction Medicine's (ASAM's) Patient Placement Criteria to determine appropriate levels and intensity of addiction treatment services. The ASAM criteria provide guidelines for continued service and transfer/discharge for those with addictive disorders. Clinical placements and treatment plans reflect assessment of the criteria's six dimensions (see Box 4-2). Patients with high potential for withdrawal, comorbid health conditions, and a poor recovery environment may require treatment in more restrictive environments. Alternatively, employed individuals with a home and family support can be treated successfully in less-intensive ambulatory settings after medical monitoring for withdrawal.

The value of the ASAM placement criteria, first released in 1991 (Hoffman et al., 1991), is supported by two decades of experience. Currently, at least 30 states mandate their use (ASAM, 2012). The current edition, *ASAM Patient Placement Criteria for the Treatment of Substance-Related Disorders*, Second Edition-Revised (Mee-Lee, 2001), includes criteria for comorbid mental health and substance-related disorders. The

BOX 4-2
Dimensions of American Society of Addiction Medicine's (ASAM's) Patient Placement Criteria

1. Acute Intoxication and/or Withdrawal Potential
2. Biomedical Conditions and Complications
3. Emotional, Behavioral, or Cognitive Conditions and Complications
4. Readiness to Change
5. Relapse, Continued Use, or Continued Problem Potential
6. Recovery Environment

SOURCE: http://www.asam.org/publications/patient-placement-criteria.

criteria, originally developed for use with adults, have been modified and updated for use with adolescents (Fishman, 2010). The continuing development and refinement of the ASAM criteria advance a paradigm shift from

- unidimensional to multidimensional assessment,
- program-driven to clinically driven treatment,
- fixed length of service to variable length of service, and
- a limited number of discrete levels of care to a continuum of care.

The ASAM criteria advocate for and provide guidelines that promote four goals. First, the criteria require individualized, assessment-driven treatment and the flexible use of a broad continuum of care. Second, the criteria encourage the use of motivational enhancement therapies in outpatient treatment, especially for those in the early stages of readiness to change, to increase access to care and reduce waits for more intensive levels of residential treatment. Third, the assessment dimensions address multiple needs of the individual (medical, psychological, social, vocational, and legal), not just alcohol and other drug use. Finally, the criteria require continual reviews of treatment plans, with modifications based on treatment response and outcomes.

In addition to state mandates to use the ASAM criteria, DoD and national health care organizations and health plans require that an ASAM level-of-care assessment guide treatment plans. The ASAM placement criteria provide a common language with which care providers and care managers can communicate about the multidimensional assessment and placement decision for those with SUDs.

Parity

The Affordable Care Act, together with the Mental Health Parity and Addiction Equity Act of 2008 (hereafter referred to as the Parity Act), is expected to enhance access to and utilization of treatment for alcohol and other drug use disorders. The Parity Act eliminates differential copayments and restrictions on mental health and addiction treatment benefits, which must be similar to benefits for other general and specialty medical care. Initial evaluations of the implementation of parity among federal employees (Goldman et al., 2006) and in Oregon (McConnell et al., 2011) found little increase in the total costs of care.

OFFICE OF NATIONAL DRUG CONTROL POLICY'S NATIONAL DRUG CONTROL STRATEGY

The Office of National Drug Control Policy (ONDCP) asserts in its 2010, 2011, and 2012 National Drug Control Strategies that addiction treatment must be integrated into mainstream health care (ONDCP, 2010, 2011, 2012). The 2012 National Drug Control Strategy's seven priorities include two that promote linkages between health care and services for alcohol and other drug use disorders.

The ONDCP strategy calls for early intervention opportunities in health care and notes that early intervention saves lives and money (ONDCP, 2012). Screening, brief intervention, and referral to treatment services are increasingly common in emergency departments and are expanding to include schools and universities as well as families involved in child welfare systems. The 2011 National Drug Control Strategy explicitly requires DoD to train health care professionals in providing evidence-based screening and interventions for alcohol and other drug use disorders for beneficiaries served by the Military Health System. Misuse and abuse of pharmaceuticals is another priority for early intervention. The 2012 National Drug Control Strategy notes that the Secure and Responsible Drug Disposal Act promotes the development of safe, easy, and affordable drug disposal options. Local authorities are encouraged to collaborate with the Drug Enforcement Agency to collect and dispose of unused and expired prescription medications.

The 2012 National Drug Control Strategy also promotes integrated treatment for SUDs in mainstream health care (ONDCP, 2012), thus supporting the Affordable Care Act's emphasis on integrated care. The Health Resources and Services Administration (HRSA) is directed to improve care for alcohol and other drug use disorders in the nation's system of community health centers. ONDCP's National Drug Control Strategy reflects a substantive change in federal policy: for the first time, addiction treatment resources are allocated to primary care settings rather than specialty clinics. The 2011 strategy also instructs federal agencies that address health care needs to meet the National Quality Forum's voluntary consensus standards for treatment of alcohol and other drug use disorders (see the next section). To help meet these standards, HRSA, the Centers for Disease Control and Prevention, and the Substance Abuse and Mental Health Services Administration must train health care practitioners to identify, diagnose, and treat SUDs.

To support and promote recovery, ONDCP created a Recovery Branch within the Office of Demand Reduction to develop a national plan for recovery-oriented systems of care. Recovery-oriented systems of care eliminate regulatory, policy, and practice barriers to recovery and celebrate and support recovery. As part of its recovery strategy, ONDCP will work with the Department of Veterans Affairs (VA) and DoD to identify "recovery support services for alcohol and drug addiction that are appropriate for active duty military, Veterans, and their families and to ensure that those services are made available to our military families to the greatest extent possible" (ONDCP, 2011, p. 42).

NATIONAL QUALITY FORUM'S VOLUNTARY CONSENSUS STANDARDS

Clear documentation of substandard care for addiction (McGlynn et al., 2003) led to the development of the first set of national standards for addiction treatment. The National Quality Forum's consensus standards for treatment of substance use conditions identify four domains (and subdomains) of expected services for addressing addiction: (1) identification of substance use conditions (screening and case finding, diagnosis and assessment), (2) initiation of and engagement in treatment (brief intervention, promoting engagement, withdrawal management), (3) therapeutic interventions to treat substance use illness (psychosocial interventions and pharmacotherapy), and (4) continuing care management of substance use illness (NQF, 2007). Box 4-3 details each subdomain contained in the voluntary consensus standards.

For the first time, a national trade organization recommended that its membership implement specific evidence-based therapies for treating tobacco, alcohol, and other drug use disorders. The standards are applicable to all members of the National Quality Forum (national consumer advocacy groups, health professional trade associations, health systems, health plans, groups that purchase health plans, pharmaceutical companies, and research institutes). Health care organizations and health plans no longer can ignore the need to better address addiction problems in primary care and acute care settings. As noted, the 2011 National Drug Control Strategy advocates for widespread adoption of the National Quality Forum standards for addiction treatment (ONDCP, 2011).

PRACTICE IMPROVEMENT EFFORTS

The Institute of Medicine's *Quality Chasm* reports challenged the U.S. health care system to adopt process improvement strategies that would reduce errors that contribute to morbidity and mortality and facilitate the adoption of evidence-based practices (IOM, 2000, 2001, 2006). The Institute for Healthcare Improvement (IHI), a leader in quality improvement for health care, works with provider and hospital systems to facilitate quality improvement at the patient-provider level by changing systems. Measurement is a key element in the IHI Model for Improvement, a simple yet powerful tool for accelerating improvement that has been used successfully by IHI and hundreds of health care organizations in many countries to

BOX 4-3
National Quality Forum's Voluntary Consensus Standards for the Treatment of Substance Use Conditions

- **Identification of Substance Use Conditions**
  - Patients in general and mental health care settings should be screened for at-risk alcohol use problems.
  - Health care providers should employ a systematic method to identify patients who use drugs.
  - Patients who have a positive screen should receive further assessment.
- **Initiation and Engagement in Treatment**
  - All patients with at-risk alcohol or tobacco use should receive a brief motivational counseling intervention.
  - Providers should promote patient initiation of care and engagement in ongoing treatment for alcohol and other drug use disorders.
  - Pharmacotherapy should be provided to manage withdrawal symptoms and consequences.
- **Therapeutic Interventions to Treat Substance Use Illness**
  - All patients should receive empirically validated psychosocial treatment interventions.
  - Pharmacotherapy should be recommended and available to all adult patients diagnosed with opioid dependence, alcohol dependence, and nicotine dependence and without contraindications. Pharmacotherapy should be linked with psychosocial treatment.
- **Continuing Care Management of Substance Use Illness**
  - Patients should be offered long-term, coordinated management of their care.

SOURCE: Adapted from NQF, 2007.

improve numerous health care processes and outcomes. For example, Mercy Hospital (Buffalo, New York) has sustained zero ventilator-associated pneumonias in the intensive care unit (ICU) by reliably implementing the IHI Ventilator Bundle, with a special focus on reducing the amount and duration of sedation for patients on ventilators in the ICU.

An example of a system quality-improvement approach applied specifically to SUD care is NIATx (formerly the Network for the Improvement of Addiction Treatment) (Capoccia et al., 2007; Gustafson and Johnson, 2012; Hoffman et al., 2008; McCarty et al., 2007b). NIATx promotes practice and system change using a simplified version of the IHI Model for Improvement. Behavioral health care organizations learn to use Plan-Do-Study-Act change cycles to reduce days to admission, improve retention in care, and reduce no-show rates. As agencies build capacity for change, they apply the model to foster the use of evidence-based practices. NIATx, like IHI, demonstrates that system change can lead to improved clinical and administrative practices. Agencies adopting process improvements have increased the use of medications for specific diagnoses, screening and brief intervention in primary care settings, and adoption of evidence-based psychosocial clinical interventions; enhanced posttreatment aftercare; and facilitated case management, wrap-around, and supportive services. See the NIATx website for case studies.[2]

To improve the effectiveness of interventions for SUDs, Humphreys and McLellan (2011) urge policy makers to implement process-focused quality improvement strategies like those of NIATx and patient-focused strategies that reward patients and practitioners for improvements. Pay-for-performance (or value-based purchasing) strategies hold promise for promoting enhanced performance during treatment and better treatment outcomes. A focus on outcomes during treatment helps providers and patients address the ongoing symptoms of SUDs and build a strong foundation for a stable recovery. A performance contracting initiative in Maine, for example, used performance-based contracting and measurement of efficiency and effectiveness to effect system improvements in access to care and retention in treatment. SUD programs entered into fee-for-service withholds with increased payments for achieving performance targets. An evaluation analysis, however, suggested that there was little improvement in outcomes and performance (Brucker and Stewart, 2011).

CLINICAL PRACTICE GUIDELINE OF THE DEPARTMENT OF VETERANS AFFAIRS AND DoD

The VA and DoD jointly issued a clinical practice guideline to standardize quality care for SUDs for veterans and military service members. The *VA/DOD Clinical Practice Guideline for Management of Substance Use Disorders* (VA and DoD, 2009) outlines principles and best practices for the treatment of SUDs, including behavioral and pharmacological interventions. It consists of five modules that address interrelated aspects of care: Screening and Initial Assessment for Substance Use, Management of SUD in Specialty SUD Care, Management of SUD in General Healthcare, Addiction-Focused Pharmacotherapy, and Stabilization and Withdrawal Management. Each module consists of a detailed decision algorithm and recommendations for each step in treatment. The decision algorithms are based on a review process that included ranking the level of evidence and achieved consensus among a panel of VA/DoD SUD experts, representatives

[2] See http://www.niatx.net (accessed May 29, 2012).

from academia, and a private-sector guideline facilitator. A detailed review of the guideline and its implementation within DoD is included in Chapter 6 of this report.

SUMMARY

Standards of care are changing to reflect research-based behavioral and pharmacological therapies. Health care reform and federal parity legislation enhance access to health insurance and mandate that commercial health plans provide similar coverage for general health care, mental health care, and care for alcohol and other drug use disorders. Advocates and policy makers have called for increased integration of addiction treatment and primary care, and DoD is uniquely positioned to take advantage of this opportunity. Greater integration of prevention and treatment services with primary care could reduce the stigma of alcohol and other drug use disorders and encourage individuals to seek care.

REFERENCES

Altice, F. L., R. D. Bruce, G. M. Lucas, P. J. Lum, P. T. Korthuis, T. P. Flanigan, C. O. Cunningham, L. E. Sullivan, P. Vergara-Rodriguez, D. A. Fiellin, A. Cajina, M. Botsko, V. Nandi, M. N. Gourevitch, and R. Finkelstein. 2011. HIV treatment outcomes among HIV-infected, opioid-dependent patients receiving buprenorphine/naloxone treatment within HIV clinical care settings: Results from a multisite study. *Journal of Acquired Immune Deficiency Syndromes* 56(Suppl. 1):S22-S32.

APA (American Psychiatric Association). 1994. *Diagnostic and statistical manual of mental disorders: DSM-IV* (4th ed.). Washington, DC: American Psychiatric Association.

ASAM (American Society of Addiction Medicine). 2012. *Patient placement criteria*. http://www.asam.org/publications/patient-placement-criteria (accessed May 29, 2012).

Barry, C. L., and H. A. Huskamp. 2011. Moving beyond parity—mental health and addiction care under the ACA. *New England Journal of Medicine* 365(11):973-975.

Brucker, D. L., and M. Stewart. 2011. Performance-based contracting within a state substance abuse treatment system: A preliminary exploration of differences in client access and client outcomes. *Journal of Behavioral Health Services & Research* 38(3):383-397.

Buck, J. A. 2011. The looming expansion and transformation of public substance abuse treatment under the Affordable Care Act. *Health Affairs* 30(8):1402-1410.

Capoccia, V. A., F. Cotter, D. H. Gustafson, E. F. Cassidy, J. H. Ford, L. Madden, B. H. Owens, S. O. Farnum, D. McCarty, and T. Molfenter. 2007. Making "stone soup": Improvements in clinic access and retention in addiction treatment. *Joint Commission Journal on Quality and Patient Safety* 33(2):95-103.

Collins, C. 2010. *Evolving models of behavioral health integration in primary care*. New York: Milbank Memorial Fund.

Fiellin, D. A., L. Weiss, M. Botsko, J. E. Egan, F. L. Altice, L. B. Bazerman, A. Chaudhry, C. O. Cunningham, M. N. Gourevitch, P. J. Lum, L. E. Sullivan, R. S. Schottenfeld, and P. G. O'Connor. 2011. Drug treatment outcomes among HIV-infected opioid-dependent patients receiving buprenorphine/naloxone. *Journal of Acquired Immune Deficiency Syndromes* 56(Suppl. 1):S33-S38.

Fishman, M. 2010. Treatment planning, matching and placement for adolescent substance abuse. In *Clinical manual of adolescent substance abuse treatment*, edited by Y. Kaminer and K. Winters. Arlington, VA: American Psychiatric Publishing. Pp. 113-135.

Garfield, R. L., S. H. Zuvekas, J. R. Lave, and J. M. Donohue. 2011. The impact of national health care reform on adults with severe mental disorders. *American Journal of Psychiatry* 168(5):486-494.

Goldman, H. H., R. G. Frank, M. A. Burnam, H. A. Huskamp, M. S. Ridgely, S. L. T. Normand, A. S. Young, C. L. Barry, V. Azzone, A. B. Busch, S. T. Azrin, G. Moran, C. Lichtenstein, and M. Blasinsky. 2006. Behavioral health insurance parity for federal employees. *New England Journal of Medicine* 354(13):1378-1386.

Gourevitch, M. N., and J. H. Arnsten. 2005. Medical complications of drug use. In *Substance abuse: A comprehensive textbook*, edited by J. H. Lowinson. Philadelphia, PA: Lippincott Williams & Wilkins.

Gustafson, D. H., and K. Johnson. 2012. *The NIATx model: Process improvement for behavioral health*. Madison, WI: Wisconsin-Madison's Center for Health Enhancement Systems Studies.

Hoffman, K. A., J. H. Ford, 2nd, D. Choi, D. H. Gustafson, and D. McCarty. 2008. Replication and sustainability of improved access and retention within the network for the improvement of addiction treatment. *Drug and Alcohol Dependence* 98(1-2):63-69.

Hoffman, N. G., J. A. Halikas, D. Mee-Lee, and R. D. Weedman. 1991. *Patient placement criteria for the treatment of psychoactive substance use disorders*. Washington, DC: ASAM.

Humphreys, K., and A. T. McLellan. 2011. A policy-oriented review of strategies for improving the outcomes of services for substance use disorder patients. *Addiction* 106:2058-2066.

IOM (Institute of Medicine). 2000. *To err is human: Building a safer health system*. Washington, DC: National Academy Press.

IOM. 2001. *Crossing the quality chasm: A new health system for the 21st century*. Washington, DC: National Academy Press.

IOM. 2006. *Improving the quality of health care for mental and substance-use conditions: Quality chasm series*. Washington, DC: The National Academies Press.

Korthuis, P. T., J. Gregg, W. E. Rogers, D. McCarty, C. Nicolaidis, and J. Boverman. 2010. Patients' reasons for choosing office-based buprenorphine: Preference for patient-centered care. *Journal of Addiction Medicine* 4(4):204-210.

Korthuis, P. T., D. A. Fiellin, R. Fu, P. J. Lum, F. L. Altice, N. Sohler, M. J. Tozzi, S. M. Asch, M. Botsko, M. Fishl, T. P. Flanigan, J. Boverman, and D. McCarty. 2011a. Improving adherence to HIV quality of care indicators in persons with opioid dependence: The role of buprenorphine. *Journal of Acquired Immune Deficiency Syndromes* 56(Suppl. 1):S83-S90.

Korthuis, P. T., M. J. Tozzi, V. Nandi, D. A. Fiellin, L. Weiss, J. E. Egan, M. Botsko, A. Acosta, M. N. Gourevitch, D. Hersh, J. Hsu, J. Boverman, and F. L. Altice. 2011b. Improved quality of life for opioid-dependent patients receiving buprenorphine treatment in HIV clinics. *Journal of Acquired Immune Deficiency Syndromes* 56(Suppl. 1):S39-S45.

Manwell, L. B., M. F. Fleming, K. Johnson, and K. L. Barry. 1998. Tobacco, alcohol, and drug use in a primary care sample: 90-day prevalence and associated factors. *Journal of Addictive Disorders* 17(1):67-81.

McCarty, D., B. E. Fuller, C. Arfken, M. Miller, E. V. Nunes, E. Edmundson, M. Copersino, A. Floyd, R. Forman, R. Laws, K. M. Magruder, M. Oyama, K. Prather, J. Sindelar, and W. W. Wendt. 2007a. Direct care workers in the national drug abuse treatment clinical trials network: Characteristics, opinions, and beliefs. *Psychiatric Services* 58(2):181-190.

McCarty, D., D. H. Gustafson, J. P. Wisdom, J. Ford, D. Choi, T. Molfenter, V. Capoccia, and F. Cotter. 2007b. The Network for the Improvement of Addiction Treatment (NIATx): Enhancing access and retention. *Drug and Alcohol Dependence* 88(2-3):138-145.

McCarty, D., K. J. McConnell, and L. A. Schmidt. 2010. Priorities for policy research on treatments for alcohol and drug use disorders. *Journal of Substance Abuse Treatment* 39(2):87-95.

McConnell, K. J., S. H. N. Gast, M. S. Ridgely, N. Wallace, N. Jacuzzi, T. Rieckmann, B. H. McFarland, and D. McCarty. 2011. Behavioral health insurance parity: Does Oregon's experience presage the national experience with the Mental Health Parity and Addiction Equity Act? *American Journal of Psychiatry* 169(1):31-38.

McGlynn, E. A., S. M. Asch, J. Adams, J. Keesey, J. Hicks, A. DeCristofaro, and E. A. Kerr. 2003. The quality of health care delivered to adults in the United States. *New England Journal of Medicine* 348(26):2635-2645.

Mee-Lee, D. 2001. *ASAM patient placement criteria for the treatment of substance-related disorders* (2nd rev. ed.). Chevy Chase, MD: ASAM.

NCQA (National Committee for Quality Assurance). 2012. *Accountable Care Organizations (ACOs).* http://www.ncqa.org/tabid/1312/Default.aspx (accessed May 29, 2012).

NQF (National Quality Forum). 2007. *National voluntary consensus standards for the treatment of substance use conditions: Evidence-based treatment practices.* Washington, DC: NQF.

O'Connor, P. G., and J. H. Samet. 2002. Substance abuse: The expanding role of general internal medicine. *Journal of General Internal Medicine* 17(5):398-399.

ONDCP (Office of National Drug Control Policy). 2010. *National drug control strategy, 2010.* Washington, DC: ONDCP.

ONDCP. 2011. *National drug control strategy, 2011.* Washington, DC: ONDCP.

ONDCP. 2012. *National drug control strategy, 2012.* Washington, DC: ONDCP.

Sommers, B. D., K. Swartz, and A. Epstein. 2011. Policy makers should prepare for major uncertainties in Medicaid enrollment, costs, and needs for physicians under health reform. *Health Affairs* 30(11):2186-2193.

VA (Department of Veterans Affairs) and DoD (Department of Defense). 2009. *VA/DoD clinical practice guideline for management of substance use disorders.* Washington, DC: VA and DoD.

Weisner, C. M., C. I. Campbell, G. T. Ray, K. Saunders, J. O. Merrill, C. Banta-Green, M. D. Sullivan, M. J. Silverberg, J. R. Mertens, D. Boudreau, and M. Von Korff. 2009. Trends in prescribed opioid therapy for non-cancer pain for individuals with prior substance use disorders. *Pain* 145(3):287-293.

5

Best Practices in Prevention, Screening, Diagnosis, and Treatment of Substance Use Disorders

This chapter reviews best practices for prevention, screening, diagnosis, and treatment of substance use disorders (SUDs). The review that follows in Chapter 6 compares current military policies and programs pertaining to SUDs with best practices as described in the scientific literature outlined here.

PREVENTION

Prevention is a key strategy for addressing substance use problems. As a first step in delaying the onset and progression of substance abuse, effective prevention has the potential to minimize the need for diagnosis, treatment, and management of SUDs and reduce the enormous social and economic costs of alcohol and other drug dependence. The 2011 National Drug Control Strategy identifies the military as an important population for the receipt of substance abuse prevention services (ONDCP, 2011b). The strategy gives priority to three objectives pertaining directly to SUD prevention within the military: community-based efforts (both on and off base); efforts with youth (i.e., military dependents); and prevention of prescription drug abuse, a growing problem in the military as well as in the general U.S. population (ONDCP, 2011b).

The major goals of prevention are to prevent or delay the onset of substance use and to delay the progression of use from experimental to regular use and dependence. The Institute of Medicine (IOM) has identified three major types of prevention activities: universal, selective, and indicated (IOM, 1994a; NRC and IOM, 2009). In the present context, universal prevention focuses on the general population or population subgroups that are not currently at high risk for SUDs. Selective prevention targets individuals and groups at greater risk of developing SUD-related problems. Finally, indicated prevention focuses on those who are already in the early stages of problematic substance use. Each type of prevention is integral to a robust and comprehensive prevention strategy.

Risk and Protective Factors for SUDs

Effective prevention programs are intended to diminish risk factors and promote protective factors for substance use. Risk factors can be divided into three categories: individual, social, and environmental. Examples include a genetic predisposition to SUD, low self-confidence, low self-efficacy, poor decision-making skills, negative peer influences, and permissive attitudes toward substance use by parents and the community, among others (Lowinson, 2005; NRC and IOM, 2000). Protective factors include, for example, having emotionally supportive parents with open communication styles who are aware of their children's potential for substance use, a strong family orientation, religion/spirituality, involvement in organized school activities, and a strong sense of connection to teachers and school. The National Institute on Drug Abuse's (NIDA's) (2009b) Prevention Research Review Work Group advocates the use of a biopsychosocial approach to identifying risk and protective factors, which involves assessing context (e.g., school, workplace, military) and stage of development (e.g., early childhood, adolescence, young adulthood) (see also NRC and IOM, 2009, and Robertson et al., 2003). This section reviews evidence on risk and protective factors for SUDs by domain (i.e., individual, social, environmental) and developmental stage (i.e., childhood, adolescence, adulthood).

Risk Factors

Most individual risk factors are identified in children and adolescents (e.g., childhood maltreatment/abuse) (Horwitz et al., 2001; Hussey et al., 2006; Mayes and Suchman, 2006; NRC and IOM, 2009; Sternberg et al., 2006; Trickett et al., 2011). Some individual risk factors, however (e.g., intimate partner violence, including physical, sexual, or emotional abuse and/or coercion and degradation) (Campbell, 2002), apply more specifically to adults. While genetic susceptibility to SUD is not modifiable, recent research on executive cognitive function and arousal mechanisms in the prefrontal cortex portions of the brain suggests that sensation seeking can be controlled and redirected by pharmacotherapeutic agents (Kalivas and Volkow, 2005). There is also evidence that prevention activities can ameliorate genetic risk (Brody et al., 2009). Social (or group) risk factors include family risk factors (e.g., modeled family drug use behavior, family management practices, family conflict, weak family bonding) (Kumpfer et al., 2003), as well as peer risk factors (e.g., peers who use substances increase risk by modeling and normalizing substance use) (Hawkins et al., 1992). Peer pressure may be especially strong among military members and their families because of the formal military structure that requires mutual support for effective functioning. Environmental risk factors include the availability of low-cost and easily accessible substances (e.g., discounted alcohol on military bases).

There are several risk factors associated specifically with military service. Examples include service-related injuries (Baker et al., 2009; Larson et al., 2012), trauma, and demands related to active duty (e.g., carrying heavy equipment; witnessing and experiencing traumatic events during deployment; being separated from family members; experiencing occupational stress and boredom when serving in isolated sites; and being the object of discriminatory treatment and, in some cases, acts of violence based on gender, race/ethnicity, or sexual orientation). Military service in general often involves exposure to stressful and traumatic events (Seal et al., 2009), and numerous studies have documented high rates of service-related mental health symptoms among military personnel, which are known to intensify the risk for substance use problems (Edlund et al., 2007; Foran et al., 2011a,b; Jakupcak et al., 2010).

The United States' current conflicts are distinguishable from those of the past by the increased length and number of deployments and the types of injuries (Tanielian et al., 2008). A recent review of substance use problems and risk factors among veterans of Operation Enduring Freedom, Operation Iraqi Freedom, and Operation New Dawn concluded that "military personnel and combat veterans have higher rates of unhealthy substance use than their age peers in the general population" (Larson et al., 2012, p. 21). The review found evidence of a positive relationship between deployment and smoking initiation and recidivism, heavy drinking, and possibly prescription drug misuse. Stress-related consequences of military service-specific conditions, such as acute stress symptoms, psychological and marital problems, and use of medication for combat stress may manifest immediately, or symptoms may be delayed, as suggested by higher rates of such problems among those with more deployments than among those with fewer (MHAT, 2006). Multiple studies have shown that deployment and combat exposure are associated with unhealthy alcohol use (Jacobson et al., 2008; Shen et al., 2012; Spera and Franklin, 2010; Wilk at al., 2010). Another IOM study currently under way is examining the physical and mental health readjustment needs of veterans of these conflicts, and should offer additional evidence on the associated types and levels of risk.[1]

---

[1]For more information, see the study website at http://www.iom.edu/Activities/Veterans/MilPersReadjustNeeds.aspx.

Certain features of military culture (e.g., drinking norms) can contribute to the initiation of problem drinking and related consequences among military personnel. For example, there may be pressure to drink excessively to prove one's toughness, perform a rite of passage, fit into a new group culture, or cope with trauma. Boredom on military bases and in deployment settings, with few recreational activities available, was highlighted as a contributor to problem drinking in presentations to the committee and during visits to military bases. Concern about family finances also is associated with problem drinking among military personnel (Foran et al., 2011a,b). Military-relevant environmental risk factors include the ready availability of alcohol on or near bases, often at reduced prices. This latter contributing factor can be effectively addressed through environmental prevention strategies, which are discussed in detail below. Finally, the strong warrior ethos in the military may be considered a risk factor for not seeking help when treatment for SUDs or other mental health problems is needed. While both male and female members of the military are at risk for substance use as a result of military-specific stressors, men (particularly those aged 25 and younger) are at greater risk of developing drug use disorders, while women are at greater risk of developing depression (Seal et al., 2009).

Compared with military service-specific risk factors among military personnel, there is a paucity of research identifying risk factors for SUDs among their spouses and children (Mansfield and Engel, 2011). Deployments, however, have a number of effects on the spouses and children of service members that may put them at risk for SUDs. Studies have shown that deployments can impact children's behavior and academic performance, spouses' stress levels, and child maltreatment rates (Chandra, 2011; Chartrand et al., 2008; Gibbs et al., 2007; Lester et al., 2010). Whether such stressors associated with military service by parents or spouses are risk factors for SUDs and other mental health problems in their dependents is not yet well documented.

Protective Factors

Compared with risk factors, less research has been conducted to identify factors that protect against the development of SUDs. Protective factors that may mediate or moderate the effects of risk exposure include resiliency, attachment, positive temperament, support (either through the family or from an external support system), and religiosity (Hawkins et al., 1992; NRC and IOM, 2000). In children, resiliency refers to the ability to thrive and exhibit positive health behaviors despite exposure to adverse living conditions (e.g., extreme poverty, crime, drugs, and abuse) (NRC and IOM, 2000; Rutter, 2006). The extent to which adult military members can be resilient to the effects of risk factors for SUDs and adverse conditions (e.g., war-related life-threatening situations) is not well understood. There is some evidence that resiliency operates through other mechanisms, including religiosity, family support, peer bonding, and parenthood (NRC and IOM, 2009). Positive temperament may enable an individual to reframe or reinterpret otherwise highly threatening situations in order to cope (e.g., functioning under fire). Finally, while lack of executive cognitive function (ECF) has been found to be a predictor of substance use and SUDs (Blume and Marlatt, 2009), it is not yet known whether the reverse is true (i.e., whether high levels of ECF can protect against the development of SUDs). Since ECF consists of a host of skills required for military members to function in the armed services—including working memory, deliberate planning, decision making, emotional regulation, and behavioral impulse control skills—it may operate indirectly as a protective factor against the development of SUDs by enhancing the ability to thrive, cope, and minimize stress.

Evidence-Based Programs and Practices

Prevention activities that reduce the incidence of one problem behavior tend to reduce other problem behaviors (Karoly et al., 1998). The initial investments in these types of interventions generally are repaid in both savings to government and benefits to society, including gains in adult employment and resulting tax revenues, as well as reductions in criminal activity and associated cost savings for arrests, judicial proceedings, probation, and incarceration (Karoly et al., 2001). Evidence-based SUD prevention programming (1) addresses the appropriate risk and protective factors for the population in question, (2) employs approaches with demonstrated effectiveness, (3) takes place at the appropriate time chronologically and developmentally, (4) makes use of proper settings and domains for delivery, and (5) manages programs effectively (ONDCP, 2001). These core elements served as the basis for the committee's assessment of the adequacy, appropriateness, and likely effectiveness of prevention programs in the various branches of the U.S. military; broader nonprogrammatic environmental prevention strategies are discussed later in this section.

Address Risk and Protective Factors

As outlined above, effective prevention programs address the risk and protective factors relevant both to the problem or issue at hand and the population(s) to be reached. Military dependents require a different set of prevention strategies from those appropriate for active duty service members, for instance. Demographic (e.g., age, race) and sociocultural (e.g., ethnicity) considerations are critical in designing effective prevention activities. Several sources (NIDA, 2009a; NRC and IOM, 2009; Robertson et al.,

2003) provide solid frameworks for identifying risk and protective factors as a component of the design and adoption of evidence-based programs.

Employ Effective Approaches

The National Registry of Evidence-based Programs and Practices (NREPP) lists SUD prevention programs determined to be evidence-based according to their readiness for dissemination and the quality of their evaluation research—specifically measurement reliability and validity; fidelity of implementation; appropriateness of analysis; and the handling of attrition, missing data, and confounding variables (SAMHSA, 2012). Programs that focus only on increasing knowledge or changing attitudes have had few effects on substance use behaviors compared with programs that focus on resistance and social/life skill building (Botvin et al., 1995). Evidence-based prevention programs often include skills particularly relevant to military members and their families, such as resisting peer pressure, avoiding high-risk situations, identifying and bonding with individuals who provide social support and a nonuse norm, and practicing emotional regulation and impulse control.

Not all prevention programs have been evaluated with all populations or in all settings. Often, prevention providers opt to adopt promising programs or approaches. Sometimes this process involves implementing programs effective in one population but not evaluated in another (e.g., adapting a program evaluated with college students for use in a military population). At other times, the process involves working with a program that is theory based, although not yet formally evaluated. Among the more prominent theories represented in evidence-based prevention efforts are social learning/cognitive theory (Bandura, 1977), attitudinal theory (Ajzen and Fishbein, 1980), and social network theory (Valente, 2010). According to the principles of participant modeling and social learning theory, program implementers must be perceived as credible role models to whom military members can relate. Use of slightly older peer leaders to assist program implementers enhances program participation and effects (Perry et al., 1986). The most effective program delivery is sequenced as the provision of general principles of the program, modeling of prevention skills, role playing or rehearsal of skills, and extended practice in real-life settings.

Take Place at the Appropriate Time

Skill development programs need to be age appropriate. Prevention programs for early childhood, for instance, should focus on parental management of children, parent-child communication, and basic health behavior (e.g., nutrition, sleep, and health care) (NRC and IOM, 2000; Shonkoff et al., 2012). Elementary school programs typically focus on building socioemotional competence and preventing conduct problems. Adolescent programs should focus on reducing risk factors and increasing protective factors, including training in resisting peer pressure, positive adult support seeking, nonuse social norms, and nonuse leisure time activities (Hansen and Graham, 1991; Wills and Vaughan, 1989). Training for adults (i.e., spouses and military members in the emerging adulthood period) should focus on brief motivational interviewing; coping skills; social support; and skills in positive parent-child communication, rule setting, and monitoring. In addition to developmental considerations, chronology is important as well; the most successful prevention efforts are reinforced over time in a variety of settings.

Make Use of Appropriate Settings

"Appropriate" settings are based on the nature of the problem/issue being addressed and the characteristics of the population being served. The setting for program delivery can be, for example, the school, the home, a religious institution, or the workplace.

Manage Programs Effectively

The most effective prevention programs provide standardized training and manualized protocols, along with specific and measurable prevention skills and goals (Mihalik et al., 2004). Standardization helps minimize program "drift" and dilution, whereas use of a general outline, procedures, or processes is not effective in changing substance use behavior (Mihalik et al., 2004)—a point that is particularly relevant given the strong empirical link between program effectiveness and implementation fidelity. Well-trained providers and consistent monitoring and program evaluation are also integral components of an evidence-based prevention strategy.

Included within this principle as well is alignment of program values and institutional values. Program buy-in, implementation, participation, and maintenance relate to whether SUD prevention is perceived to enhance military functioning and promote individual warrior fitness. Important factors include (1) an environment supportive of the delivery of prevention programs (in terms of allocation of time and availability of qualified implementers), (2) social environmental norms consistent with nonuse, (3) supportive (versus punitive) policies that link directly and clearly to prevention programs, and (4) reinforcement of nonuse behaviors and practices.

Environmental Strategies

Beyond prevention programs and efforts aimed at impacting individual behavior, the military is uniquely positioned to implement more overarching systems-level, or environmental, prevention strategies that affect the community at large. Environmental prevention strategies are directed at community norms and policy regulations. This section describes best practices in environmental prevention efforts for SUDs applicable in military settings.

Alcohol

A number of strategies based on sound theory and with proven effectiveness exist to control alcohol use and related problems at the population level. These strategies are "environmental" because they work by decreasing the availability or appeal of alcohol or illicit drugs (including prescription drugs) in the community rather than attempting to change individual behavior. These strategies lead to decreases in consumption and minimization or prevention of alcohol-related problems. Several reviews of these policies are available in the scientific literature (e.g., Babor et al., 2010a,b; Saltz et al., 2010; Wagenaar et al., 2009; WHO, 2009), some of which are addressed specifically to policy makers, including those in charge of developing and implementing health policies in the U.S. armed forces.

In the alcohol field, Babor and colleagues (2010a) discuss seven policy approaches, four of which are environmental and can be used by the U.S. armed forces to address alcohol consumption and related problems among military personnel. (An additional approach discussed by these authors—advertising regulation—affects military personnel but cannot be changed by the military.)

The first of these four pertinent approaches is controlling affordability through pricing and taxation. The evidence in this area clearly indicates that higher prices lead to a decrease in alcohol consumption (Chisholm et al., 2004; Wagenaar et al., 2009).

The second approach is restricting the availability of alcohol available for purchase (Chaloupka et al., 2002; Stockwell and Gruenewald, 2004). Consistent enforcement of the legal drinking age is a key strategy that falls under this approach and is highly effective in reducing alcohol consumption in this age group (Wagenaar and Toomey, 2002).

The third environmental prevention approach involves altering the context in which alcohol is consumed. Best practices in this area entail "server intervention" strategies, or training bar staff and liquor and convenience store employees in responsible beverage service (e.g., requiring age identification, recognizing potential problems, and exercising increased responsibility in selling alcohol and serving alcoholic beverages) and in the management and prevention of aggressive and/or problematic patrons, who may or may not be intoxicated (Babor et al., 2010a; Graham, 2000; Graham and Homel, 2008; Graham et al., 2005). Dram shop liability laws—the U.S. laws that hold bar owners responsible for injuries caused to a third party by someone who was sold or served alcohol when intoxicated—are also effective in modifying drinking contexts (Rammohan et al., 2011).

The fourth approach is directed at preventing impaired driving. While policies reflecting this approach were developed to respond to drinking and driving, many of them can also be used to prevent driving under the influence of other drugs, including prescription drugs. Drinking and driving countermeasures are among the most effective population-level control policies in the alcohol field. Enforcement of these policies contributed to a decrease in alcohol-related traffic fatalities from a high of 59.5 percent of all traffic fatalities in 1982 to 32 percent in 2009 (National Highway Traffic Safety Administration, 2009). Sobriety checkpoints and random breath testing are two of the most effective policies in this area. Their effectiveness, however, is associated with the frequency of their implementation and consistency in advertising (i.e., alerting drivers in the community to the existence—although not the location—of checkpoints and random breath testing). Also relevant for the military is enforcement of blood alcohol content (BAC) limits and administrative license suspension. There is some evidence that the lower the BAC limit, the more effective it can be, although BAC limits lower than .02 are difficult to enforce (Babor et al., 2010a). Two rigorous evaluations of these types of environmental initiatives found significant reductions in alcohol-related traffic accidents, assaults involving alcohol, amount or quantity of drinking, and driving while intoxicated in intervention compared with control communities (Holder et al., 2000; Treno et al., 2007). Appendix I summarizes policy-relevant strategies discussed by Babor and colleagues (2010a) for the prevention of alcohol-related problems by category and strength of evidentiary support.

Other Drugs

Use of illicit drugs and abuse of prescription drugs continue to be a major public health problem in the United States. Prescription drug abuse, one of the major concerns that prompted this study, is a vexing problem among military personnel. As in the alcohol field, there are environmental, population-level approaches that can be useful in the prevention of drug use and abuse. Babor and colleagues (2010b) discuss various approaches, one of which is pertinent to the U.S. military to address concerns related to prescription drug abuse. This approach is what Babor and colleagues (2010b) call "prescription regimes," which involve controlling the safety, storage, and distribution of prescription drugs to prevent or minimize their diversion to the black market for illicit use and abuse. Some of these measures entail tight regulation of prescription dispensation and control and over-the-counter sales, physician education, and enforcement of prescription regulations.

In the context of the increasing incidence of prescription drug problems in both the military and civilian sectors, the Office of National Drug Control Policy's (ONDCP's) four major strategies also provide best practices in environmental prevention that correspond with the prescription regimes of Babor et al. (2010b) (ONDCP, 2012). The first strategy is education. While ONDCP's 2011 Prescription Drug Abuse Prevention Plan focuses on parent, child, and patient education (ONDCP, 2011a), also critical is provider education regarding responsible prescribing practices and alternative pain medications with lower dependence potential. The second strategy is monitoring, which involves the implementation of prescription drug monitoring programs. In the military setting specifically, it is critically important that monitoring systems be capable of sharing data across branches and with state monitoring programs to prevent the practice of "doctor shopping." The third strategy in ONDCP's prevention plan is disposal, which entails "convenient and environmentally responsible prescription drug disposal programs to help decrease the supply of unused prescription drugs in the home" (ONDCP, 2012, p. 1). Finally, proper enforcement of policies and laws is necessary to ensure consistent implementation and maximum effectiveness.

Summary

In conclusion, SUD prevention in the military is a complex issue. Changing attitudes about acceptable alcohol and other drug use is central to changing drinking and drug using behavior. Intensive antismoking campaigns of the past several decades—entailing a combination of higher prices (through taxation) (Chaloupka et al., 2012); restrictions on where use is permitted; and above all, changed social norms about smoking—have resulted in major reductions in smoking initiation and tobacco use. Structural measures can impact alcohol use problems, illicit drug use, and prescription drug problems. Environmental strategies for these problems, as discussed above, are available and effective. Partnerships within the larger communities in which military bases are located are also integral to a solid environmental prevention strategy (e.g., Spoth et al., 2011). The military has a unique opportunity to communicate consistent messages about drinking (clearly the most prevalent substance use problem in the military, about which great ambivalence persists at the highest levels), illicit drug use, and nonmedical use of prescription drugs, as well as to control the environmental factors that drive both heavy drinking and prescription drug misuse through such measures as restricting availability, increasing cost, and limiting permitted times and locations for the use of legal drugs.

SCREENING, DIAGNOSIS, AND TREATMENT

While the prevention of SUDs is the foundation of any good strategy for addressing the problem, a comprehensive strategy must also include evidence-based screening mechanisms to identify at-risk and existing users, validated diagnostic instruments with which to obtain accurate diagnoses, and empirically supported treatment approaches for effective rehabilitation.

Screening

As discussed previously, selective and indicated prevention each involve the identification of particular target groups (e.g., high-risk individuals), which is frequently accomplished through screening. Screening can detect both health problems and risk factors, the latter of which is particularly useful for these groups. As a strategy for universal prevention, screening must be linked to effective subsequent interventions. False-positive and false-negative cases each carry undesirable consequences (e.g., unnecessary anxiety and medical expenditure for the former, missed opportunities for intervention for the latter), and effort should therefore be made to minimize error.

Awareness of the limitations of screening has led the public health sector to develop a series of parameters to guide screening activities (Gray, 2001; Wilson and Jungner, 1968), including guidelines to identify the populations that should be screened and the diseases that should be screened for, performance standards for screening tests, and guidance on how performance should be assessed. Because screening for disease can be costly, inconvenient, and not always reliable, guidelines for effective screening identify situations in which screening is advantageous and will promote and protect health in the population. Classic criteria for evaluating screening programs emphasize the need for screening to focus on important health problems, link to diagnosis and treatment, have acceptable screening procedures, attend to costs, and be a continuous activity (Wilson and Jungner, 1968). The United Kingdom's National Screening Committee added three additional criteria to be considered (Muir Gray, 2004): potential harm caused by screening, the strength of the evidence with which to evaluate success, and the opportunity costs associated with screening.

Disease Characteristics

Screening should focus on serious health problems that are highly prevalent in the target population. Preclinical symptoms or behaviors also should be highly prevalent in the population, and this preclinical phase should be long and clearly detectable. Treatment should exist, and should be more effective if initiated at an early stage (Hennekens et al., 1987). Altogether, SUDs affect about 10 percent of the U.S. adult population, and the prevalence of these disorders is higher among young people (SAMHSA, 2010), who make up a large percentage of the armed forces. The preclinical phase of SUDs is also highly prevalent and of long duration, and therefore highly detectable by the use and abuse of alcohol and/or other drugs or by the presence of recognizable behavioral, interpersonal, work-related, and health-related problems (e.g., drinking and driving, family problems, work absenteeism). There is evidence that early intervention (e.g., brief intervention based on motivational interviews) can be effective in changing the course of some of these problems, especially those that are alcohol related (Ahmadi and Green, 2011).

Cultural Acceptance

Acceptance among the population being screened is fundamental to successful screening. Cultural and social acceptance hinges on the extent to which the population sees the focus of the screening as a real problem and on the characteristics of the screening procedures (e.g., how long they last; how physiologically, psychologically, and/or socially invasive they are). Screening for alcohol and other drug problems can pose major challenges. The problems are stigmatized and may be perceived as moral weaknesses rather than health problems. Questions about alcohol and illicit drug use can be experienced as invasive and may result in underreporting. In the United States, although these challenges can be present in some population groups, they do not pose considerable barriers to the implementation of screening for risky drinking, prescription drug abuse, and illicit drug use. Screening for alcohol and other drug problems can be conducted effectively with a few brief questions. Screening for drug use can be accomplished relatively easily through urinalysis.

Cost-Effectiveness

The cost-effectiveness of screening encompasses the type of screening procedure being employed, the length of screening, the background of the personnel administering the screening, and the type of health problem under focus. Screening for alcohol and other drug use does not involve complex procedures, can be done rapidly with just a few questions, and can be conducted by lay personnel. Alcohol- and other drug-dependent individuals overutilize health services because they are usually in poor health, have a higher risk of injuries that may require medical care, and may develop a number of health problems (e.g., ulcer, cancer, liver cirrhosis) that are costly to treat (Mertens et al., 2005; Weisner and Matzger, 2002). Screening for SUDs is therefore cost-effective because it can circumvent costly overutilization of services.

Characteristics of Screening Tests

The ideal screening test should be brief, safe, noninvasive, inexpensive, and easy to administer and should carry no negative or legal consequences. Screening tests should have high validity, meaning they should measure what they purport to measure. In the case of alcohol and other drug use, screening should identify as "positive" those individuals who are engaging in risky (e.g., binge) drinking or other drug use (e.g., abuse of opioid prescription drugs), and as "negative" those individuals who are abstainers or normal drinkers or do not use illicit drugs or abuse prescription drugs. The sensitivity of a test (its ability to identify as true positives all of those individuals who are positive) and its specificity (its ability to identify as negative all of those individuals who are negative) reflect its validity. Ideally, these two aspects of the test should be as high as possible (e.g., above 90 percent). For alcohol and other drug screening, sensitivity is most important because the consequences of a false negative are great. Screening programs also are highly dependent on positive yield, or the proportion of individuals identified as positive by the test who are actually positive. Positive yield provides an assessment of the extent to which the test will be able to identify those who must be identified if the screening program is to be successful. These are the individuals who have preclinical disease or, in the case of alcohol and other drugs, show risky alcohol or other drug intake that puts them at risk for developing a substance use–related health problem or dependence in the future. A low predictive positive yield indicates that the screening procedure will have too many false positives, which will lead to too many second-level diagnostic procedures for false-positive individuals (Aschengrau and Seage, 2008).

Screening Tests for Alcohol and Other Drugs

Many valid and reliable screening tests are available for alcohol and other drug use (Babor and Kadden, 2005). Most are self-administered and require 1-5 minutes to complete. They can be used in a variety of health care settings, such as primary care offices and emergency rooms. Because they are brief, most can be added to more extensive and intensive health assessments. The U.S. military, for instance, uses the Alcohol Use Disorders Identification Test (AUDIT)-C as part of its Pre-Deployment Health Assessment (completed 60 days prior to deployment). The AUDIT-C is also part of the *Clinical Practice Guideline for Management of Substance Use Disorders* of the Department of Veterans Affairs and Department of Defense (VA and DoD, 2009).

Besides self-report, screening tests for drug use include urinalysis and other biological methods, such as cheek swabbing or hair analysis. Urinalysis is an attractive screening option because it is independent of self-report. The circumstances in which most screening for drug use takes place (e.g., pre-employment testing) are not conducive to self-disclosure of drug use. Subjects therefore may underreport or deny use, thereby invalidating screening efforts. However, urinalysis also has a number of limitations. It is highly dependent on laboratory standards related to chain of custody, quality control, validity (sensitivity and specificity) and reliability of testing procedures, and confidentiality of results. Further, a positive test does not provide information about chronicity, frequency, and/or quantity of use; the presence of drug dependence; and in the case of prescription drugs, whether the drug was taken under medical order. Similarly, a negative test does not mean that drug use is absent. A negative test can occur because the drug was taken in a small enough dosage to be undetected, because the drug taken had already been eliminated from the body when the specimen was collected, or because the testing method was not sensitive enough to detect the presence of the drug. Urine drug screening would optimally take place in conjunction with education and treatment.

Screening and Brief Intervention

In the United States, the National Institute on Alcohol Abuse and Alcoholism (NIAAA) has sponsored the development of evidence-based screening, brief intervention, and referral to treatment (SBIRT) protocols. SBIRT includes screening with an evidence-based screener for at-risk drinking; providing a brief intervention; and, for those whose problems are more severe, referring to specialty substance use treatment. The evidence-based guidelines developed by NIAAA define "risky" drinking as having more than 4 drinks for men and more than 3 drinks for women on any given day. Also, men should not have more than 14 drinks and women not more than 7 drinks per week (NIAAA, 2005). SBIRT has been shown to be an efficacious, cost-effective intervention across heterogeneous populations (Bertholet et al., 2005; Kaner et al., 2009). It has been implemented in many different types of health care settings, including primary care and emergency room settings.

Different organizations (e.g., the Centers for Disease Control and Prevention [CDC], NIAAA, the World Health Organization [WHO]) suggest different lengths of time for the SBIRT process or do not specify a length of time. The times specified, however, are all brief—between 5 and 20 minutes. SBIRT has been shown to be effective when conducted by both physicians and nonphysician providers (Babor et al., 2006; Ockene et al., 1999; Reiff-Hekking et al., 2005). It can serve as an intervention to decrease the problem in those who are experiencing at-risk substance use and as an early case-finding intervention in those whose problem is beginning to become more severe.

Diagnosis

Diagnosis is another essential part of a comprehensive response to alcohol and other drug problems. Diagnostic procedures for SUDs in the United States are guided by the *Diagnostic and Statistical Manual of Mental Disorders, Fourth Edition, Text Revision* (DSM-IV-TR) of the American Psychiatric Association (APA) (2000), which contains standardized diagnostic criteria for a number of alcohol- and other drug-related conditions. Of interest in the present context are the DSM-IV-TR diagnoses of "abuse" and "dependence" (see also Chapter 2). Abuse is defined in a previous IOM report as "a level of drug use that typically leads to adverse consequences (physical or psychological). Drug use at this level is not necessarily associated with any particular frequency but is associated with use in quantities sufficient to result in some toxicity to the user, and the patterns of use usually have some characteristics of psychopathological behavior" (IOM, 1994b, p. 2). The same report defines dependence as "a level of drug use that has significant adverse physical and psychological consequences. This level of use is characterized by the consumption of toxic doses of the substance that impair the user's ability to function and is also characterized by a compulsive desire to use a drug repeatedly" (IOM, 1994b, p. 2).

The DSM-IV-TR diagnoses of abuse and dependence are based on the presence of specific indicators within a 12-month period. Substance dependence is "a maladaptive pattern of substance use, leading to clinically significant impairment or distress" (APA, 2000, p. 128). In order to be diagnosed as having substance dependence, the individual should have 3 or more of the following indicators: (1) tolerance; (2) withdrawal; (3) more substance use than intended; (4) desire or unsuccessful efforts to decrease use; (5) significant amount of time spent related to the substance use; (6) social, occupational, or recreational activities are given up or reduced due to substance use; and (7) use is continued despite knowledge of having a persistent or recurrent physical or psychological problem (APA, 2000). The diagnosis of substance abuse should be made only in the absence of a diagnosis of substance dependence. To be diagnosed with substance abuse, the individual should have one or more of the following indicators: (1) recurrent substance use resulting in a failure to fulfill major role obligations; (2) recurrent substance use in situations in which it is physically hazardous; (3) recurrent substance-related legal problems; and (4) continued substance use despite having persistent or recurrent social or interpersonal problems (APA, 2000). As discussed in Chapter 2, the APA began to reexamine the diagnostic criteria for abuse and dependence in preparation for DSM-5. A website describes in detail the activities that have taken place as part of this effort and the proposed changes that will likely be included in DSM-5 (APA, 2012).

Standardized diagnostic procedures that are valid and reliable and reflect the latest research findings can be implemented in a busy clinical setting by professionals with various levels of training and with different backgrounds. Such standardization should not be seen as a luxury that can be implemented only by academic settings or specialized treatment facilities. Rather, this standardization is necessary for the development of accurate diagnoses, the collection of valid and reliable data on clients, and the administration of effective treatments. Standardization also is a necessary first step for the evaluation of treatment protocols. Without such evaluation, changes in service provision cannot be implemented in a rational manner so as to provide the maximum benefit to patients.

Treatment

Standards and expectations for the treatment of alcohol and other drug use disorders are changing. In the second decade of the 21st century, three environmental forces may reshape treatment services. First, as summarized in Chapter 4, health care reform and federal parity legislation enhance access to health insurance and mandate that commercial health plans provide similar coverage for general health, mental health, and SUDs. Second, standards of care continually evolve as research-based behavioral and pharmacological therapies emerge. Finally, advocates and policy makers have called for increased integration of addiction treatment and primary care (Treatment Research Institute, 2010). These influences enhance the capacity of primary care to screen, diagnose, and intervene for patients with SUDs of all levels of severity.

To integrate substance abuse treatment into primary care, however, systems of care must address four limitations:

1. Current capacity—Most primary care settings are unprepared to screen for, assess, and treat SUDs, especially among women and men whose disorders are severe.
2. Inadequate reimbursement—Productivity expectations, procedure codes, and reimbursement rates do not reflect the time required to address SUDs.
3. Workforce skills and abilities—Few primary care practitioners have specialty training in addressing SUDs.

4. Integration strategies—Strategies to link primary care and specialty care for SUDs need to be developed and tested.

In addition, patients with comorbid serious mental illnesses often require specialty treatment services and cannot be given sufficient attention in the primary care setting.

The IOM's *Quality Chasm* reports challenge the U.S. health care system to adopt evidence-based practices and to make process improvements to reduce the morbidity and mortality related to the delivery of health care (IOM, 2000, 2001). A subsequent IOM report extends the *Quality Chasm* recommendations to address treatment for alcohol, other drug, and mental health disorders and the integration of these services into the medical mainstream (IOM, 2006). If this is to be accomplished, change at the system level will be necessary.

The implementation of evidence-based pharmacological and behavioral therapies for alcohol and other drug use disorders is a major challenge for both policy makers and treatment providers (McCarty et al., 2010). While evidence from research demonstrates the effectiveness of evidence-based therapies for the treatment of SUDs, many practitioners do not use evidence-based treatments routinely or have adopted eclectic treatment approaches (Miller et al., 2006). Some variation in treatment approaches is to be expected and reflects patient-centered or personalized medicine; variability among patients inhibits the adoption of condition-specific practice guidelines. Patients present with a mix of comorbidities and other psychosocial and environmental factors that influence the treatment approach and their response to treatment. Research-based practice guidelines, moreover, generally are based on carefully selected research samples that exclude many complex patients, and therapists may be uncomfortable with generalizing them to apply to specific patients.

A clinical challenge for patient-centered care, then, is maintaining the effective elements of evidence-based treatment while adapting therapies for particular patients. Results of many studies suggest that general therapist skills have more influence on outcomes than specific treatments (Blatt et al., 1996; Crits-Christoph and Mintz, 1991; Luborsky et al., 1997). Experience enhances therapists' effectiveness (Kivlighan and Kivlighan, 2009; Mallinckrodt and Nelson, 1991; Mayfield et al., 1999). Therapeutic effectiveness may also be linked to the measurement of treatment effects during treatment (outcome-informed treatment) (Duncan et al., 2003; Miller et al., 2003, 2005). Outcome-informed techniques can quickly clarify the effects of a modified treatment for a particular patient and guide the therapist's search for an effective intervention. Outcome-informed techniques can therefore improve treatment outcomes (Brown, 2004; Lambert, 2005). Likewise, tools that measure the therapeutic alliance help clarify for the therapist when the patient's perceptions of care delivery point to a negative or ineffective status (Duncan et al., 2003; Miller et al., 2003, 2005). In quality improvement circles, the importance of measurement is well understood; the operational mantra is, "You can't improve what you don't measure."

Higher-quality behavioral health provider systems (e.g., university-based care systems, credibly funded research treatment centers) promote fidelity and reduce competency drift (i.e., the reduction of clinical sharpness and skill level posttraining). They do so through specific improvement strategies in three best-practice domains as recommended by the National Institutes of Health's Behavior Change Consortium (Bellg et al., 2004) and outlined in Table 5-1.

In summary, the best-practice principles and factors for high-quality delivery of SUD treatment at the provider-patient level include the use of evidence-based treatments specific to SUDs. Practitioners need to have skills and demonstrated competency in all of the evidence-based approaches to be effective with their treatment population. Implementation of treatment approaches also should be adapted to the patient's specific need and stage of treatment.

Improving the Delivery and Organization of Care

SUD is often a chronic illness and needs to be treated with a system of care structured similarly to the systems of care for other chronic medical illnesses (e.g., diabetes, asthma, high blood pressure) (McLellan et al., 2000). SUD patients are treated with different levels of care based on variations in the level of protection from the outside environment and in the level of service intensity (Mee-Lee, 2001). Environmental protection and service intensity are assessed independently and drive decisions on treatment placement and needed services. Treatment plans may require creative flexibility. When health care benefits do not pay for residential care, for example, an intensive outpatient program can provide needed services while alcohol- and drug-free housing provides environmental protection.

The quality of the care delivery system or a treatment program is important to patient-level outcomes; a fragmented or broken delivery system reduces the effectiveness of treatment at the patient-provider level. To frame best practices for a SUD care delivery system, the committee referenced the principles laid out in Treatment Improvement Protocol No. 47, *Substance Abuse: Clinical Issues in Intensive Outpatient Treatment*, authored by the Center for Substance Abuse Treatment (CSAT) (2006). These principles are based on an integration of the findings from evidence-based research and on expert opinion where there was a gap in the research.

TABLE 5-1 Best-Practice Domains and Recommendations of the National Institutes of Health's Behavior Change Consortium

Goals	Strategies
Domain: Provider training	
• Standardize training for all provider types	• Use standardized training manuals, materials, resources, field guides, structured practice and role playing; standardized patients; same instructors/supervisors; video training
• Ensure the acquisition of provider skills	• Observe implementation of interventions with standardized patients or role playing; score providers according to a checklist; conduct debriefings; administer written pre- and posttraining examinations; certify skills during and after training
• Identify and have processes to minimize "competency drift" in provider skills	• Conduct booster sessions; conduct in vivo observations scored against a standard checklist; supervise; obtain provider self-reports; conduct patient exit interviews or obtain feedback
• Accommodate differences in providers' backgrounds with respect to skill expectations and roles	• Have certified or established professional supervisors for provider training; monitor patient dropouts and treatment effectiveness
Domain: Delivery of treatment	
• Control for provider variability	• Assess patient perceptions of providers through questionnaires, and give feedback to providers; audiotape sessions, and have different supervisors review; monitor patient complaints; have providers work with all treatment populations served
• Reduce ineffective variation within treatments	• Use scripted protocols, treatment manual; have supervisors rate audiotapes, videotapes
• Ensure adherence to evidence-based treatment protocols	• Audiotape or videotape encounters, and review with providers; randomly monitor audio or videotapes for adherence to protocols; have providers complete a checklist of intervention components
Domain: Receipt of treatment and enactment of treatment skills	
• Ensure patients' comprehension and acquisition of skills	• Have providers review participants' homework, self-monitoring logs; assess, measure participants' performance; have structured interviews with patients; use questionnaires; use hypothetical scenarios to test patients
• Ensure patients' ability to perform new skills	• Collect patient self-monitoring, self-report data; use behavioral outcome measures

SOURCE: Adapted from Bellg et al., 2004.

The delivery system approach presented in Table 5-2 is based on the committee's operationalization of the CSAT principles.

Transitions to different levels of care are most successful when they occur between settings of care that employ similar philosophies and can transfer client records efficiently. A step down or step up in treatment intensity within the same program or through referral to a nonaffiliated provider can be disruptive for the patient and lead to dropping out of treatment (CSAT, 2006). Mee-Lee and Shulman (2003) suggest that an effective continuum of care successfully transitions the patient to the next level of care; successful transition is defined as the patient remaining engaged in treatment posttransition and not dropping out during the critical transition period. Transitioning to a different level of care also requires a clear delineation of the appropriate clinical characteristics of the patient to ensure that they match the new level of care.

Given that SUD is often a chronic illness, long-term monitoring supports maintenance of recovery (Dennis et al., 2003; McKay et al., 2005; Scott et al., 2005); however, research has not determined an optimal duration for long-term monitoring. An analysis of 1,271 admissions to a publicly funded treatment center found that 47 percent of the sample achieved 12 months of continuous sobriety within 3 years of entering the study (Dennis et al., 2005). The mean time from first treatment to last use was 9 years, and increased for men, individuals who began using at a younger age, and participants with comorbid mental illnesses (Dennis et al., 2005). On the other hand, physician assistance programs and other assistance programs for professionals often require 5 years of continuous monitoring (McLellan et al., 2008). What is important is that treatment systems be structured to monitor a patient as long as possible and in the same objective manner as is applied to other chronic conditions. An ideal care delivery system is comprehensive and includes long-term services in addition to preventive services, community or workplace initiatives, primary care screening and brief interventions, and specialized treatment services (McLellan, 2002). In some systems, primary care physicians assume the role of screening, brief intervention, referral, and long-term monitoring of abstinence from substance use. In general medical practices, however, the engagement of primary care physicians in best-practice treatment for alcohol use disorders was found to be very low (rates of adherence to treatment guidelines were 10.5 percent for these disorders versus 57.7 percent for depression and 64.7 percent for hypertension) (McGlynn et al., 2003). Specialty programs therefore may need to assume the role and accountability for long-term recovery monitoring.

TABLE 5-2 A Delivery System Approach Based on the Center for Substance Abuse Treatment's (CSAT's) Treatment Improvement Protocol No. 47

CSAT Principle	Delivery System Approach
1. Having the ability to make effective connections and treatment readily available	• Crisis assessments available 24/7 • Screening, brief intervention, and referral to treatment (SBIRT) approaches adopted in various medical settings; use of peers
2. Enabling easy treatment entry	• Crisis assessments 24/7 • Wide geographic coverage • Access standards and time frames from assessment to start of treatment
3. Building on existing motivation (i.e., treatment system is able to handle and manage unwilling patients' entry into treatment)	• Manualized readiness for treatment interviews and rating scales • Legal system, job jeopardy or support systems mandates • Staff competencies in behavioral techniques for working through treatment resistance (e.g., motivational interviewing) • Policies and program philosophy that promote a safe harbor that reduces stigma and maintains necessary confidentiality
4. Building an enhanced therapeutic alliance	• Staff trained in engagement techniques • Measurement of the therapeutic alliance by accountable provider/program • Use of recovered peers
5. Offering appropriate treatment that is patient specific and not a singular provider approach	• Move away from set program protocols and time frames • Individualized treatment plans and treatments • Adjunctive services to match the specific needs of special populations (e.g., pregnant or newly delivered mothers—skill building in parenting)
6. Providing ongoing care through a continuum and extending into the long-term sobriety period	• Multiple levels of the care system (inpatient, residential, partial hospitalization, intensive outpatient, outpatient sessions, community support systems such as Alcoholics Anonymous [AA], long-term case management, primary care physician monitoring, alumni groups) • System that facilitates interconnectivity and collaboration necessary to create seamless care
7. Having the ability to address the multiple needs of the patient, not just the substance use disorder	• Psychiatric services (high psychiatric comorbidity) • Linkage to employee assistance programs (EAPs) and employment, financial, child care services

continued

TABLE 5-2 Continued

8. Retaining the patient in treatment for an adequate time period and facilitating continuous long-term connections to support recovery	• Use of level-of-care guidelines (e.g., American Society of Addiction Medicine [ASAM] Patient Placement Criteria) • Treatment program protocols that incorporate linkages to community supports during the treatment process, long-term case management, alumni groups, linkages to primary care provider (PCP) as a monitoring system • Measurement of long-term engagement with the treatment and case management support system
9. During the treatment process, continuously assessing and modifying the treatment plan as necessary to ensure that the treatment is effective and meets the patient's changing needs	• Program treatment protocols • Use of objective tools and benchmarks to measure progress • Systematic reassessments during the treatment process within a level of care and upon transition to the next level of care
10. Using a treatment system that monitors for abstinence and expects successful management of treatment relapses	• Repeated drug and breathalyzer testing • Use of use-limiting medications (e.g., antabuse, naltrexone) • Treatment program rules that do not discharge because of use during treatment but use it as a treatment opportunity
11. Using mutual-help and other community-based supports	• Treatment protocols that incorporate use of community support groups during the treatment process (AA, Narcotics Anonymous [NA], other 12-step programs, Web-based social networking programs)
12. Successfully and appropriately engaging families, employers, and significant others	• Family therapy as a standard part of treatment protocols and expectations • Appropriate incorporation of employer and/or EAP for work reentry
13. Using mutual-help and other community-based supports	• Linkage of patients to community-based supports prior to discharge • Use of Web-based social networks and gaming approaches to facilitate engagement
14. Educating and promoting knowledgeable empowerment with respect to substance use, recovery, and relapse for patients and families	• Education sessions as part of the treatment approach, with homework and testing of skills • Patient self-report surveys focused on the perception of confidence in new skills

SOURCE: CSAT, 2006.

Behavioral Therapies

A substantial body of research supports the use of behavioral therapies for treating SUDs. Various approaches have emerged from empirical research as effective for treatment of SUDs, including contingency management and community reinforcement, cognitive-behavioral therapy, family and couples therapy, motivational therapy, and 12-step facilitation (Carroll, 2005; Carroll and Onken, 2005; Moos, 2007). A meta-analysis of treatment interventions for alcohol use disorders suggested that the psychosocial interventions with the most consistent evidence of effectiveness include brief interventions based on motivational enhancement therapy, social skills training, community reinforcement approaches, behavior contracting, and behavioral marital therapy (Miller and Wilbourne, 2002). A recent meta-analysis comparing effectiveness between psychosocial treatments for alcohol use disorders found that therapies on average had no difference in effect sizes when compared with one another, suggesting that while each of these treatments has demonstrated effectiveness when compared to control or non-treatment conditions, the relative effectiveness of these types of treatments is more or less equivalent (Imel et al., 2008). For other substance abuse beyond just alcohol, a meta-analysis of 34 treatments for SUDs found that psychosocial treatments had a moderate effect size (comparable to those of other efficacious psychiatric interventions); contingency management had the greatest effect sizes; and interventions for cannabis use were the most efficacious (Dutra et al., 2008). The therapeutic approaches that have consistently garnered the most empirical support are briefly reviewed in this section. As discussed earlier in this chapter, it should also be noted that the skill and experience of the therapist are presumably at least as important as the particular therapy that is delivered, a finding that is further supported by the Imel et al. (2008) meta-analysis.

Contingency management is a treatment approach based on operant conditioning theory and the principle that future behavior is based on the positive or negative consequences of past behavior. Positive (drug effects) and negative (withdrawal symptoms) reinforcers support continued substance use. To reinforce abstinence, other rewards are introduced. The challenge is to identify for a desired behavior a reward that is practical and sufficiently powerful. Recent effectiveness trials within the Clinical Trials Network confirm the value of providing inexpensive incentives for abstinence (contingency management) among stimulant users in outpatient (Petry et al., 2005) and methadone (Peirce et al., 2006) treatment settings. A Cochrane review of randomized controlled trials found that incorporating some form of contingency management or community reinforcement approach was associated with slightly better outcomes and improved retention in care among patients with stimulant use disorders (Knapp et al.,

2007). A meta-analysis of psychosocial treatments for SUDs also demonstrated that studies with contingency management interventions had greater effect sizes compared with studies that incorporated cognitive-behavioral therapy and relapse prevention approaches (Dutra et al., 2008). While the greatest effect sizes were seen in studies that incorporated both cognitive-behavioral therapy and contingency management approaches, this finding is limited because only two studies in the review incorporated both of these approaches.

Cognitive-behavioral therapy, based on social learning models, generally focuses on helping patients understand what factors contribute to and reinforce their substance use (Carroll, 2005). Skills training with the goal of increasing the patient's coping skills is an integral component of this therapy. A recent review of the literature showed that cognitive-behavioral therapy is more effective than very minimal treatments or controls, but is essentially equivalent in effectiveness to other active treatments (Morgenstern and McKay, 2007). The combination of cognitive-behavioral therapy and the use of medication (naltrexone) for alcohol dependence was tested in a national randomized controlled trial and found to be more effective than cognitive-behavioral therapy combined with a placebo (Anton et al., 2006).

Family and couples therapy generally entails including family members in every stage of treatment—the intake interview, counseling sessions, observed medication, and recovery management. Research documents the value of family involvement in treatment and attests to the need for family-based treatments for adolescent drug abuse (Rowe, 2012; Rowe and Liddle, 2003). For couples, a 2008 meta-analysis found that behavioral couples therapy showed better outcomes than individual-based treatments for those with alcohol and other drug dependence (Powers et al., 2008).

Research has shown mixed results for motivational approaches such as motivational interviewing and motivational enhancement therapy (Morgenstern and McKay, 2007). A recent Cochrane review found that motivational interviewing was associated with reductions in substance use compared with no-treatment controls, but there was no significant difference between motivational interviewing and treatment as usual (Smedslund et al., 2011). Similarly, a multisite randomized controlled trial found that motivational interviewing improved retention in care for both alcohol and other drug use disorders but had no significant effect on substance use outcomes (Carroll et al., 2006). Motivational enhancement therapy appears to be more effective in alcohol abusers than in those with more severe alcohol dependence and in those who are more hostile or angry when they enter treatment (Allen et al., 1998). Research results may not translate to all populations, however. While motivational enhancement therapy has been found to enhance outcomes in Spanish-speaking individuals (Carroll et al.,

2009), a recent Clinical Trials Network study found that it was not efficacious for African Americans seeking outpatient substance abuse treatment (Montgomery et al., 2011). More research is needed to determine how motivational interventions and other types of therapeutic interventions compare in effectiveness and to define this effectiveness more clearly with different patient populations.

Finally, 12-step facilitation therapy is based on the behavioral, spiritual, and cognitive principles of 12-step groups such as Alcoholics Anonymous (AA) and Narcotics Anonymous (NA). Abstinence is a key component of the approach, as is active participation in peer support groups. Most of the literature on the effectiveness of the 12-step approach compares the therapy with other treatment interventions. Results have been mixed but generally have shown that 12-step facilitation therapy yields effects similar to those of other treatment modalities (Morgenstern and McKay, 2007).

Pharmacotherapies

Six medications have been approved by the Food and Drug Administration (FDA) for maintenance treatment or relapse prevention after withdrawal from dependence on either opioids (buprenorphine, methadone, naltrexone, extended-release naltrexone) or alcohol (acamprosate, disulfiram, naltrexone, extended-release naltrexone). Randomized controlled trials have shown enhanced outcomes when medication is combined with psychosocial therapy for the treatment of alcohol and opioid use disorders (Anton et al., 2006). In trials completed within the Clinical Trials Network, (1) community-based addiction treatment services used buprenorphine safely (Amass et al., 2004); (2) a buprenorphine detoxification protocol was superior to a clonidine detoxification protocol for opioid dependence (Ling et al., 2005); (3) opioid-dependent adolescents and young adults responded well to buprenorphine and were less likely to use opioids while on medication (Woody et al., 2008); and (4) individuals dependent on prescription opioids were less likely to use opioids while taking buprenorphine (Weiss et al., 2011). Cochrane reviews found that methadone maintenance (Mattick et al., 2009) and buprenorphine (Mattick et al., 2008) enhance treatment outcomes for opioid dependence.

As an often chronic relapsing disorder, SUDs may require ongoing pharmacotherapy. Pharmacotherapy for opioid dependence can use an agonist (e.g., methadone) or an antagonist (e.g., naltrexone) medication. An assessment of methadone treatment found that at least 2 years was required to achieve sustained prevention of relapse to use of illicit opiates (Ball and Ross, 1991; IOM, 1995). Shorter-term treatments have shown high relapse rates (Simpson et al., 1997). Long-term treatment is probably also required for buprenorphine and extended-release naltrexone, although long-term outcomes have not yet been assessed for these medications. However, opioid-positive urine tests declined with longer duration of buprenorphine treatment among patients dependent on prescription opioids (Weiss et al., 2011). A critical issue for pharmacotherapy involving naltrexone is that acute withdrawal treatment is the first part of therapy, not the last (Kosten and O'Connor, 2003). The utility of naltrexone in its oral or sustained-release injectable form is limited by relatively poor compliance in the general population (Stine et al., 2004). The more structured environment of the armed forces may reinforce compliance with these blocking agents and could be used to enhance treatment outcomes, but this has not yet been studied. In another structured context, the use of extended-release naltrexone in criminal justice populations reduced relapse to use of illicit opioids (Coviello et al., 2010, 2012). The major problem with naltrexone is that opioid analgesics will be ineffective for patients taking this medication, who will then require alternative pain management strategies (Center for Substance Abuse Treatment, 2009, Chapters 4 and 5). Medication-assisted treatment, moreover, appears to be more effective when combined with psychosocial interventions for opioid maintenance treatment (Amato et al., 2008).

Withdrawal from alcohol can be treated successfully with a variety of medications; preventing delirium tremens is essential since this is a medical emergency with potential mortality (Kosten and O'Connor, 2003). Treating alcoholism then requires follow-up care. Three medications are FDA approved for this purpose—naltrexone, acamprosate, and disulfiram. They work best in patients who have already completed withdrawal treatment and have been alcohol free for about 5 days.

Cochrane reviews document the effectiveness of naltrexone (Rösner et al., 2010b; Srisurapanont and Jarusuraisin, 2005) and acamprosate (Rösner, 2011; Rösner et al., 2010a) for the treatment of alcohol dependence. The reviews observe that the moderate to small effect sizes associated with the use of medication-assisted treatment are noteworthy because medications reduce the risk of relapse despite the chronic nature of alcohol and other drug use disorders (Rösner, 2011; Rösner et al., 2010b). Duration of therapy remains an important issue for these maintenance treatments, but one study found that a year of naltrexone maintenance provided better outcomes than only 3 months, while discontinuing naltrexone even after 9 months of treatment led to relapse within 3 months of discontinuation (Krystal et al., 2001). Sustained medication treatment is as essential for alcoholism as it is for hypertension, diabetes, or other medical disorders.

Evidence-Based Practices: Integrated Substance Abuse and Mental Health Care

Comorbidity of PTSD and SUDs is a major concern in both military and community samples (Brady et al., 2009; Kessler et al., 1995). This common comorbidity is associated with substantial psychiatric and functional impairment (Ouimette and Brown, 2002). Veterans from Iraq and Afghanistan have high rates of both of these disorders (Erbes et al., 2007; Seal et al., 2007, 2009, 2011; VHA Office of Public Health and Environmental Hazards, 2008). An estimated 20 percent of veterans who receive treatment services for PTSD through a VA medical center have a comorbid SUD (Jacobsen et al., 2001). A recent RAND Corporation study of Iraq and Afghanistan veterans diagnosed with PTSD found binge alcohol abuse rates that were twice the community rate for young adult men (Tanielian et al., 2008). The study also found that tobacco smoking occurred in 50 percent of these veterans, a rate 2.5 times greater than the community rate. Opiate abuse was detected in 9 percent—three times the community rate. Efforts of both the military and the VA provide help with these problems.

Many individuals with PTSD use alcohol, sedatives, and opiates in an attempt to reduce the chronic state of hyperarousal. Continued use of these substances may lead to SUDs. Individuals with SUDs also are at greater risk for developing PTSD because of presumed increased exposure to stressful events as a consequence of their SUD lifestyle. Gender differences have been found across several nonveteran samples, with drug abuse appearing to put women at greater risk than men for developing PTSD (Hien et al., 2010).

Addiction represents a possible physiological complication of chronic nonmalignant pain treatment with opioids. A structured evidence-based review of 67 studies found that among patients with chronic nonmalignant pain exposed to chronic opioid therapy, 3.2 percent developed abuse and addiction, while 11.5 percent developed aberrant drug-related behaviors (Fishbain et al., 2008). Published rates of abuse and/or addiction in chronic pain populations are estimated to be approximately 10 percent, ranging from 3 percent to 18 percent (Adams et al., 2001; Brown et al., 1996; Manchikanti et al., 2004; Martell et al., 2007). Treatment for comorbid opioid use disorder within the context of comprehensive PTSD therapy involves medical withdrawal (detoxification) and/or maintenance therapy using either a full opioid agonist (methadone) or a partial agonist (buprenorphine). These treatments are needed to reduce tolerance and hyperalgesia, as these complications of chronic opiate treatment often worsen the symptoms of PTSD and undermine its most effective treatments. Innovative approaches for detoxification include buprenorphine.

Pharmacotherapy is used to address both PTSD and alcohol use disorders. These medications include antidepressants, anticonvulsants, and antipsychotic medications (Back et al., 2006; Brady et al., 2000; Davidson, 2000; Marshall et al., 2001; Petrakis et al., 2006; Tucker et al., 2001). A recent case study (Back et al., 2012) found exposure therapy (progressive exposure to anxiety stimulus) combined with naltrexone to be more effective in alcoholism comorbid with PTSD than either therapy alone.

Psychotherapy remains one of the primary modes of treatment for those with comorbid PTSD and SUDs, especially as medications have limited effectiveness (IOM, 2007; Najavits et al., 2008). There are various psychotherapies for PTSD and SUDs, singularly and collectively, and a substantial number of outcome studies on such models have been conducted (Amaro et al., 2007; Carroll and Onken, 2005; Foa et al., 2008; Morrissey et al., 2005; Najavits et al., 2008).

SUMMARY

The best practices laid out in this chapter for SUD prevention, screening, diagnosis, and treatment reflect the current literature in each of these areas. While the evidence base is constantly evolving, foundational concepts remain consistent. Evidence-based SUD prevention programs and practices address risk and protective factors, use approaches with demonstrated effectiveness, are age and developmentally appropriate, take place in suitable settings, and manage programs effectively. Best practice in SUD prevention also involves the inclusion of environmental strategies that affect whole communities on a systems-wide versus individual level. Effective SUD screening programs and practices focus on prevalent disease characteristics and are culturally acceptable and cost-effective. The best screening tests are brief, safe, noninvasive, inexpensive, easy to administer, and carry no negative or legal consequences. Diagnosis follows from positive screens and involves the implementation of standardized procedures that are both valid and reliable, can be used in busy clinical settings by professionals with various levels of training and different backgrounds, and reflect the latest research findings. Best practices in SUD treatment involve both the systems of care in which treatment is provided as well as the types of therapies employed; the delivery and organization of care for SUDs must be in line with current health care reform and federal parity legislation and make use of the most up to date behavioral and pharmacological therapies.

REFERENCES

Adams, N. J., M. B. Plane, M. F. Fleming, M. P. Mundt, L. A. Saunders, and E. A. Stauffacher. 2001. Opioids and the treatment of chronic pain in a primary care sample. *Journal of Pain and Symptom Management* 22(3):791-796.

Ahmadi, H., and S. L. Green. 2011. Screening, brief intervention, and referral to treatment for military spouses experiencing alcohol and substance use disorders: A literature review. *Journal of Clinical Psychology in Medical Settings* 18(2):129-136.

Ajzen, I., and M. Fishbein. 1980. *Understanding attitudes and predicting social behavior.* Englewood Cliffs, NJ: Prentice-Hall.

Allen, J., R. F. Anton, T. F. Babor, J. Carbonari, K. M. Carroll, G. J. Connors, N. L. Cooney, F. K. Del Boca, C. C. DiClemente, D. Donovan, R. M. Kadden, M. Litt, R. Longabaugh, M. Mattson, W. R. Miller, C. L. Randall, B. J. Rounsaville, R. G. Rychtarik, R. L. Stout, J. S. Tonigan, P. W. Wirtz, and A. Zweben. 1998. Matching alcoholism treatments to client heterogeneity: Project MATCH three-year drinking outcomes. *Alcoholism: Clinical and Experimental Research* 22(6):1300-1311.

Amaro, H., J. Dai, S. Arevalo, A. Acevedo, A. Matsumoto, R. Nieves, and G. Prado. 2007. Effects of integrated trauma treatment on outcomes in a racially/ethnically diverse sample of women in urban community-based substance abuse treatment. *Journal of Urban Health* 84(4):508-522.

Amass, L., W. Ling, T. E. Freese, C. Reiber, J. J. Annon, A. J. Cohen, D. McCarty, M. S. Reid, L. S. Brown, Jr., C. Clark, D. M. Ziedonis, J. Krejci, S. Stine, T. Winhusen, G. Brigham, D. Babcock, J. A. Muir, B. J. Buchan, and T. Horton. 2004. Bringing buprenorphine-naloxone detoxification to community treatment providers: The NIDA clinical trials network field experience. *American Journal on Addictions* 13(Suppl. 1):S42-S66.

Amato, L., S. Minozzi, M. Davoli, S. Vecchi, M. M. F. Ferri, and S. Mayet. 2008. Psychosocial combined with agonist maintenance treatments versus agonist maintenance treatments alone for treatment of opioid dependence. *Cochrane Database of Systematic Reviews* 4.

Anton, R. F., S. S. O'Malley, D. A. Ciraulo, R. A. Cisler, D. Couper, D. M. Donovan, D. R. Gastfriend, J. D. Hosking, B. A. Johnson, J. S. LoCastro, R. Longabaugh, B. J. Mason, M. E. Mattson, W. R. Miller, H. M. Pettinati, C. L. Randall, R. Swift, R. D. Weiss, L. D. Williams, A. Zweben, and C. S. R. Group. 2006. Combined pharmacotherapies and behavioral interventions for alcohol dependence: The combine study: A randomized controlled trial. *Journal of the American Medical Association* 295(17):2003-2017.

APA (American Psychiatric Association). 2000. *Diagnostic and statistical manual of mental disorders, fourth edition, text revision (DSM-IV-TR).* Washington, DC: American Psychiatric Association.

APA. 2012. *DSM-5: The future of psychiatric diagnosis.* http://www.dsm5.org/Pages/Default.aspx (accessed May 28, 2012).

Aschengrau, A., and G. R. Seage. 2008. *Essentials of epidemiology in public health* (2nd ed.). Sudbury, MA: Jones and Bartlett Publishers.

Babor, T. F., and R. M. Kadden. 2005. Screening and interventions for alcohol and drug problems in medical settings: What works? *Journal of Trauma* 59(3):S80-S87.

Babor, T. F., J. C. Higgens-Biddle, D. Dauser, J. A. Burleson, G. A. Zarkin, and J. Bray. 2006. Brief interventions for at-risk drinking: Patient outcomes and cost-effectiveness in managed care organizations. *Alcohol and Alcoholism* 41(6):624-631.

Babor, T. F., R. Caetano, S. Casswell, G. Edwards, N. Giesbrecht, K. Graham, J. Grube, L. Hill, H. Holder, R. Homel, M. Livingston, E. Osterberg, J. Rehm, R. Room, and I. Rossow. 2010a. *Alcohol: No ordinary commodity: Research and public policy.* Oxford: Oxford University Press.

Babor, T., J. Caulkins, G. Edwards, B. Fischer, D. Foxcroft, K. Humphreys, I. Obot, J. Rehm, P. Reuter, R. Room, I. Rossow, and J. Strang. 2010b. *Drug policy and the public good.* Oxford: Oxford University Press.

Back, S. E., K. T. Brady, S. C. Sonne, and M. L. Verduin. 2006. Symptom improvement in co-occurring PTSD and alcohol dependence. *Journal of Nervous and Mental Disease* 194(9):690-696.

Back, S. E., T. Killeen, E. B. Foa, E. J. Santa Ana, D. F. Gros, and K. T. Brady. 2012. Use of an integrated therapy with prolonged exposure to treat PTSD and comorbid alcohol dependence in an Iraq veteran. *American Journal of Psychiatry* 169(7):688-691.

Baker, D. G., P. Heppner, N. Afari, S. Nunnink, M. Kilmer, A. Simmons, L. Harder, and B. Bosse. 2009. Trauma exposure, branch of service, and physical injury in relation to mental health among US veterans returning from Iraq and Afghanistan. *Military Medicine* 174(8):773-778.

Ball, J. C., and A. Ross. 1991. *The effectiveness of methadone maintenance treatment: Patients, programs, services, and outcome*. New York: Springer-Verlag.

Bandura, A. 1977. *Social learning theory*. Englewood Cliffs, NJ: Prentice Hall.

Becker, C. B., C. Zayfert, and E. Anderson. 2004. A survey of psychologists' attitudes towards and utilization of exposure therapy for PTSD. *Behaviour Research and Therapy* 42(3):277-292.

Bellg, A. J., B. Resnick, D. S. Minicucci, G. Ogedegbe, D. Ernst, B. Borrelli, J. Hecht, M. Ory, D. Orwig, and S. Czajkowski. 2004. Enhancing treatment fidelity in health behavior change studies: Best practices and recommendations from the nih behavior change consortium. *Health Psychology* 23(5):443-451.

Bertholet, N., J.-B. Daeppen, V. Wietlisbach, M. Fleming, and B. Burnand. 2005. Reduction of alcohol consumption by brief alcohol intervention in primary care: Systematic review and meta-analysis. *Archives of Internal Medicine* 165(9):986-995.

Blatt, S. J., C. A. Sanislow, III, D. C. Zuroff, and P. A. Pilkonis. 1996. Characteristics of effective therapists: Further analyses of data from the National Institute of Mental Health treatment of depression collaborative research program. *Journal of Consulting and Clinical Psychology* 64(6):1276-1284.

Blume, A. W., and G. A. Marlatt. 2009. The role of executive cognitive functions in changing substance use: What we know and what we need to know. *Annals of Behavior Medicine* 37(2):117-125.

Botvin, G. J., E. Baker, L. Dusenbury, E. M. Botvin, and T. Diaz. 1995. Long-term follow-up results of a randomized drug abuse prevention trial in a white middle-class population. *Journal of the American Medical Association* 273(14):1106-1112.

Brady, K., T. Pearlstein, G. M. Asnis, D. Baker, B. Rothbaum, C. R. Sikes, and G. M. Farfel. 2000. Efficacy and safety of sertraline treatment of posttraumatic stress disorder: A randomized controlled trial. *Journal of the American Medical Association* 283(14):1837-1844.

Brady, K. T., P. Tuerk, S. E. Back, M. E. Saladin, A. E. Waldrop, and H. Myrick. 2009. Combat posttraumatic stress disorder, substance use disorders, and traumatic brain injury. *Journal of Addiction Medicine* 3(4):179-188.

Brody, G. H., Y. F. Chen, S. R. H. Beach, R. A. Philibert, and S. M. Kogan. 2009. Participation in a family-centered prevention program decreases genetic risk for adolescents' risky behaviors. *Pediatrics* 124(3):911-917.

Brown, J. M. 2004. The effectiveness of treatment. In *The essential handbook of treatment and prevention of alcohol problems*, edited by N. Heather and T. Stockwell. London: John Wiley and Sons, Ltd. Pp. 9-20.

Brown, R. L., J. J. Patterson, L. A. Rounds, and O. Papasouliotis. 1996. Substance abuse among patients with chronic back pain. *Journal of Family Practice* 43(2):152-160.

Campbell, J. 2002. Health consequences of intimate partner violence. *Lancet* 359(9314):1331-1336.

Carroll, K. M. 2005. Recent advances in the psychotherapy of addictive disorders. *Current Psychiatry Reports* 7(5):329-336.

Carroll, K. M., and L. S. Onken. 2005. Behavioral therapies for drug abuse. *American Journal of Psychiatry* 162(8):1452-1460.

Carroll, K. M., S. A. Ball, C. Nich, S. Martino, T. L. Frankforter, C. Farentinos, L. E. Kunkel, S. K. Mikulich-Gilbertson, J. Morgenstern, J. L. Obert, D. Polcin, N. Snead, and G. E. Woody. 2006. Motivational interviewing to improve treatment engagement and outcome in individuals seeking treatment for substance abuse: A multisite effectiveness study. *Drug and Alcohol Dependence* 81(3):301-312.

Carroll, K. M., S. Martino, S. A. Ball, C. Nich, T. Frankforter, L. M. Anez, M. Paris, L. Suarez-Morales, J. Szapocznik, W. R. Miller, C. Rosa, J. Matthews, and C. Farentinos. 2009. A multisite randomized effectiveness trial of motivational enhancement therapy for Spanish-speaking substance users. *Journal of Consulting and Clinical Psychology* 77(5):993-999.

Center for Substance Abuse Treatment. 2006. *Substance abuse: Clinical issues in intensive outpatient treatment. Treatment Improvement Protocol (TIP) series* 47. Rockville, MD: Substance Abuse and Mental Health Services Administration.

Center for Substance Abuse Treatment. 2009. *Incorporating alcohol pharmacotherapies into medical practice.* Rockville, MD: Substance Abuse and Mental Health Services Administration.

Chaloupka, F. J., M. Grossman, and H. Saffer. 2002. The effects of price on alcohol consumption and alcohol-related problems. *Alcohol Research & Health* 26(1):22-34.

Chaloupka, F. J., A. Yurekli, and G. T. Fong. 2012. Tobacco taxes as a tobacco control strategy. *Tobacco Control* 21(2):172-180.

Chandra, A. 2011. *Views from the homefront: The experiences of youth and spouses from military families.* Santa Monica, CA: RAND Corporation.

Chartrand, M. M., D. A. Frank, L. F. White, and T. R. Shope. 2008. Effect of parents' wartime deployment on the behavior of young children in military families. *Archives of Pediatrics and Adolescent Medicine* 162(11):1009-1014.

Chisholm, D., J. Rehm, M. Van Ommeren, and M. Monteiro. 2004. Reducing the global burden of hazardous alcohol use: A comparative cost-effectiveness analysis. *Journal of Studies on Alcohol* 65(6):782-793.

Coviello, D. M., J. W. Cornish, K. G. Lynch, A. I. Alterman, and C. P. O'Brien. 2010. A randomized trial of oral naltrexone for treating opioid-dependent offenders. *American Journal on Addictions* 19(5):422-432.

Coviello, D. M., J. W. Cornish, K. G. Lynch, T. Y. Boney, C. A. Clark, J. D. Lee, P. D. Friedmann, E. V. Nunes, T. W. Kinlock, M. S. Gordon, R. P. Schwartz, E. S. Nuwayser, and C. P. O'Brien. 2012. A multisite pilot study of extended-release injectable naltrexone treatment for previously opioid-dependent parolees and probationers. *Substance Abuse* 33(1):48-59.

Crits-Christoph, P., and J. Mintz. 1991. Implications of therapist effects for the design and analysis of comparative studies of psychotherapies. *Journal of Consulting and Clinical Psychology* 59(1):20-26.

Davidson, J. R. T. 2000. Pharmacotherapy of posttraumatic stress disorder: Treatment options, long-term follow-up, and predictors of outcome. *Journal of Clinical Psychiatry* 61(Suppl. 5):52-59.

Dennis, M., C. K. Scott, and R. Funk. 2003. An experimental evaluation of recovery management checkups (RMC) for people with chronic substance use disorders. *Evaluation and Program Planning* 26(3):339-352.

Dennis, M. L., C. K. Scott, R. Funk, and M. A. Foss. 2005. The duration and correlates of addiction and treatment careers. *Journal of Substance Abuse Treatment* 28(Suppl. 1):S51-S62.

Duncan, B. L., S. D. Miller, J. A. Sparks, D. A. Claud, L. R. Reynolds, J. Brown, and L. D. Johnson. 2003. The session rating scale: Preliminary psychometric properties of a "working" alliance measure. *Journal of Brief Therapy* 3(1):3-11.

Dutra, L., G. Stathopoulou, S. L. Basden, T. M. Leyro, M. B. Powers, and M. W. Otto. 2008. A meta-analytic review of psychosocial interventions for substance use disorders. *American Journal of Psychiatry* 165(2):179-187.

Edlund, M. J., D. Steffick, T. Hudson, K. M. Harris, and M. Sullivan. 2007. Risk factors for clinically recognized opioid abuse and dependence among veterans using opioids for chronic non-cancer pain. *Pain* 129(3):355-362.

Erbes, C., J. Westermeyer, B. Engdahl, and E. Johnsen. 2007. Post-traumatic stress disorder and service utilization in a sample of service members from Iraq and Afghanistan. *Military Medicine* 172(4):359-363.

Fishbain, D. A., B. Cole, J. Lewis, H. L. Rosomoff, and R. S. Rosomoff. 2008. What percentage of chronic nonmalignant pain patients exposed to chronic opioid analgesic therapy develop abuse/addiction and/or aberrant drug-related behaviors? A structured evidence-based review. *Pain Medicine* 9(4):444-459.

Foa, E. B., T. M. Keane, M. J. Friedman, and J. Cohen. 2008. *Effective treatments for PTSD: Practice guidelines from the International Society for Traumatic Stress Studies* (2nd ed.). New York: Guilford Press.

Foran, H., A. Smith Slep, and R. Heyman. 2011a. Hazardous alcohol use among active duty Air Force personnel: Identifying unique risk and promotive factors. *Psychology of Addictive Behaviors* 25(1):28-40.

Foran, H. M., R. E. Heyman, and A. M. S. Slep. 2011b. Hazardous drinking and military community functioning: Identifying mediating risk factors. *Journal of Consulting & Clinical Psychology* 79(4):521-532.

Gibbs, D. A., S. L. Martin, L. L. Kupper, and R. E. Johnson. 2007. Child maltreatment in enlisted soldiers' families during combat-related deployments. *Journal of the American Medical Association* 298(5):528-535.

Graham, K. 2000. Preventive interventions for on-premise drinking: A promising but under-researched area of prevention. *Contemporary Drug Problems* 27(3):593-668.

Graham, K., and R. Homel. 2008. *Raising the bar: Preventing aggression in and around bars, clubs and pubs.* Abingdon, UK: Willan Publishing.

Graham, K., S. Bernards, D. W. Osgood, R. Homel, and J. Purcell. 2005. Guardians and handlers: The role of bar staff in preventing and managing aggression. *Addiction* 100(6):755-766.

Gray, B. T. 2001. A factor analytic study of the Substance Abuse Subtle Screening Inventory (SASSI). *Educational and Psychological Measurement* 61(1):102-118.

Hansen, W. B., and J. W. Graham. 1991. Preventing alcohol, marijuana, and cigarette use among adolescents: Peer pressure resistance training versus establishing conservative norms. *Preventive Medicine* 20(3):414-430.

Hawkins, J. D., R. F. Catalano, and J. Y. Miller. 1992. Risk and protective factors for alcohol and other drug problems in adolescence and early adulthood: Implications for substance abuse prevention. *Psychological Bulletin* 112(1):64-105.

Hennekens, C. H., J. E. Buring, and S. L. Mayrent. 1987. *Epidemiology in medicine* (1st ed.). Philadelphia, PA: Lippincott Williams and Wilkins.

Hien, D. A., A. N. C. Campbell, L. M. Ruglass, M. C. Hu, and T. Killeen. 2010. The role of alcohol misuse in PTSD outcomes for women in community treatment: A secondary analysis of NIDA's Women and Trauma Study. *Drug and Alcohol Dependence* 111(1-2):114-119.

Holder, H. D., P. J. Gruenewald, W. R. Ponicki, A. J. Treno, J. W. Grube, R. F. Saltz, R. B. Voas, R. Reynolds, J. Davis, L. Sanchez, G. Gaumont, and P. Roeper. 2000. Effect of community-based interventions on high-risk drinking and alcohol-related injuries. *Journal of the American Medical Association* 284(18):2341-2347.

Horwitz, A. V., C. S. Widom, J. McLaughlin, and H. R. White. 2001. The impact of childhood abuse and neglect on adult mental health: A prospective study. *Journal of Health and Social Behavior* 42(2):184-201.

Hughes, C. E., and A. Stevens. 2010. What can we learn from the Portuguese decriminalization of illicit drugs? *British Journal of Criminology* 50(6):999-1022.

Hussey, J. M., J. J. Chang, and J. B. Kotch. 2006. Child maltreatment in the United States: Prevalence, risk factors, and adolescent health consequences. *Pediatrics* 118(3):933-942.

Imel, Z. E., B. E. Wampold, S. D. Miller, and R. R. Fleming. 2008. Distinction without a difference: Direct comparisons of psychotherapies for alcohol use disorders. *Psychology of Addictive Behaviors* 22(4):533-543.

IOM (Institute of Medicine). 1994a. *Reducing risks for mental disorders: Frontiers for preventive intervention research*. Washington, DC: National Academy Press.

IOM. 1994b. *Under the influence? Drugs and the American work force: Summary: Conclusion and recommendations*. Washington, DC: National Academy Press.

IOM. 1995. *Federal regulation of methadone treatment*. Washington, DC: National Academy Press.

IOM. 2000. *To err is human: Building a safer health system*. Washington, DC: National Academy Press.

IOM. 2001. *Crossing the quality chasm: A new health system for the 21st century*. Washington, DC: National Academy Press.

IOM. 2006. *Improving the quality of health care for mental and substance-use conditions: Quality chasm series*. Washington, DC: The National Academies Press.

IOM. 2007. *Treatment of PTSD: An assessment of the evidence*. Washington, DC: The National Academies Press.

Jacobsen, L. K., S. M. Southwick, and T. R. Kosten. 2001. Substance use disorders in patients with posttraumatic stress disorder: A review of the literature. *American Journal of Psychiatry* 158(8):1184-1190.

Jacobson, I. G., M. A. K. Ryan, T. I. Hooper, T. C. Smith, P. J. Amoroso, E. J. Boyko, G. D. Gackstetter, T. S. Wells, and N. S. Bell. 2008. Alcohol use and alcohol-related problems before and after military combat deployment. *Journal of the American Medical Association* 300(6):663-675.

Jakupcak, M., M. T. Tull, M. J. McDermott, D. Kaysen, S. Hunt, and T. Simpson. 2010. PTSD symptom clusters in relationship to alcohol misuse among Iraq and Afghanistan war veterans seeking post-deployment VA health care. *Addictive Behaviors* 35(9):840-843.

Kalivas, P. W., and N. D. Volkow. 2005. The neural basis of addiction: A pathology of motivation and choice. *American Journal of Psychiatry* 162(8):1403-1413.

Kaner, E. F. S., H. O. Dickinson, F. R. Beyer, F. Campbell, C. Schlesinger, N. Heather, J. B. Saunders, B. Burnand, and E. D. Pienaar. 2009. Effectiveness of brief alcohol interventions in primary care populations. *Cochrane Database of Systematic Reviews* 1.

Karoly, L. A., P. W. Greenwood, S. S. Everingham, J. Hoube, M. R. Kilburn, C. P. Rydell, M. Sanders, and J. Chiesa. 1998. *Investing in our children: What we know and don't know about the costs and benefits of early childhood interventions*. Santa Monica, CA: RAND Corporation.

Karoly, L. A., M. R. Kilburn, J. H. Bigelow, J. P. Caulkins, and J. S. Cannon. 2001. *Assessing costs and benefits of early childhood intervention programs: Overview and application to the starting early starting smart program*. Seattle, WA: Casey Family Programs and Santa Monica, CA: RAND Corporation.

Kessler, R. C., A. Sonnega, E. Bromet, M. Hughes, and C. B. Nelson. 1995. Posttraumatic stress disorder in the National Comorbidity Survey. *Archives of General Psychiatry* 52(12):1048-1060.

Kivlighan, D. M., Jr., and D. M. Kivlighan, III. 2009. Training related changes in the ways that group trainees structure their knowledge of group counseling leader interventions. *Group Dynamics* 13(3):190-204.

Knapp, W. P., B. Soares, M. Farrel, and M. S. Lima. 2007. Psychosocial interventions for cocaine and psychostimulant amphetamines related disorders. *Cochrane Database of Systematic Reviews* 3.

Kosten, T. R., and P. G. O'Connor. 2003. Management of drug and alcohol withdrawal. *New England Journal of Medicine* 348(18):1786-1795.

Krystal, J. H., J. A. Cramer, W. F. Krol, G. F. Kirk, and R. A. Rosenheck. 2001. Naltrexone in the treatment of alcohol dependence. *New England Journal of Medicine* 345(24):1734-1739.

Kumpfer, K. L., R. Alvarado, and H. O. Whiteside. 2003. Family-based interventions for substance use and misuse prevention. *Substance Use and Misuse* 38(11-13):1759-1787, 1916.

Lambert, M. J. 2005. Early response in psychotherapy: Further evidence for the importance of common factors rather than "placebo effects." *Journal of Clinical Psychology* 61(7):855-869.

Larson, M. J., N. R. Wooten, R. S. Adams, and E. L. Merrick. 2012. Military combat deployments and substance use: Review and future directions. *Journal of Social Work Practice in the Addictions* 12(1):6-27.

Lester, P., K. Peterson, J. Reeves, L. Knauss, D. Glover, C. Mogil, N. Duan, W. Saltzman, R. Pynoos, K. Wilt, and W. Beardslee. 2010. The long war and parental combat deployment: Effects on military children and at-home spouses. *Journal of the American Academy of Child and Adolescent Psychiatry* 49(4):310-320.

Ling, W., L. Amass, S. Shoptaw, J. J. Annon, M. Hillhouse, D. Babcock, G. Brigham, J. Harrer, M. Reid, J. Muir, B. Buchan, D. Orr, G. Woody, J. Krejci, and D. Ziedonis. 2005. A multi-center randomized trial of buprenorphine-naloxone versus clonidine for opioid detoxification: Findings from the National Institute on Drug Abuse Clinical Trials Network. *Addiction* 100(8):1090-1100.

Lowinson, J. H., ed. 2005. *Substance abuse: A comprehensive textbook*. Philadelphia, PA: Lippincott Williams & Wilkins.

Luborsky, L., A. T. McLellan, L. Diguer, G. Woody, and D. A. Seligman. 1997. The psychotherapist matters: Comparison of outcomes across twenty-two therapists and seven patient samples. *Clinical Psychology: Science and Practice* 4(1):53-65.

Mallinckrodt, B., and M. L. Nelson. 1991. Counselor training level and the formation of the psychotherapeutic working alliance. *Journal of Counseling Psychology* 38(2):133-138.

Manchikanti, L., K. S. Damron, C. D. McManus, and R. C. Barnhill. 2004. Patterns of illicit drug use and opioid abuse in patients with chronic pain at initial evaluation: A prospective, observational study. *Pain Physician* 7(4):431-437.

Mansfield, A. J., and C. C. Engel. 2011. Understanding substance use in military spouses. *Journal of Clinical Psychology in Medical Settings* 18(2):198-199.

Marshall, R. D., K. L. Beebe, M. Oldham, and R. Zaninelli. 2001. Efficacy and safety of paroxetine treatment for chronic PTSD: A fixed-dose, placebo-controlled study. *American Journal of Psychiatry* 158(12):1982-1988.

Martell, B. A., P. G. O'Connor, R. D. Kerns, W. C. Becker, K. H. Morales, T. R. Kosten, and D. A. Fiellin. 2007. Systematic review: Opioid treatment for chronic back pain: Prevalence, efficacy, and association with addiction. *Annals of Internal Medicine* 146(2):116-127.

Mattick, R. P., J. Kimber, C. Breen, and M. Davoli. 2008. Buprenorphine maintenance versus placebo or methadone maintenance for opioid dependence. *Cochrane Database of Systematic Reviews (Online)* 2.

Mattick, R. P., C. Breen, J. Kimber, and M. Davoli. 2009. Methadone maintenance therapy versus no opioid replacement therapy for opioid dependence. *Cochrane Database of Systematic Reviews* 3.

Mayes, L. C., and N. Suchman. 2006. Developmental pathways to substance abuse. In *Developmental psychopathology: Risk, disorder, and adaptation* (Vol. 3), edited by D. Cicchetti and D. Cohen. New York: Wiley. Pp. 599-619.

Mayfield, W. A., C. M. Kardash, and D. M. Kivlighan, Jr. 1999. Differences in experienced and novice counselors' knowledge structures about clients: Implications for case conceptualization. *Journal of Counseling Psychology* 46(4):504-514.

McCarty, D., K. J. McConnell, and L. A. Schmidt. 2010. Priorities for policy research on treatments for alcohol and drug use disorders. *Journal of Substance Abuse Treatment* 39(2):87-95.

McGlynn, E. A., S. M. Asch, J. Adams, J. Keesey, J. Hicks, A. DeCristofaro, and E. A. Kerr. 2003. The quality of health care delivered to adults in the United States. *New England Journal of Medicine* 348(26):2635-2645.

McKay, J. R., K. G. Lynch, D. S. Shepard, and H. M. Pettinati. 2005. The effectiveness of telephone-based continuing care for alcohol and cocaine dependence: 24-month outcomes. *Archives of General Psychiatry* 62(2):199-207.

McLellan, A. T. 2002. Have we evaluated addiction treatment correctly? Implications from a chronic care perspective. *Addiction* 97(3):249-252.

McLellan, A. T., D. C. Lewis, C. P. O'Brien, and H. D. Kleber. 2000. Drug dependence, a chronic medical illness. *Journal of the American Medical Association* 284(13):1689-1695.

McLellan, A. T., G. S. Skipper, M. Campbell, and R. L. DuPont. 2008. Five year outcomes in a cohort study of physicians treated for substance use disorders in the United States. *British Medical Journal* 337(7679):1154-1156.

Mee-Lee, D. 2001. *ASAM patient placement criteria for the treatment of substance-related disorders*. (2nd rev. ed.). Chevy Chase, MD: American Society of Addiction Medicine.

Mee-Lee, D., and G. D. Shulman. 2003. The ASAM placement criteria and matching patients to treatment. In *Principles of addiction medicine* (3rd ed.), edited by A. W. Graham, T. K. Schultz, M. F. Mayo-Smith, R. K. Ries, and B. B. Wilford. Chevy Chase, MD: American Society of Addiction Medicine. Pp. 453-465.

Mertens, J. R., C. Weisner, G. T. Ray, B. Fireman, and K. Walsh. 2005. Hazardous drinkers and drug users in HMO primary care: Prevalence, medical conditions, and costs. *Alcoholism: Clinical and Experimental Research* 29(6):989-998.

MHAT (Mental Health Advisory Team). 2006. *Mental Health Advisory Team (MHAT) IV, Operation Iraqi Freedom 05-07*. Washington, DC: Office of the Surgeon, Multinational Force-Iraq and Office of the Surgeon General, United States Army Medical Command.

Mihalik, S., A. Fagan, K. Irwin, D. Ballard, and D. Elliot. 2004. *Blueprints for violence prevention*. Boulder, CO: Center for the Study and Prevention of Violence.

Miller, S. D., B. L. Duncan, J. Brown, J. A. Sparks, and D. A. Claud. 2003. The outcome rating scale: A preliminary study of the reliability, validity, and feasibility of a brief visual analog measure. *Journal of Brief Therapy* 2(2):91-100.

Miller, S. D., D. Mee-Lee, W. Plum, and M. A. Hubble. 2005. Making treatment count: Client-directed outcome-informed clinical work with problem drinkers. In *Handbook of clinical family therapy*, edited by J. Lebow. Hoboken, NJ: John Wiley & Sons. Pp. 281-308.

Miller, W. R., and P. L. Wilbourne. 2002. Mesa grande: A methodological analysis of clinical trials of treatments for alcohol use disorders. *Addiction* 97(3):265-277.

Miller, W. R., J. L. Sorensen, J. A. Selzer, and G. S. Brigham. 2006. Disseminating evidence-based practices in substance abuse treatment: A review with suggestions. *Journal of Substance Abuse Treatment* 31(1):25-39.

Montgomery, L., A. K. Burlew, A. S. Kosinski, and A. A. Forcehimes. 2011. Motivational enhancement therapy for African American substance users: A randomized clinical trial. *Cultural Diversity and Ethnic Minority Psychology* 17(4):357-365.

Moos, R. H. 2007. Theory-based active ingredients of effective treatments for substance use disorders. *Drug and Alcohol Dependence* 88(2-3):109-121.

Morgenstern, J., and J. R. McKay. 2007. Rethinking the paradigms that inform behavioral treatment research for substance use disorders. *Addiction* 102(9):1377-1389.

Morrissey, J. P., E. W. Jackson, A. R. Ellis, H. Amaro, V. B. Brown, and L. M. Najavits. 2005. Twelve-month outcomes of trauma-informed interventions for women with co-occurring disorders. *Psychiatric Services* 56(10):1213-1222.

Muir Gray, J. A. 2004. New concepts in screening. *British Journal of General Practice* 54(501):292-298.

Najavits, L. M., D. Ryngala, S. E. Back, E. Bolton, K. T. Mueser, and K. T. Brady. 2008. Treatment for PTSD and comorbid disorders: A review of the literature. In *Effective treatments for PTSD: Practice guidelines from the International Society for Traumatic Stress Studies* (2nd ed.), edited by E. B. Foa, T. M. Keane, M. J. Friedman, and J. Cohen. New York: Guilford Press. Pp. 508-535.

National Highway Traffic Safety Administration. 2009. *Traffic Safety Facts 2009: A Compilation of Motor Vehicle Crash Data from the Fatality Analysis Reporting System and the General Estimates System, Early Edition.* Washington, DC: U.S. Department of Transportation.

NIAAA (National Institute on Alcohol Abuse and Alcoholism). 2005. *Helping patients who drink too much: A clinician's guide.* Bethesda, MD: NIAAA.

NIDA (National Institute on Drug Abuse). 2009a. *Principles of drug addiction treatments.* NIH Publication Number: 09-4180. Bethesda, MD: NIDA.

NIDA. 2009b. *Review of the prevention research portfolio.* Bethesda, MD: NIDA.

NRC (National Research Council) and IOM. 2000. *From neurons to neighborhoods: The science of early childhood development.* Washington, DC: National Academy Press.

NRC and IOM. 2009. *Preventing mental, emotional, and behavioral disorders among young people: Progress and possibilities.* Washington, DC: The National Academies Press.

Ockene, J. K., A. Adams, T. G. Hurley, E. V. Wheeler, and J. R. Hebert. 1999. Brief physician- and nurse practitioner-delivered counseling for high-risk drinkers: Does it work? *Archives of Internal Medicine* 159(18):2198-2205.

ONDCP (Office of National Drug Control Policy). 2001. *Evidence-based principles for substance abuse prevention.* Washington, DC: ONDCP. https://www.ncjrs.gov/ondcppubs/publications/prevent/evidence_based_eng.html (accessed August 6, 2012).

ONDCP. 2011a. *Epidemic: Responding to America's prescription drug abuse crisis.* Washington, DC: ONDCP.

ONDCP. 2011b. *National drug control strategy, 2011.* Washington, DC: ONDCP.

ONDCP. 2012. *Prescription drug abuse.* Washington, DC: ONDCP. http://www.whitehouse.gov/ondcp/prescription-drug-abuse (accessed August 7, 2012).

Ouimette, P., and P. J. Brown. 2002. *Trauma and substance abuse: Causes, consequences, and treatment of comorbid disorders.* Washington, DC: American Psychological Association Press.

Peirce, J. M., N. M. Petry, M. L. Stitzer, J. Blaine, S. Kellogg, F. Satterfield, M. Schwartz, J. Krasnansky, E. Pencer, L. Silva-Vazquez, K. C. Kirby, C. Royer-Malvestuto, J. M. Roll, A. Cohen, M. L. Copersino, K. Kolodner, and R. Li. 2006. Effects of lower-cost incentives on stimulant abstinence in methadone maintenance treatment: A national drug abuse treatment clinical trials network study. *Archives of General Psychiatry* 63(2):201-208.

Perry, C. L., K.-I. Klepp, A. Halper, K. G. Hawkins, and D. M. Murray. 1986. A process evaluation study of peer leaders in health education. *Journal of School Health* 56(2):62-67.

Petrakis, I. L., J. Poling, C. Levinson, C. Nich, K. Carroll, E. Ralevski, and B. Rounsaville. 2006. Naltrexone and disulfiram in patients with alcohol dependence and comorbid post-traumatic stress disorder. *Biological Psychiatry* 60(7):777-783.

Petry, N. M., S. M. Alessi, J. Marx, M. Austin, and M. Tardif. 2005. Vouchers versus prizes: Contingency management treatment of substance abusers in community settings. *Journal of Consulting and Clinical Psychology* 73(6):1005-1014.

Powers, M. B., E. Vedel, and P. M. G. Emmelkamp. 2008. Behavioral couples therapy (BCT) for alcohol and drug use disorders: A meta-analysis. *Clinical Psychology Review* 28(6):952-962.

Rammohan, V., R. A. Hahn, R. Elder, R. Brewer, J. Fielding, T. S. Naimi, T. L. Toomey, and S. K. Chattopadhyay. 2011. Effects of dram shop liability and enhanced over-service law enforcement initiatives on excessive alcohol consumption and related harms: Two community guide systematic reviews. *American Journal of Preventive Medicine* 41(3):334-343.

Reiff-Hekking, S., J. K. Ockene, T. G. Hurley, and G. W. Reed. 2005. Brief physician and nurse practitioner-delivered counseling for high-risk drinking. Results at 12-month follow-up. *Journal of General Internal Medicine* 20(1):7-13.

Robertson, E. B., S. L. David, and S. A. Rao. 2003. *Preventing drug use among children and adolescents: A research-based guide for parents, educators, and community leaders* (2nd ed.). Rockville, MD: NIDA.

Rösner, S. 2011. Review: Acamprosate increases abstinence in patients with alcohol dependence. *Annals of Internal Medicine* 154(2):JC1-10.

Rösner, S., A. Hackl-Herrwerth, S. Leucht, P. Lehert, S. Vecchi, and M. Soyka. 2010a. Acamprosate for alcohol dependence. *Cochrane Database of Systematic Reviews (Online)* 9.

Rösner, S., A. Hackl-Herrwerth, S. Leucht, S. Vecchi, M. Srisurapanont, and M. Soyka. 2010b. Opioid antagonists for alcohol dependence. *Cochrane Database of Systematic Reviews* 12.

Rowe, C. L. 2012. Family therapy for drug abuse: Review and updates 2003-2010. *Journal of Marital and Family Therapy* 38(1):59-81.

Rowe, C. L., and H. A. Liddle. 2003. Substance abuse. *Journal of Marital and Family Therapy* 29(1):97-120.

Rutter, M. 2006. Implications of resilience concepts for scientific understanding. *Annals of the New York Academy of Sciences* 1094:1-12.

Saltz, R. F., M. J. Paschall, R. P. McGaffigan, and P. M. Nygaard. 2010. Alcohol risk management in college settings: The safer California universities randomized trial. *American Journal of Preventive Medicine* 39(6):491-499.

SAMHSA (Substance Abuse and Mental Health Services Administration). 2010. *Results from the 2009 National Survey on Drug Use and Health: Mental health findings.* NSDUH Series H-39. Rockville, MD: Office of Applied Studies.

SAMHSA. 2012. *NREPP's quality of research.* http://www.nrepp.samhsa.gov/ReviewQOR.aspx (accessed May 28, 2012).

Scott, C. K., M. L. Dennis, and M. A. Foss. 2005. Utilizing recovery management checkups to shorten the cycle of relapse, treatment reentry, and recovery. *Drug & Alcohol Dependence* 78(3):325-338.

Seal, K. H., D. Bertenthal, C. R. Miner, S. Sen, and C. Marmar. 2007. Bringing the war back home mental health disorders among 103,788 US veterans returning from Iraq and Afghanistan seen at Department of Veterans Affairs facilities. *Archives of International Medicine* 167(5):476-482.

Seal, K. H., T. J. Metzler, K. S. Gima, D. Bertenthal, S. Maguen, and C. R. Marmar. 2009. Trends and risk factors for mental health diagnoses among Iraq and Afghanistan veterans using Department of Veterans Affairs health care, 2002-2008. *American Journal of Public Health* 99(9):1651-1658.

Seal, K. H., G. Cohen, A. Waldrop, B. E. Cohen, S. Maguen, and L. Ren. 2011. Substance use disorders in Iraq and Afghanistan veterans in VA healthcare, 2001-2010: Implications for screening, diagnosis and treatment. *Drug and Alcohol Dependence* 116(1-3):93-101.

Shen, Y.-C., J. Arkes, and T. V. Williams. 2012. Effects of Iraq/Afghanistan deployments on major depression and substance use disorder: Analysis of active duty personnel in the US military. *American Journal of Public Health* 102(S1):S80-S87.

Shonkoff, J. P., L. Richter, J. van der Gaag, and Z. A. Bhutta. 2012. An integrated scientific framework for child survival and early childhood development. *Pediatrics* 129(2):e460-e472.

Simpson, D. D., G. W. Joe, G. A. Rowan-Szal, and J. M. Greener. 1997. Drug abuse treatment process components that improve retention. *Journal of Substance Abuse Treatment* 14(6):565-572.

Smedslund, G., R. C. Berg, K. T. Hammerstrøm, A. Steiro, K. A. Leiknes, H. M. Dahl, and K. Karlsen. 2011. Motivational interviewing for substance abuse. *Cochrane Database of Systematic Reviews* 5.

Spera, C., and K. Franklin. 2010. Reducing drinking among junior enlisted Air Force members in five communities: Early findings of the EUDL program's influence on self-reported drinking behaviors. *Journal of Studies on Alcohol and Drugs* 71(3):373-383.

Spoth, R. L., L. M. Schainker, and S. HillerSturmhöefel. 2011. Translating family-focused prevention science into public health impact: Illustrations from partnership-based research. *Alcohol Research and Health* 34(2):188-203.

Srisurapanont, M., and N. Jarusuraisin. 2005. Opioid antagonists for alcohol dependence. *Cochrane Database of Systematic Reviews* 1.

Sternberg, K. J., L. P. Baradaran, C. B. Abbott, M. E. Lamb, and E. Guterman. 2006. Type of violence, age, and gender differences in the effects of family violence on children's behavior problems: A mega-analysis. *Developmental Review* 26(1):89-112.

Stine, S. M., M. K. Greenwald, and T. R. Kosten. 2004. Pharmacologic interventions for opioid addiction. In *Principles of addiction medicine* (3rd ed.), edited by S. T. Graham, M. Mayo-Smith, R. K. Ries, and B. B. Wilford. Chevy Chase, MD: American Society of Addiction Medicine. Pp. 735-748.

Stockwell, T., and P.J. Gruenewald. 2004. Controls on the physical availability of alcohol. In *The essential handbook of treatment and prevention of alcohol problems*, edited by N. Heather and T. Stockwell. Chichester, UK: Wiley and Sons. Pp. 213-233.

Tanielian, T. L., L. Jaycox, T. L. Schell, G. N. Marshall, M. A. Burnam, C. Eibner, B. R. Karney, L. S. Meredith, J. S. Ringel, and M. E. Vaiana. 2008. *Invisible wounds of war: Summary and recommendations for addressing psychological and cognitive injuries.* Santa Monica, CA: RAND Corporation, Center for Military Health Policy Research.

Treatment Research Institute. 2010. *Integrating appropriate services for substance use conditions in health care settings: An issue brief on lessons learned and challenges ahead.* Philadelphia, PA: Forum on Integration, Treatment Research Institute.

Treno, A. J., P. J. Gruenewald, J. P. Lee, and L. G. Remer. 2007. The sacramento neighborhood alcohol prevention project: Outcomes from a community prevention trial. *Journal of Studies on Alcohol and Drugs* 68(2):197-207.

Trickett, P. K., J. G. Noll, and F. W. Putnam. 2011. The impact of sexual abuse on female development: Lessons from a multigenerational, longitudinal research study. *Development and Psychopathology* 23(02):453-476.

Tucker, P., R. Zaninelli, R. Yehuda, L. Ruggiero, K. Dillingham, and C. D. Pitts. 2001. Paroxetine in the treatment of chronic posttraumatic stress disorder: Results of a placebo-controlled, flexible-dosage trial. *Journal of Clinical Psychiatry* 62(11):860-868.

VA (Department of Veterans Affairs) and DoD (Department of Defense). 2009. *VA/DoD clinical practice guideline for management of substance use disorders.* Washington, DC: VA and DoD.

Valente, T. W. 2010. *Social networks and health: Models, methods, and applications.* Oxford, UK: Oxford University Press.

VHA (Veterans Health Administration) Office of Public Health and Environmental Hazards. 2008. *Analysis of VA health care utilization among US Global War on Terrorism (GWOT) veterans: Operation Enduring Freedom/Operation Iraqi Freedom.* Washington, DC: VHA.

Wagenaar, A. C., and T. L. Toomey. 2002. Effects of minimum drinking age laws: Review and analyses of the literature from 1960 to 2000. *Journal of Studies on Alcohol* 14(Suppl.):206-225.

Wagenaar, A. C., M. J. Salois, and K. A. Komro. 2009. Effects of beverage alcohol price and tax levels on drinking: A meta-analysis of 1003 estimates from 112 studies. *Addiction* 104(2):179-190.

Weisner, C., and H. Matzger. 2002. A prospective study of the factors influencing entry to alcohol and drug treatment. *Journal of Behavioral Health Services and Research* 29(2):126-137.

Weiss, R. D., J. S. Potter, D. A. Fiellin, M. Byrne, H. S. Connery, W. Dickinson, J. Gardin, M. L. Griffin, M. N. Gourevitch, D. L. Haller, A. L. Hasson, Z. Huang, P. Jacobs, A. S. Kosinski, R. Lindblad, E. F. McCance-Katz, S. E. Provost, J. Selzer, E. C. Somoza, S. C. Sonne, and W. Ling. 2011. Adjunctive counseling during brief and extended buprenorphine-naloxone treatment for prescription opioid dependence: A 2-phase randomized controlled trial. *Archives of General Psychiatry* 68(12):1238-1246.

WHO (World Health Organization). 2009. *Global health risks: Mortality and burden of disease attributable to selected major risks.* Geneva, Switzerland: World Health Organization.

Wilk, J. E., P. D. Bliese, P.Y. Kim, J.L. Thomas, D. McGurk, and C.W. Hoge. 2010. Relationship of combat experiences to alcohol misuse among U.S. soldiers returning from the Iraq war. *Drug and Alcohol Dependence* 108(1-2):115-121.

Wills, T. A., and R. Vaughan. 1989. Social support and substance use in early adolescence. *Journal of Behavioral Medicine* 12(4):321-339.

Wilson, J. M. G., and G. Jungner. 1968. *Principles and practice of screening for disease.* Geneva, Switzerland: World Health Organization.

Woody, G. E., S. A. Poole, G. Subramaniam, K. Dugosh, M. Bogenschutz, P. Abbott, A. Patkar, M. Publicker, K. McCain, J. S. Potter, R. Forman, V. Vetter, L. McNicholas, J. Blaine, K. G. Lynch, and P. Fudala. 2008. Extended vs. short-term buprenorphine-naloxone for treatment of opioid-addicted youth a randomized trial. *Journal of the American Medical Association* 300(17):2003-2011.

6

Policies and Programs on Substance Use Disorders

The committee's comprehensive review of the policies and programs on substance use disorders (SUDs) of the Department of Defense (DoD) and the branches built on DoD's *Comprehensive Plan on Prevention, Diagnosis, and Treatment of Substance Use Disorders and Disposition of Substance Abuse Offenders in the Armed Forces* (*Comprehensive Plan*) (DoD, 2011b). The committee's review responded to two requirements in its statement of task:

- an assessment of the adequacy and appropriateness of protocols used by the Military Health System relevant to the prevention, diagnosis, treatment, and management of SUDs in members of the armed forces; and
- an assessment of the adequacy of the prevention, diagnosis, treatment, and management of SUDs for dependents of members of the armed forces, whether such dependents suffer from their own SUD or because of the SUD of a member of the armed forces.

This chapter summarizes and assesses the policies relating to SUDs of DoD and each of the branches and comments on their adequacy and appropriateness. Box 6-1 lists the SUD policies reviewed. Note that while DoD-level policies apply to each of the individual branches, branch-level policies apply only within that branch. The chapter also highlights strengths and identifies areas for improvement within selected SUD prevention, screening, diagnosis, and treatment programs of DoD and the branches (see Appendix D for detail on these programs). The chapter concludes with a discussion

BOX 6-1
Policies and Directives Related to Substance Use Disorders

Department of Defense (DoD)	
DODD 1010.1	Military Personnel Drug Abuse Testing Program
DODD 1010.4	Drug and Alcohol Abuse by DoD Personnel
DODI 1010.6	Rehabilitation and Referral Services for Alcohol and Drug Abusers
DODD 1010.9	DoD Civilian Employee Drug Abuse Testing Program
DODI 6490.03	Deployment Health
DODI 6490.08	Command Notification Requirements to Dispel Stigma in Providing Mental Health Care to Service Members
Department of Veterans Affairs (VA)/ DoD	VA/DoD Clinical Practice Guideline: Management of Substance Use Disorders (2009)
Air Force	
AFI 44-121	Alcohol and Drug Abuse Prevention and Treatment (ADAPT) Program
AFI 44-172	Medical Operations: Mental Health
Army	
AR 600-85	The Army Substance Abuse Program
ALARACT 062/2011	Changes to Length of Authorized Duration of Controlled Substances Prescriptions in MEDCOM Regulation 40-51
Navy	
OPNAV 5350.4D	Navy Alcohol and Drug Abuse Prevention and Control
SECNAVINST 5300.28E	Military Substance Abuse Prevention and Control
BUMEDINST 5350.4	Navy Medicine Alcohol and Drug Prevention Program
BUMEDINST 5353.3	Use of Disulfiram (Antabuse)
BUMEDINST 5353.4A	Standards for Provision of Substance Related Disorder Treatment Services
Marine Corps	
NAVMC 2931	Marine Corps Drug and Alcohol Abuse, Prevention, and Treatment Programs
MCO 5300.17	Marine Corps Substance Abuse Program

of the committee's key findings regarding the programs and policies that address prevention, screening, diagnosis, treatment, and management of SUDs within the armed forces. Other findings on access to and utilization of programs and the TRICARE benefit used to provide SUD coverage for military dependents and on the adequacy of the workforce are presented in Chapters 7 and 8, respectively. The review of programs and policies in this chapter and Appendix D, along with the findings presented in Chapters 7 and 8, serves as a foundation for the conclusions and recommendations presented in Chapter 9.

DEPARTMENT OF DEFENSE

This section reviews the policies outlined in DoD's Comprehensive Plan, and others the committee identified, pertaining to SUD prevention, screening, diagnosis, and treatment at the DoD-wide level.

Prevention

The committee made use of the best-practice elements for SUD prevention discussed in Chapter 5 to assess the adequacy and appropriateness of DoD and branch SUD policies and programs. In summary, evidence-based SUD prevention (1) addresses the appropriate risk and protective factors for the population in question, (2) employs approaches with demonstrated effectiveness, (3) takes place at the appropriate time chronologically and developmentally, (4) makes use of proper settings and domains for delivery, and (5) manages programs effectively (Office of National Drug Control Policy, 2001).

Two DoD policies—DODD 1010.1 and DODD 1010.4 (DoD, 1994, 1997)—articulate DoD's interest in preventing and eliminating alcohol and other drug abuse and dependence in service members and employees because the disorders are incompatible with readiness. As a result, DoD seeks to "deter and identify drug and alcohol abuse and dependence," and will not take into service military personnel or hire civilians who present with these disorders (DoD, 1997). The policies call for the provision of education to ensure that personnel understand the implications of not adhering to DoD alcohol and other drug use policies.

DODD 1010.1 guides the Military and Civilian Drug Testing Program and requires urinalysis screening to detect illicit drug use among active duty service members. Urinalysis screening deters drug use because of the consequences of positive results. However, use of random urinalysis to deter drug use has limitations, as use of substances not included in the testing panel or not included on a routine basis may not be detected. In addition, if the screening is not performed randomly or is anticipated, individuals can avoid use of substances prior to being screened. DODD 1010.1 and DODD 1010.4 provide little or no guidance for other prevention strategies (e.g., large-scale efforts to educate individuals on the risks and health consequences of alcohol and other drug use, indicated prevention programs for those identified as at risk, prevention efforts aimed at military families, environmental prevention strategies). The policies do not appear to provide a clear strategy for preventing risky alcohol use and the potential development of alcohol use disorders. While some branches have policies that address these additional prevention strategies, they are not covered by overarching DoD policies.

The detailed review and assessment of DoD-wide prevention programs in Appendix D reveals that aside from drug testing, DoD relies heavily on campaign-style prevention programs (e.g., That Guy, the national Red Ribbon campaign). The National Institute on Drug Abuse (NIDA) has sponsored research on media campaigns to prevent drug use in youth and found that theory-based and evidence-based media campaigns can be effective in this population (Crano and Burgoon, 2002), but the effectiveness of campaign activities within the military is unknown. Moreover, campaign implementation varies across branches and bases, and participation requirements are unspecified. Overall, DoD delegates to the individual branches authority for implementing prevention for service members and their families, and the committee observed inconsistent implementation among the branches.

Monitoring for Prescription Drug Abuse

According to the ONDCP, the abuse of controlled prescription drugs such as pain relievers, central nervous system depressants, and stimulants is the nation's fastest-growing drug problem. Although such prescription drugs have legitimate medical uses, they also pose the potential for abuse and addiction and may be diverted for nonmedical, illicit use. While it was outside the scope of the committee's charge to study all the DoD and branch policies and programs related to the prescribing of controlled substances, the committee believes that the rising rates of prescription drug abuse in the military (as reviewed in Chapter 2) make it necessary to understand the DoD and branch policies and practices aimed at preventing the abuse of controlled substances prescribed to service members.

In both the civilian sector and the military, there are far-ranging programs and guidelines designed to ameliorate prescription drug abuse. These include diversion control activities of the Drug Enforcement Administration of the U.S. Department of Justice (GAO, 2011); education programs for primary care physicians and other specialists who prescribe these powerful medications; and additional guidelines for physicians to follow (Chou et al., 2009) when prescribing these medications that recommend a thorough patient history to assess the risk of prescribing controlled substances to the patient (i.e., to identify any current or prior alcohol or other drug misuse), as well as frequent patient contact, monitoring, and urine screening when prescribing to high-risk patients. While the committee was concerned with the abuse of prescription pain medications among members of the armed forces, the problem is also increasing in civilian populations (Compton and Volkow, 2006).

Although its review was limited, the committee learned through testimony, an examination of the literature, and site visits about several resources intended to encourage responsible prescribing within DoD. The committee heard testimony from pain management specialists who identified far-reaching changes being planned to revolutionize pain management in the military.[1] These changes include state-of-the-art interventions in theater and on the battlefield so that the wounded warrior is not started on high continuous doses of morphine, as well as expansion of multidisciplinary pain clinics that rely on physical therapy, strengthening, exercise, yoga, and cognitive-behavioral techniques to help the wounded cope with chronic pain and recondition the body rather than dull the pain with medications. The committee learned about the following resources aimed specifically at creating a military medical practice environment that reduces the risk of prescription drug abuse and diversion:

- a Department of Veterans Affairs (VA) and DoD clinical practice guideline for opioid therapy;
- recent development of pain management specialty services;
- the Army pain management task force;
- new policy guidance and policy changes on prescriptions for certain substances;
- expansion of the random urinalysis drug testing program to include additional prescribed medications; and
- special initiatives and reporting programs of DoD's Pharmacoeconomic Center (PEC).

With regard to clinical practice guidelines, the committee learned that, to address pain management practices, the VA and DoD have jointly published the *VA/DoD Clinical Practice Guideline for Management of Opioid Therapy for Chronic Pain* (VA and DoD, 2010). The committee found this guideline to be in line with other accepted guidelines (Chou et al., 2009) and comprehensive in its approach to managing pain and addressing aberrant behaviors of abuse and diversion. The extent of implementation of this

[1] Personal communication, Lt. Col. Kevin Galloway, Army Pain Management Task Force and Col. Chester Buckenmaier, M.D., Walter Reed Army Medical Center, July 19, 2011.

relatively new guideline at the provider level is unknown, and likely varies across installations and clinic settings.

During its site visits, the committee observed the recent development of pain management specialty services at some military treatment facilities but also learned that only a handful of pain specialists (frequently anesthesiologists) are currently serving in the armed forces.[2] The integration of these services with substance abuse programs, as was observed at Fort Belvoir's newly opened residential treatment center for substance abuse, demonstrates that the Army is beginning to address the issue of prescribing practices that contribute to the development of physical dependence and tolerance to pain medication, raising the risk of abuse. Because of the limited number of pain specialists, however, specialty pain clinics and pain management services are not available at all locations.

To help improve the quality of treatment for wounded warriors with chronic pain and simultaneously address concerns about prescription drug abuse and other problems arising from overreliance or sole reliance on prescription pain medications, the Army pain management task force was created to review current practices and policies and develop recommendations. The task force's final report, published in May 2010, articulates a strategy for controlling and preventing opiate abuse that is science-based (U.S. Army, 2010). The committee found that one focus and four objectives laid out in the task force report are relevant to the prevention of opiate abuse. The one focus is for the armed forces to implement a drug abuse assessment strategy to ensure the efficacy of its pain treatment program, which in turn will reduce aberrant behavior, abuse, and addiction to overprescribed opioids. The four objectives include developing a patient-centric approach to injury recovery and rehabilitation, satisfaction, and pain control, with greater attention to controlling opioids and minimizing abuse. The Army is also developing an electronic pain order set for managing patients and mitigating the risk of prescription drug abuse and dependence in pain patients, focusing on controlled substances for chronic pain. Finally, the Army will identify substance abuse patients in Warrior Transition Units by embedding the necessary resources to develop and implement a coordinated care and monitoring plan. In the committee's view, these recommendations will encourage practice and research advances in pain management and have the potential to prevent the misuse and abuse of prescription pain medications.

Additional actions by the Army and DoD are aimed at tackling prescription drug abuse in the military. These actions include a recent change in policy to set limits on the length of prescriptions and the quantity dispensed for controlled substances (U.S. Army, 2011a), which has the potential to

---

[2] Personal communication, Ben Krepps, M.D., Director of the Pain Clinic at Fort Belvoir Community Hospital, November 15, 2011.

decrease ready access to some of the most commonly abused medications. The Army recently published policy guidance to caution providers about prescribing certain medications for the treatment of posttraumatic stress disorder (PTSD), specifically citing the lack of evidence for effectiveness of benzodiazepines and the risk for abuse of these substances (U.S. Army, 2012). In May 2012, DoD also implemented new practices for its urinalysis drug testing programs to screen for some of the most commonly abused prescription medications (e.g., hydrocodone, benzodiazepines). The new limits on the length of prescriptions for controlled medications, coupled with urinalysis for some of these substances, demonstrate that DoD, and particularly the Army, are undertaking new tactics to deter prescription drug misuse and abuse. However, it remains to be seen whether these new measures will affect the prevalence of prescription drug abuse in the military.

To monitor the use of prescription drugs, PEC has developed tools for use by installations and clinicians in identifying aberrant use and prescription patterns that increase the risk or are indicative of an SUD or diversion activity. The tools permit close monitoring when controlled substances are being prescribed for individuals with known SUDs and can also help identify high-risk behaviors of individuals with no known SUD who may need to be assessed for patterns that may lead to an SUD. PEC aims to "improve the clinical, economic and humanistic outcomes of drug therapy in support of the readiness and managed healthcare mission of the Military Health System" (DoD, 2012, p. 1). It conducts research and operates programs to monitor the prescription drug use behavior of persons identified by medical providers as exhibiting drug-seeking behavior or having a high risk of harming themselves through their drug use. Among the programs PEC operates are (1) the Prescription Restriction Program, (2) the Military Treatment Facility Lock-in Edit, (3) the Deployment Prescription Medication Analysis Reporting Tool (PMART), (4) the Warrior Transition Unit (WTU)-MART, and (5) the Controlled Drug Management Analysis and Reporting Tool (CD-MART).

The committee finds that PEC's activities are comprehensive. In addition to the aforementioned deployment and controlled medication monitoring and reporting tools, PEC provides a full program of DoD prescription management support services, including pharmacoeconomic analysis and support for and/or collaboration with the DoD Pharmacy & Therapeutics Committee, the Pharmacy Operations Center, and the VA/DoD Clinical Practice Guidelines workgroup.

The reporting tools made available to clinicians and pharmacies through Deployment PMART, WTU-MART, and CD-MART appear to be as comprehensive and detailed as those of any state prescription monitoring program, and in fact are quite complete in that they contain all mail order and retail pharmacy claims and prescriptions dispensed through the VA to service members. A recent report by the Defense Health Board (2011), however, found limitations to the PEC data systems. Specifically, the systems do not include in-theater pharmacy data in settings where there are no electronic medical records. Nor are they equipped to assess illicit activity on the part of service members who obtain prescriptions from civilian providers and pay out of pocket to obtain the medications from retail pharmacies.

The Prescription Restriction program gives military medical providers the ability to restrict patients to a specific pharmacy(ies) and/or provider(s) and restrict the dispensing of controlled medications from mail order and retail pharmacies. Currently the system is unable to restrict controlled medications to a specific provider and pharmacy simultaneously. Addressing this limitation might encourage more medical providers to adopt restrictions on controlled substances for more service members. As is the case with all prescription reporting tools, the key to effectiveness is adoption and use by medical providers.

Screening, Diagnosis, and Treatment

Urinalysis screening is the primary DoD strategy for identification of drug use; alcohol-related incidents are a primary source of referral for alcohol misuse screening at substance abuse clinics; and deployment health assessments (reviewed in Appendix D) are used to identify alcohol misuse in deployed service members who self-report such misuse. Beyond random urinalysis screening programs, Command may order a urinalysis screen or a breath test when performance suggests drug or alcohol use. Individual branch policies detail responsibilities for conducting and supervising random and Command screening, as well as the consequences of positive screens. DoD policies do not appear to recognize or address the limitations of urinalysis screening in identifying the extent of drug use, and fail to acknowledge that the screening identifies only the drugs tested for and miss drug use when a screen is not used or is unavailable. Several other screening programs and efforts, including the deployment health assessments, Military Pathways, and Military OneSource, are reviewed in Appendix D.

The *Comprehensive Plan* (DoD, 2011b) identifies four policies with elements pertinent to SUD diagnosis: DODD 1010.1, DODD 1010.4, DODI 1010.6, and DODI 6490.03 (DoD, 1985, 1994, 1997, 2011b). DODD 1010.4 uses the American Psychiatric Association's (2000) *Diagnostic and Statistical Manual of Mental Disorders, Fourth Edition, Text Revision* (DSM-IV-TR) to define alcohol dependence, alcoholism, and drug dependence. This policy appropriately classifies drug and alcohol dependence as chronic psychiatric conditions that affect both individuals and families and recognizes the need for periodic assessments of alcohol and other drug use. The practice of making SUD diagnoses, however, varies from branch to branch.

DODI 6490.08 (DoD, 2011a) clarifies DoD policy regarding the responsibility of health care providers to notify Command of potential SUDs. It is intended "to foster a culture of support in the provision of mental health care and voluntarily sought substance abuse education to military personnel in order to dispel the stigma of seeking mental health care and/or substance misuse education services" (DoD, 2011a, p. 2). The instruction directs health care providers to "follow a presumption that they are not to notify a Service member's commander when the Service member obtains mental health care or substance abuse education services" (p. 2). This policy update could support implementation of routine screening and brief interventions in health care settings and substantially enhance the capacity of DoD and the armed forces for early intervention prior to the development of severe and disabling SUDs.

To provide an additional screening resource, the Military Pathways program, sponsored by DoD, was designed to encourage help seeking and reduce stigma for mental health disorders (including depression, PTSD, and alcohol abuse) for military populations. The Web-based program, developed by the nonprofit organization Screening for Mental Health, utilizes a "video doctor" that is meant to simulate a doctor-patient conversation and provide screening, brief advice, and referral to appropriate resources if indicated (Screening for Mental Health, 2012). Participation in the screening is anonymous and accessible to anyone (including reserve component members and dependents) through the Military Pathways website. While an evaluation of this program's effectiveness has not been published, the concept for the program is based on research that has documented the benefit of video doctor screening and brief counseling services (Humphreys et al., 2011; Jackson et al., 2011; Tsoh et al., 2010). This screening program is an example of DoD's utilizing new technology to help address the mental health needs of service members and their families. See Appendix D for further review of Military Pathways.

DoD policies DODI 1010.6 and DODD 1010.4 and the *VA/DoD Clinical Practice Guideline for Management of Substance Use Disorders* (VA and DoD, 2009) address treatment for SUDs. These policies encompass the components of health care delivery systems: patient-provider relationships, delivery of care, organizational functioning, and health care policy and regulation (Berwick, 2002) (see Chapter 5 for detail). Most policies are applicable to all active duty military personnel. Branch policies cover the governance structure for the delivery of SUD treatment; the philosophy and principles of treatment (e.g., SUD is often a chronic and relapsing disorder); and the training, certification, credentialing, and accreditation requirements for providers of care and facilities.

DODI 1010.6 addresses organizational and regulatory requirements. It outlines a governance structure with representation from the Air Force, Army, Navy, and Marine Corps and, by invitation, the VA. Constituting this governance structure is the DoD Joint-Service and VA Oversight Committee, which is responsible for coordinating policies and resources among the DoD branches and making recommendations on treatment and policy issues of joint interest. The Office of the Assistant Secretary of Defense for Health Affairs chairs this committee. DODI 1010.6 states that SUD staff members should be under the direct supervision of personnel qualified to evaluate their performance. However, the policy is vague with respect to how provider performance is to be rated or measured. The policy language implies that supervisors assess performance qualitatively; it does not describe quantitative measures of clinical effectiveness (e.g., Brief Addiction Monitor [BAM] score change or effect size, treatment adherence rates).

DoD appears to be moving toward an "umbrella structure" to connect the branches and the VA (i.e., a high-level set of policies establishing the basic governance structure, SUD treatment philosophy, and best treatment practices). This coordinated approach produced policies for DoD and VA sharing of resources under Public Law 96-22 (which created centers for PTSD counseling for Vietnam Veterans) and facilitates the standardization of basic quality structural requirements (e.g., each program must have a standard operating procedure). Current governance policies, however, allow variation among the branches in key areas (e.g., SUD program evaluations and policies related to the commander's role in treatment decisions). This "umbrella structure" could be instrumental in driving coordination and enhanced consistency across all DoD components, including consistent implementation of measures of system/program effectiveness, performance, and efficiency. Coordination creates the opportunity to build comparability in processes and measurement across DoD and VA SUD services. Better management and analysis may support more rapid system improvements and increased efficiencies.

The *VA/DoD Clinical Practice Guideline for Management of Substance Use Disorders* (VA and DoD, 2009) (see Chapter 4) provides guiding principles; it does not prevent providers from using clinical judgment. Updating of the guideline is stated as a goal; however, no timeline is given for any updating activity. Work on developing and implementing the guideline is intended to inform areas for future research and the optimal allocation of VA/DoD resources. Systematic measurement of treatment outcomes, provider capabilities, program implementation, and system performance supports continuous improvement, care responsive to patient needs, and enhanced effectiveness. DoD and VA policies and the Clinical Practice Guideline include recommendations for clinical measurement using validated tools for assessment and measurement of treatment progress: the

Alcohol Use Disorders Identification Test (AUDIT)-C for assessment and the VA's BAM for tracking treatment progress.

The VA/DoD Clinical Practice Guideline, DoD policies (DODD 1010.9, DODI 1010.6), and branch policies generally are aligned with the best-practice principles discussed in Chapter 5 regarding detailed decision support algorithms incorporating evidence-based practices for assessments, psychotherapies, pharmacotherapies, withdrawal management, medical setting management, and management by specialty. The level of detail guides treatment choices and practices in key areas (e.g., use of validated tools for assessment and tracking of treatment response [see Chapter 5]). Individual branch policies, however, typically are silent on the use of the VA/DoD Clinical Practice Guideline. Staff training requirements are addressed in the umbrella DoD policy (DODI 1010.6) (DoD, 1985), with additional detail being provided in Army, Navy, Marine Corps, and Air Force policies. Best training practices that promote fidelity (see Chapter 5) consist of manualized training and demonstration of knowledge and/or competency with the use of a standard written examination, as well as supervision by trained instructors in clinical settings. See Chapter 8 for more detail on SUD staff training and credentialing within DoD programs.

Despite general alignment with best practices, the committee noted omissions and deviations. DODD 1010.9, for example, allows branches and programs to use idiosyncratic evaluations and metrics. Quality improvement initiatives usually rely on standardized measures of process and outcomes. The Comprehensive Plan came to similar findings that policies do not address standardization of data and outcome measures (DoD, 2011b). The lack of standardized outcome measures and benchmarks or a system that promotes the development of measures will undoubtedly lead to difficulties in evaluating program effectiveness and impact. Having a set of basic metrics that reflect the overarching goals of SUD treatment (e.g., sobriety, stabilization, and functionality) would be a good starting point. Some branches of the military (e.g., the Marine Corps) have begun outlining performance measures for SUD programs in their policies. Another area of omission within the policies is the absence of systems for measuring the clinical effectiveness of providers at both the provider population and individual case levels. As described in Chapter 5, the use of outcome measurement to demonstrate clinical effectiveness improves clinical competency and population outcomes. The policies contain references to the use of tracking tools to monitor the response to treatment, but there is no reference to aggregating these outcomes to measure the effectiveness of individual providers or programs. Finally, although the VA/DoD Clinical Practice Guideline is applicable to all branches of the military, the lack of reference to the guideline in branch-specific policies raises questions about the degree of its adoption. The *Comprehensive Plan* came to similar findings that policies do not address the level to which the Clinical Practice Guideline is implemented (DoD, 2011b). During site visits to branch SUD programs and interviews with staff at treatment sites, the committee observed wide variation in the adoption of the Clinical Practice Guideline and variations in the implementation of umbrella DoD policies.

In summary, the VA/DoD Clinical Practice Guideline and DoD/branch policies include many best practices and processes for SUD screening, diagnosis, and treatment: central governance through the DoD Joint-Service and VA Oversight Committee; a structure for accountability within the different branches of the military; well-written practice guidelines; and policies at the DoD level and within the branches that, in the aggregate, align with best practices. At the same time, increased standardization of training requirements and evaluation measures would enhance DoD's ability to monitor and manage SUD services.

AIR FORCE

Air Force Instruction (AFI) 44-121 covers various aspects of SUD care in this branch (U.S. Air Force, 2011). Section 3C covers eligibility, identification, and referral; 3D covers targeted and secondary prevention and education; and 3F (Clinical Care in Tiers II and III) covers documentation, assessment, and program completion. Regarding eligibility, the policy identifies Air Force members, dependents, and retirees as eligible for treatment under TRICARE; other employees can be seen by Alcohol and Drug Abuse Prevention and Treatment (ADAPT) personnel.

Prevention

Air Force prevention policy (AFI 44-121) uses programs, activities, and outreach to build individual and unit resiliency in the general military population and targeted high-risk groups (U.S. Air Force, 2011). The Drug Demand Reduction Program (urinalysis screens to prevent illicit drug use), the Resiliency Element (community programming to enhance resiliency and reduce the incidence of family abuse and neglect), and the ADAPT program collaborate to develop and implement prevention programs at the installation level. The policy includes educational outreach to train health care providers and individuals in leadership roles to recognize risk factors, serve as role models, and provide support for prevention.

Air Force prevention programs promote military readiness, health, and wellness and minimize the negative consequences of substance misuse and abuse. The primary source of prevention services is the ADAPT program. ADAPT prevention programs are stipulated at two levels, or tiers. Tier I includes prevention and education for general military populations, delivered through a variety of channels that are tailored to the specific needs of each installation and specific groups (e.g., military members, leaders, family members, youth). Channels include population-based and community outreach through the Culture of Responsible Choices (CoRC), Enforcing Underage Drinking Laws (EUDL), Drug Education for Youth (DEFY), and Adolescent Substance Abuse Counseling (ASAC) programs for youth, as well as programs that reach military members and their families, including the recently developed New Orientation to Reduce Threats to Health from Secretive Problems That Affect Readiness (NORTH STAR) program (see Appendix D for program descriptions).

AFI 44-121 requires that at least four groups of military members receive prevention education. First, for service members on their first duty assignments, prevention focuses on responsible behavior, healthy alternatives to substance use, consequences of use, and techniques for dealing with peer acceptance. Second, for service members in grades E1-E4 on a second assignment or permanent change of station, the same set of prevention concerns is addressed within 60 days after change of station. Third, health care professionals who provide direct patient care receive training in prevention, as well as substance use identification and diagnosis and treatment of substance abuse. Fourth, for Airman Leadership School or Non-Commissioned Officer Academy students who are being trained for leadership roles, education and training emphasize leadership in delivering prevention, identification and referral of substance abusers, and education and counseling processes. Tier II includes screening, assessment, education, brief preventive counseling, and feedback to individuals or groups identified as at higher risk for substance abuse than the general military population.

Two Air Force prevention initiatives could be considered potential models for improving program standardization across the branches—the CoRC and NORTH STAR programs. The logic model or flow pattern used in the CoRC program starts with annual training of leadership (i.e., commanders and health care providers) in prevention programs. Program implementation sequentially targets service members and their families, military bases, and finally surrounding communities. Although there are no published studies on the efficacy of CoRC, it specifies a clear chain of command regarding leadership, training, responsibility for implementation, and dissemination from the base to the surrounding community. CoRC provides a good model for standardizing prevention training and delivery across the military branches, and should be evaluated to determine its efficacy.

NORTH STAR, a randomized controlled trial of 24 Air Force bases and more than 50,000 active duty military members, funded by DoD and the Department of Agriculture, provides "a community-based framework for the prevention of family maltreatment, suicidality and substance problems" (Heyman et al., 2011, p. 85). It is an integrated delivery system involving commanders and providers partnered with Air Force community action and information boards at each of the 10 major Commands (Heyman et al., 2011). Using a guide on evidence-based programs that are rated according to evaluation outcomes and targeted risk and protective factors, the partners at each Command selected the programs that matched their specific risk and protective factor profiles. The guide also reviews training, implementation, and survey evaluation protocols. The use of a framework, delivery system, and guide to select prevention programs that fit a particular base's risk and protective factor profile is based on extensive community-based prevention research strategies that have been evaluated in civilian populations (Heyman and Smith Slep, 2001; Pentz, 2003; Riggs et al., 2009). Initial results of the NORTH STAR program suggest significant reductions in alcohol abuse among military members and reduced prescription drug use after controlling for level of integrated delivery system functioning and Command support (Heyman et al., 2011). Training and programs are manualized, and individual bases can select from a menu of evidence-based programs tailored to their needs.

The EUDL program should be noted as a promising example of the implementation of environmental prevention strategies to reduce underage drinking in service members. In this discretionary grant program, "funds were used in each community to form a broad-based coalition, with the responsibility of implementing a set of environmental strategies to reduce drinking and associated alcohol-related misconducts among Air Force members, with a focus on the underage active duty population" (Spera et al., 2012, p. 513). The results of a recent evaluation demonstrated the effectiveness of the environmental strategies employed (Spera and Franklin, 2010; Spera et al., 2012). This program is further reviewed in Appendix D.

Screening, Diagnosis, and Treatment

Unit commanders, first sergeants, substance abuse counselors, and military medical professionals encourage self-identification of alcohol and other drug problems. Commanders may grant limited protection to individuals who self-identify and may not use self-disclosure against those individuals in personnel actions. Air Force policy provides incentives to encourage members to seek help for problems with substances. Self-identification is reserved for members who are not currently under investigation or pending action as a result of an alcohol- or other drug-related incident (U.S. Air Force, 2011).

Commanders are required to refer service members for an assessment if there is suspicion that substance use led to problematic behavior (e.g., driving under the influence/driving while intoxicated, public intoxication, drunk and disorderly conduct, spouse/child abuse and maltreatment, underage drinking). Blood alcohol tests should be conducted as soon as possible after an instance of problematic behavior to determine alcohol involvement. Commanders are required to contact ADAPT for assessment of SUDs within 7 days of a potential alcohol- or other drug-related incident. In the case of driving-under-the-influence/driving-while-intoxicated offenses, commanders are required to contact ADAPT within 24 hours, but no later than the next duty day. Members who return from deployment because of problematic behavior must be assessed at the nearest ADAPT program. Air Force policy requires commanders or first sergeants to "actively participate" on the treatment team "by providing input to treatment decisions" (U.S. Air Force, 2011). Health care providers can also identify substance abuse. They are required to notify unit commanders and the ADAPT program manager when a service member is observed, identified, or suspected to be under the influence of alcohol or other drugs; receives treatment for an injury or illness that may be the result of substance use; is suspected of abusing substances; or is admitted as a patient for alcohol or other drug detoxification.

In the committee's review of Air Force programming, the Behavioral Health Optimization Program (BHOP) stood out as a useful model for integrating behavioral health with primary care services. The Air Force recognizes that the primary care work setting differs substantially from specialty behavioral health care and requires a different practice pattern and pace. The BHOP training is designed to prepare behavioral health consultants to work effectively in the primary care setting. A study on the initial implementation of BHOP showed high levels of satisfaction among patients and primary care providers at pilot sites with integrated behavioral health care (Runyan et al., 2003). BHOP is an important step toward fully integrated care, particularly as it evolves from identification and referral to specialty care to include the provision of early and brief intervention for SUDs by primary care providers. BHOP may be a model for expanding integrated care in all military treatment facilities.

Individuals referred to ADAPT complete a detailed computerized assessment with the Substance Use Assessment Tool (SUAT). The use of this tool is standardized across all Air Force ADAPT sites, and contains validated screening tools to assess for SUD. The committee heard during its site visit to Keesler Air Force Base that use of the SUAT allows service members to complete a detailed assessment without having to spend hours being interviewed by a licensed clinician. Once the SUAT has been completed, a licensed clinician reviews the results and meets with the service member to ask follow-up questions and determine an appropriate diagnosis (the SUAT even provides a diagnostic impression as part of its results). After reviewing the content of the SUAT, the committee found it to be comprehensive and based on the use of validated screening instruments (see Appendix D for further review of the SUAT).

Individuals identified with high-risk alcohol and other drug use who do not meet the requirements for an SUD diagnosis are targeted for secondary prevention and educational activities—Alcohol Brief Counseling (ABC) (see Appendix D) and education on Air Force and DoD policies related to alcohol use, plus educational modules covering anger management, assertive communication, changing self-talk, sleep enhancement, and other areas. The ABC counseling sessions last 45 minutes and are usually offered one to four times per week, depending on the individual's needs and risk level. ADAPT counselors use motivational interviewing techniques to provide individual feedback based on what was found during the SUAT initial assessment.

Overall, AFI 44-121 is comprehensive. Encouragement of self-identification is a plus, particularly the recognition that commanders should support self-disclosure; that self-disclosure should not be used against service members in personnel actions; and that when self-disclosure occurs, Command should contact ADAPT for an assessment. On the other hand, encouraging medical personnel to communicate with commanders and ADAPT personnel if alcohol and other drug problems are suspected may be necessary for commanders to assess fitness and readiness for military duty, but it also removes confidentiality from the identification and treatment process and may ultimately inhibit self-disclosure. Moreover, targeted prevention education and brief counseling for those suspected of high-risk alcohol and other drug use is appropriate, but "high-risk" is not defined. Further, the policy requires that treatment or prevention counseling for all clients be based on a thorough assessment (e.g., the SUAT, a clinical interview, and the collection of collateral data as appropriate) and determination of risk and be tailored to the individual; however, it fails to identify specific procedures for conducting a standardized initial assessment and making a subsequent diagnosis.

Clinical services are required for service members medically diagnosed with substance abuse or dependence. The level and intensity of care are determined by the ADAPT program manager using the American Society of Addiction Medicine (ASAM) Patient Placement Criteria. The Air Force's philosophy is to place personnel with substance abuse problems in the least intensive or restrictive treatment environment that is appropriate to their therapeutic needs. Depending on the service member's needs, variable lengths of stay or durations of treatment are provided within an array of treatment settings. For example, individuals may be placed in short-term outpatient or intensive outpatient programs at their local base, referred to a partial hospitalization program, or entered into an inpatient residential treatment program with a variable length of stay. Regardless of the level or intensity of care, programs are tailored to meet the specific needs of the individual.

ARMY

Army Regulation (AR) 600-85 (U.S. Army, 2009) guides the implementation of the Army Substance Abuse Program (ASAP). AR 600-85 "provides comprehensive alcohol and drug abuse prevention and control policies, procedures, and responsibilities for Soldiers of all components, Army civilian corps members, and other personnel eligible for Army Substance Abuse Program (ASAP) services" (U.S. Army, 2009, p. 1). The regulation's 18 chapters and 8 appendixes specify the purpose and authority of the regulation; articulate staffing roles and responsibilities; review the policies for alcohol and other drug testing for officers, soldiers, and civilian employees; and list services available for civilian corps members, family members, and retirees. The regulation also addresses procedures for identification, referral, and evaluation of individuals with suspected SUDs; describes the rehabilitation procedures and programs for prevention, education, and training; and specifies legal and administrative procedures. Drug testing standards are listed, and the risk reduction program is described. Chapters also detail procedures for program evaluation, data collection, and record keeping. The regulation concludes with descriptions of services for the Army National Guard and Army Reserve, a review of Army awards and campaigns, and guidance for resource management.

The Army Center for Substance Abuse Programs manages the ASAP services as part of its mission "to strengthen the overall fitness and effectiveness of the Army and to enhance the combat readiness of its personnel and units by eliminating alcohol and/or other drug abuse" (U.S. Army, 2009, p. 104). Located within the Army's Human Resources Policy Directorate, ASAP is a Command program that emphasizes readiness and personal responsibility. ASAP provides prevention (education, deterrence, identification/detection, referral, and risk reduction programs) and treatment (screening and rehabilitation) services. Box 6-2 summarizes ASAP's prevention and treatment capabilities.

ASAP prevention and treatment services are currently in transition. In October 2010, personnel, resources, and equipment used for screening and rehabilitation services in ASAP were transferred from Medical Command (MEDCOM) to Installation Management Command (IMCOM) to consolidate the program's prevention and rehabilitation services within one Command. Services are being reengineered "to promote a full spectrum of care based on a public health model."[3] The committee's discussions with ASAP staff during site visits to the Fort Belvoir and Fort Hood Army bases revealed strong support for the consolidation of prevention and treat-

[3]Personal communication, Col. John Stasinos, Addiction Medicine Consultant for the Army Office of the Surgeon General, November 15, 2011.

BOX 6-2
Army Substance Abuse Program (ASAP)
Prevention and Treatment Capabilities

Prevention

- Education and training—Instruction for soldiers to increase knowledge, skills, and/or experience.
- Deterrence—Actions to dissuade soldiers from abusing or misusing substances. Random drug testing is the primary deterrence activity.
- Identification/detection—Identification of soldiers as potential substance abusers through self-identification, Command identification, drug testing identification, medical identification, or investigation or apprehension identification.
- Referral—Self-referral and Command referral to ASAP.
- Risk reduction—Analysis of behavioral risk data to identify units with high-risk profiles and provide prevention interventions to mitigate high-risk behaviors.

Treatment

- Screening—Individual biopsychosocial evaluation interviews to determine whether soldiers need to be referred to treatment.
- Rehabilitation—Clinical intervention to either return soldiers to full duty or identify soldiers who cannot be rehabilitated successfully.

SOURCE: Adapted from U.S. Army, 2009.

ment services. The ASAP staff acknowledged, however, that under the new structure, it is more difficult to coordinate treatment for SUDs with other medical care. ASAP no longer has access to a scheduling and tracking database previously used to track compliance with treatment requirements. In addition, the medical record permits limited documentation of ASAP care because of concern about the confidentiality of alcohol and other drug abuse records (42 *Code of Federal Regulations* [CFR] Part 2). During the transition period from MEDCOM to IMCOM, moreover, attrition of clinical staff has exacerbated the need to hire additional clinicians.

Prevention

ASAP prevention, education, and training services are intended to prevent, deter, and reduce alcohol and other drug abuse and to provide soldiers with prevention and awareness training (U.S. Army, 2009). Prevention and awareness training includes information on "a) ASAP policies and services, b) consequences of alcohol and other drug abuse, and c) incompatibility of alcohol and other drug abuse with physical and mental fitness, combat readiness, Army Values, and the Warrior Ethos" (U.S. Army, 2009, p. 55). Training to sustain and improve prevention counseling and training also is emphasized as a mission-wide effort. Specifically, the policy requires cooperation and partnerships with the installation and local communities and the availability of information about counseling and other substance abuse services at the installation. Deglamorization of alcohol is viewed as essential, and marketing and promotion of practices that glamorize alcohol use are prohibited. Commanders and supervisors are trained to identify early substance abuse problems among their personnel. The Army Training System incorporates alcohol and other drug abuse education and is compatible with the indoctrination of recruits in standards of discipline, performance, and behavior.

Drug testing is part of the prevention program, with detailed requirements for urine sample collection, screening of tests, breath testing, and personnel training. The policy extends substance abuse awareness training to all civilian employees and drug testing to those in designated positions (e.g., Department of Transportation [DOT] personnel). Prevention programs are encouraged for families, retirees, and off-duty contract personnel and their families, as well as for K-12 schools associated with military installations. ASAP is specifically authorized to purchase promotional items to encourage prevention (e.g., T-shirts, mugs, pens), particularly in connection with prevention campaigns (e.g., Red Ribbon Week, Warrior Pride, National Alcohol Awareness month). However, the committee did not identify any published peer-reviewed articles evaluating the effectiveness of these prevention campaigns and activities in military populations. Training in healthy life choices, responsible decision making, Army values, and alternatives to alcohol all reinforce the mission of preventing alcohol and other drug abuse. ASAP establishes goals and milestones in annual prevention plans and evaluates methods and outcomes of prevention activities. (The committee did not receive copies of evaluation reports or data on outcomes of prevention services.) Army policy states that prevention programs must be science based and focuses on deterrence through drug testing and law enforcement (i.e., eliminating supplies of illegal drugs, enforcing laws on driving under the influence and underage drinking).

Screening, Diagnosis, and Treatment

Chapter 7 of AR 600-85 addresses identification, referral, and evaluation of substance use, abuse, and dependence (U.S. Army, 2009). The policy notes (Chapter 7, section I) that substance abuse and dependence are preventable and treatable and states that military personnel who abuse alcohol should receive education, counseling, and rehabilitation services. Self-identification is the preferred mode of identification, but Command referral is more common. Positive identification of alcohol abuse and dependence requires referral to ASAP in order to return the service member to "full duty status." Although DoD policies identify alcohol and other drug abuse and dependence as chronic conditions, AR 600-85 permits only "one period of rehabilitation" per alcohol incident. In exceptional cases, commanders may recommend a second period of rehabilitation. Any alcohol-related incidents occurring after two rehabilitation periods require separation. According to the policy, soldiers identified as drug abusers are referred to ASAP, and a diagnosis of drug dependence leads to detoxification and treatment while separation procedures are initiated. AR 600-85 (U.S. Army, 2009, p. 47) asserts that soldiers diagnosed as drug dependent "generally, do not have potential for continued military service and should not be retained."

AR 600-85 describes six different methods of identification of alcohol and other drug abuse and dependence: (1) voluntary (self-referral), (2) Command referral, (3) drug testing, (4) alcohol testing, (5) medical referral, and (6) investigation and apprehension. As noted, voluntary disclosure is the preferred method of identification, and commanders must be involved in the process of evaluation. Commanders should encourage self-identification and avoid actions that would discourage personnel from seeking help. Civilian employees and family members seeking help should be offered employee assistance program evaluation. Commander identification, drug and alcohol testing identification, and identification through investigation and/or apprehension lead to referral to ASAP. Referrals to ASAP are required within 5 duty days of receipt of test results. If identification occurs during a routine medical screening, the provider should refer the soldier to ASAP and notify the commander. In the case of identification of a problem in a civilian employee or family member, the referral should be to the employee assistance program.

Overall, the methods of identification described in the policy are comprehensive, and the emphasis on encouraging self-referral is constructive. The specification of the number of days within which referral to the ASAP program should be made strengthens the policy. Still, the policy is vague regarding identification methods, especially during routine medical exams. As suggested above, commander involvement and disclosure of self-referral to commanders by health care providers may discourage rather than encourage self-disclosure because it gives commanders access to in-depth confidential information about soldiers' alcohol and other drug abuse and dependence.

Chapter 8 outlines the rehabilitation services provided through ASAP. AR 600-85 requires the unit commander to participate in the treatment team and support the rehabilitation process. The goal of rehabilitation is to (1) return the soldier to full duty as soon as possible, and (2) identify soldiers for separation who cannot be rehabilitated with ASAP services. ASAP rehabilitation services include four elements: (1) identification and referral, (2) biopsychosocial assessments and Command consultation, (3) rehabilitation and follow-up, and (4) mandatory monthly alcohol and drug testing for soldiers enrolled in the rehabilitation program. Specific rehabilitation services include Level I (nonresidential outpatient rehabilitation) and Level II (partial inpatient and residential treatment). Level I services require a minimum of 30 days and a maximum of 360 days of participation. Education services may be provided as appropriate. Level II services provide intensive partial residential treatment programs of varying lengths and a 1-year period of mandatory nonresidential follow-up for individuals who do not respond favorably to outpatient treatment. Participating soldiers are encouraged to attend self-help groups, and the rehabilitation plan must "specify an appropriate number of meetings per week the client will be encouraged to attend" (U.S. Army, 2009, p. 53). AR 600-85 does not describe the content of Level I and Level II services and is silent on the use of evidence-based behavioral and pharmacological therapies. While the policy identifies the need for an in-depth biopsychosocial interview, it does not specify how this interview should be conducted. The regulations require that ASAP clinical providers have a master's degree in social work or psychology from an accredited university.

AR 600-85 underscores the importance of Command. Commanders can make decisions about who should be evaluated, how evaluation and rehabilitation will take place, and whether soldiers can remain in the service.

The Confidential Alcohol Treatment and Education Pilot (CATEP) permits soldiers to self-refer to ASAP (if not involved in an alcohol incident) and receive confidential treatment without Command notification. The pilot initiative seeks to engage soldiers in alcohol treatment at earlier stages of the disorder. CATEP began in July 2009 and is now at six Army sites across the United States. Soldiers in CATEP are not subject to negative personnel actions (i.e., barred, flagged), and those who fail treatment will not be administratively separated. Enrollment in CATEP treatment does not count toward the number of trials of rehabilitation allowed per military career.[4] This small but promising program emphasizes confidential alcohol treatment. Soldiers seeking services for drug use many not enroll in CATEP. CATEP appears to be worthy of expansion within the Army and could be

[4]Personal communication, Col. Charles S. Milliken, M.D., Walter Reed Army Institute of Research, May 3, 2011.

considered as a strategy for addressing misuse of prescription opioids in addition to alcohol.

The committee also interviewed several staff at the Fort Hood pilot Intensive Outpatient Program (IOP) (see Appendix A for the committee's site visit agenda). The IOP, which opened in February 2010, provides more intensive care than is typically available from ASAP clinics. The program also treats soldiers with comorbid mental health disorders and SUDs. The Fort Hood pilot IOP provides ASAM Level II.5 care as a 4-week day treatment program. It provides both group and individual therapy sessions using cognitive-behavioral therapies and eye movement desensitization and reprogramming therapy (DCoE, 2011). While the IOP program was initially created to provide intensive outpatient-level care, the actual level of care provided is partial hospitalization; the program's name is therefore being changed. To enroll in the program, patients must have a primary diagnosis of SUD, and their commander must support their participation. The primary substance of abuse is alcohol, but the program addresses both alcohol and other drug use disorders. Currently, staff conduct follow-up interviews to assess patient outcomes at 30, 60, and 90 days after treatment completion. Typically, 70 percent of patients reached remain on active duty after completing treatment. Continuing care includes regular appointments for acudetox and eye movement treatments. Anecdotal evidence suggests that soldiers—at least those that continue in the Army rather than being administratively separated—continue to do well after completing the program. The Fort Hood IOP pilot may be an excellent model for expansion and adoption at other bases.

The committee also visited the Army SUD treatment programs at Fort Belvoir. The Co-Occurring Program is housed at the DeWitt Army Hospital within the Warrior Transition Brigade (WTB). Once enrolled in the WTB, soldiers are engaged in care for 18 to 24 months, but they must have complex case management needs in order to be enrolled. Program personnel reported that two-thirds of the Fort Belvoir WTB population has been diagnosed with a mental health condition rather than a physical health condition or injury, which necessitates access to mental health care within the WTB. The Co-Occurring Program provides several treatment tracks: strictly substance abuse treatment, no substance abuse treatment, and treatment of substance abuse with a comorbid anxiety or other mood disorder. The length of stay is typically 4 to 6 weeks, and most referrals come from the national capital area. Upon completion of the program, soldiers return to ASAP at their individual unit for follow-up care. The program will be using the Parent Management Training Oregon model and Seeking Safety as part of its treatment programming. All patients receiving any level of treatment in the Co-Occurring Program must also be enrolled in ASAP. The committee heard testimony that psychiatrists involved in patient care often walk a fine line with respect to how much information to share with the patient's commander, depending particularly on how receptive commanders are to helping their soldiers get the care they need.

NAVY

Navy Instructions 5350.4D (U.S. Navy, 2009) and 5300.28E (U.S. Navy, 2011) govern the Navy's Alcohol and Drug Abuse Prevention and Control programs and establish policies and procedures for the prevention and control of alcohol and other drug abuse within the Department of the Navy (U.S. Navy, 2011). Navy Bureau of Medicine (BUMED) Instruction 5353.4A operationalizes the standards for provision of SUD treatment services (U.S. Navy, 1999). Two additional BUMED instructions detail the operation of BUMED's Alcohol and Drug Prevention Program (U.S. Navy, 2009) and provide guidance on the use of disulfiram (Antabuse) for the treatment of alcohol dependence (U.S. Navy, 1990).

Prevention

Navy Instruction 5340.4D states that alcohol and other drug abuse undermines combat readiness and interferes with maintaining high standards of performance and military discipline. Specific attention is given to responsible drinking by those of legal age (21 and over) who choose to drink (U.S. Navy, 2009). Navy policy supports those who choose not to drink and does not condone drinking during working hours (except in the case of special authorized occasions). Prevention is focused on enhanced detection, deterrence, prevention, and education within a Command climate of "zero tolerance" for drug use. The Navy's urinalysis program detects and deters the use of illegal drugs. Enlisted recruits, officer candidates, midshipmen, and officers in pre-Fleet assignment or entry programs also complete alcohol and other drug abuse prevention education programs. Alcohol and other drug abuse prevention curricula must be included in General Military Training.

Responsibilities of different Command levels include ensuring that education and training in alcohol and other drug use prevention are carried out effectively and maintaining data on all related activities. Senior personnel act as alcohol and drug control officers (ADCOs) and provide guidance to drug and alcohol program advisors (DAPAs). DAPAs manage the substance abuse prevention program and conduct prevention education courses: Alcohol-AWARE, Personal Responsibility and Values Education and Training, Alcohol and Drug Abuse Management Seminar for Leaders/Supervisors, and Skills for Life. Courses are provided for multiple levels of Command to ensure clear and consistent delivery of the prevention messages.

In May 2011, a policy update (SECNAVINST 5300.28E) expanded the role of drug testing to include commonly abused prescription drugs (U.S. Navy, 2011). Guidance issued in March 2012 specifies testing practices for synthetic compounds (e.g., Spice and bath salts) using the Navy's steroid testing model (U.S. Navy, 2012a). To address alcohol abuse, current policy under SECNAVINST 5300.28E stipulates that breath testing may be used as a prevention strategy, and the Navy planned to roll out an alcohol breath testing program in late 2012 (U.S. Navy, 2012b). Random breath testing will be conducted aboard Navy ships, and positive tests will lead to referral to the Navy Substance Abuse Rehabilitation Program (SARP). The updated policies and programs reflect the Navy's leadership in implementing strategies to deter alcohol, prescription drug, and designer drug abuse. It remains to be seen whether these new measures will be effective.

SECNAVINST 5300.28E further stipulates that prevention programs should be directed toward known SUD threats in a geographic area or Command. The programs may include threat assessment, policy development and implementation, public information activities, education and training, deglamorization messages, and evaluations tailored to individual Commands (U.S. Navy, 2011).

Navy prevention policies appear to focus primarily on drug testing procedures and contain little guidance or information on other prevention activities. The committee's review of Navy material and information, however, indicated that the Navy has the largest number of formal and established prevention programs among the armed forces (see Appendix D for detail on these programs). Although they are not described in policy, the Navy provides a wide range of prevention services beyond the urinalysis drug screening program.

Screening, Diagnosis, and Treatment

OPNAVINST 5350.4D recognizes that alcohol abuse and dependence are preventable and treatable (U.S. Navy, 2009). SECNAVINST 5300.28E (U.S. Navy, 2011) states that alcohol and other drug abuse is incompatible with high performance standards, readiness, discipline, and military missions, and that drug-dependent individuals should not be inducted into the Navy or Marine Corps. The policy states that military members who are diagnosed as drug dependent should be disciplined and separated, as should those who are involved in an "alcohol-related incident" after entering treatment. Any alcohol-related incident after two treatment periods triggers separation. Military personnel receive detoxification and limited treatment prior to separation. Exceptions are made for those with a "high probability of successful treatment." SECNAVINST 5300.28E, however, does not identify specific evidence-based prevention and treatment services, when and how interventions should be implemented, or what type(s) of personnel should provide such services.

The Navy encourages both Command and self-referrals for alcohol misuse, abuse, and dependence. Self-referral cannot be associated with an alcohol-related incident. Command referral can be based on personal observation of behavior or a change in job performance. If the service member is involved in an alcohol-related incident (e.g., driving under the influence, alcohol-related arrest, alcohol-related domestic violence, drunkenness), screening is required. After assessment within SARP, Command receives results and treatment recommendations.

Urinalysis is the main drug testing program in the Navy. The policy provides guidance on response to a positive drug screen, an alcohol incident such as impaired driving, or a positive alcohol blood level while on duty. But the policy tends to perceive substance use as a personnel-related rather than a health-related issue. It does not specify how screening should be conducted or who should conduct it, and there is no mention of targeted prevention for high-risk users or the types of treatment offered. The policy defines alcohol abuse and dependence and drug abuse and dependence based on standard criteria in DSM-IV-TR (APA, 2000). It also defines alcohol incidence, anabolic steroids, controlled substances, driving under the influence/driving while intoxicated, drug abuse paraphernalia, drug trafficking, inhalant abuse, and other relevant terms.

Navy policy has positive characteristics, including recognition that alcohol abuse and dependence are preventable and treatable; encouragement of self-referral; and recommendation for assessment, diagnosis, and treatment. As with Air Force and Army policies, however, Command involvement in screening and treatment may severely inhibit self-disclosure of alcohol problems. The Navy SARP program that the committee visited on the San Diego Naval Base used evidence-based treatments. It utilized identifiable definitions of treatment failure and conducted periodic evaluations to understand its successes and areas in which improvements were needed. The San Diego SARP has an expressed focus on assessing depression, PTSD, and other psychiatric comorbidities among the patients it treats. Information was presented to the committee on the capacity of the program to provide dual-disorder treatment based on Dual Diagnosis Capability in Addiction Treatment (DDCAT) scoring. The DDCAT scoring, however, is based on self-report rather than an external assessment. All SARPs encourage aftercare. Unlike other branches, the Navy has a specialized aftercare program, My Ongoing Recovery Experience (MORE), that uses telephone and Web-based follow-up to support service members in maintaining their recovery (see Appendix D for further review of the Navy MORE program). By utilizing MORE to provide ongoing follow-up and recovery support,

Navy SARP counselors can focus more of their time on providing screening and treatment services.

Overall, the committee finds Navy SARPs to be comprehensive treatment programs that offer several therapeutic interventions with varying levels of intensity depending on the ASAM Patient Placement Criteria (Levels 0.5 to IV). Besides treatment, SARP activities appropriately encompass prevention, early indicated intervention, screening and diagnosis, and aftercare. Evidence-based practices are applied throughout. The effectiveness of treatment is monitored, although no assessment of effectiveness with state-of-the-art randomized techniques has been conducted. The committee was particularly impressed with the focus, breadth, supervision, and operation of the SARP prevention, screening, diagnostic, and treatment services.

MARINE CORPS

Two policies guide SUD prevention, screening, diagnosis, and treatment for the Marine Corps: NAVMC 2931 and MCO 5300.17. Unlike the other military branches, the Marine Corps does not have its own Medical Command and therefore receives medical services through the Navy.

Prevention

Marine Corps prevention awareness and education training policy has two stated goals: (1) to enhance mission readiness and (2) to provide knowledge of the effects of substance abuse to assist individuals in making responsible decisions (U.S. Marine Corps, 2011). Training military and civilian supervisors in the importance of eliminating alcohol abuse and illegal drug use is a secondary purpose of prevention policy. While the primary emphasis of Marine Corps prevention policy is information and knowledge transmission, the policy also recognizes the importance of using this information to clarify personal values, improve decision making, and understand alternative lifestyle choices that do not depend on alcohol and other drug use.

Marine policy mandates prevention awareness education and training for Marines at all levels at least annually. The committee, however, did not receive data on the proportion of Marines who receive this education and training or on how it is delivered (e.g., whether prevention is embedded in other aspects of Marine education and training or is addressed separately). Initial training for officer candidates and recruits includes alcohol and other drug abuse prevention as part of the core training curriculum. Training consists of information and guided discussion on the progressive nature and risks of alcohol and other drug abuse (i.e., domestic abuse, sexual assault, and financial difficulties). Specific information on alcohol describes alcohol metabolism and physiological effects, defines and outlines effects of blood alcohol levels, and identifies factors that influence these levels. Supervisors have key roles in setting positive examples in prevention and referral of abusers to treatment, as well as in supporting alternative, nondrinking recreational activities, including tutoring in the community, coaching sports, and volunteering for fire and rescue services. The essential elements of Marine Corps prevention policy are aggressive random urinalysis testing, random vehicle inspections, and use of drug detection dogs. The policies also actively endorse nondrinking and non-drug-using norms (e.g., no drinking contests, no alcoholic beverages as gifts or prizes, food and nonalcoholic beverages made readily available). Deterrence is a key prevention policy goal, although it is unclear to what extent these measures are employed consistently on the ground or have been evaluated for effectiveness.

Screening, Diagnosis, and Treatment

Two Marine Corps policies address prevention and treatment for alcohol and drug use, abuse, and dependence (MCO 5300.17 and NAVMC 2931). MCO 5300.17 identifies prevention, timely identification, and education and/or treatment, as well as "appropriate discipline or other administrative actions" (which may include restoration to full duty or separation), as key elements of Marine substance abuse programs (U.S. Marine Corps, 2011). The policy specifies that the wrongful use of drugs may result in prosecution and administrative action. The Personal and Family Readiness Division prepares a prevention plan covering training curricula and materials and assesses effectiveness, hosts conferences and working groups on substance abuse programs, conducts research and provides evidence-based models for prevention and treatment services, and evaluates programs. Commanders are intimately involved in responding to alcohol and drug use incidents and problems. They are directed to refer service members to prevention and intervention services and designate a substance abuse control officer (SACO). SACOs refer personnel for screening, maintain records of personnel with alcohol and other drug problems, ensure annual drug screening and proper implementation of screening, and conduct substance abuse prevention education. Medical officers (e.g., physicians, clinical psychologists) are responsible for diagnosis and for all aspects of treatment.

Chapter 2 of MCO 5300.17 addresses substance abuse prevention. Item 4 (Chapter 2) covers the drug testing program, designed to inspect personnel and assess Command readiness. Urinalysis testing is random and applied to all personnel. Commanders may order a drug test if there is suspicion of drug use. If a urine test is positive for one or more illicit drugs and other evidence corroborates drug use, commanders commence separation proceedings. NAVMC form 11700 guides assessments for SUDs—the signs and symptoms of abuse and dependence that constitute DSM-IV-TR criteria for abuse and dependence. Items listed on NAVMC form 11700, however, do not appear to come from a recognized standardized psychiatric interview with known psychometric properties. If screening rules out the need for a more complete assessment, the Marine receives early intervention and returns to duty. If a more complete assessment is necessary, it is conducted by a counselor (who becomes the Marine's case manager) using NAVMC form 11692. The counselor conducts a detailed assessment of cultural and family background, education and work, military experience, socialization, self-concept and communication, financial status, spirituality, and emotional and behavioral areas. Form 11692, however, does not incorporate a standardized diagnostic instrument with which to identify alcohol and other drug abuse or dependence. Diagnosis appears to occur in a nonstandardized manner or with NAVMC form 11700. NAVMC 2931, which describes procedures for drug and alcohol prevention and treatment programs, contains several forms used in comprehensive assessments of alcohol and other drug use and related problems. Although the forms cover signs and symptoms of abuse and dependence (e.g., withdrawal, job and financial problems), the questions in these areas do not appear to come from standardized screening interviews or psychiatric interviews designed to provide DSM diagnoses. Despite the wide array of assessments described in the policies, screening and diagnostic procedures fail to take advantage of standardized screening instruments or psychiatric interviews to reach DSM diagnoses.

Chapter 3 of MCO 5300.17 addresses substance abuse treatment provided by a physician or clinical psychologist. The Substance Abuse Counseling Center (SACC) provides alcohol and drug abuse treatment that includes screening, early intervention, biopsychosocial assessment, and treatment. The vast majority of Marines (approximately 90 percent) who receive treatment from the Marine Corps program have been identified either by Command or through the screening process. Very few Marines self-refer to treatment because of the belief that there will be consequences for their job position if they admit to needing help (as discussed further in Chapter 7). Moreover, according to information the committee received during its site visit to Camp Pendleton, the identification of problems is highly variable, depending on the SACOs and particular commanders. Once a Marine has been identified for treatment, the treatment program follows ASAM's Patient Placement Criteria, including early intervention and outpatient and intensive outpatient treatment.

The committee had concerns regarding several elements of the Marine Corps' substance abuse program. First, there is no uniformity in treatment programs or modalities across sites. For instance, the Marines Alcohol

Awareness Course is used only at Camp Pendleton. The majority of SACCs utilize the Impact as an indicated prevention program, but treatment modalities vary from site to site; some use 12-step programs, others use motivational interviewing, and so on. Second, Marines ordered to treatment are given mandatory orders to attend or face separation, but there are no data on whether mandatory treatment ensures treatment "success." In the case of alcohol abuse/dependence, separation decisions are made following treatment. Marines who self-refer for treatment for drug abuse/dependence and receive a diagnosis of abuse are processed for separation without treatment and are subject to disciplinary action; those who receive a diagnosis of dependence are processed for administrative separation, but are offered treatment and are exempt from disciplinary action. Third, it is unclear whether the Marine Corps' 58 substance use counselors make use of evidence-based treatments. Fourth, aftercare is insufficient; it serves more as administrative monitoring than recovery support. Finally, while treatment programs are accredited by the Commission on Accreditation of Rehabilitation Facilities, they have not been internally evaluated.

Because the Marines work with the Navy for many of their services, they share many of the same strengths and weaknesses. Marine policies, however, have additional weaknesses. They do not require measurement of clinical outcomes or provision of relapse treatment. Further, SUD treatment in the Marine Corps does not use a multidisciplinary team approach, nor does it employ master's-level counselors with SUD training, relying instead on certified substance abuse counselors to provide counseling and group therapy. Only two of the Marine Corps programs offer integrated traumatic brain injury (TBI)/PTSD treatment, and they are provided by the Navy (Camp Pendleton and Naval Medical Center Portsmouth).

SUD POLICIES AND PROGRAMS FOR MILITARY DEPENDENTS IN THE DIRECT CARE SYSTEM

Dependents of military members include adult spouses and children who may have their own needs for SUD care. Dependents who enroll in the TRICARE Prime program have the option at the commander's discretion to use medical and behavioral care in the direct care system (see Chapter 3 for a description of TRICARE benefit programs); however, dependents who require behavioral health services, including SUD treatment, make use of civilian providers paid through a TRICARE benefit. The committee's findings on the adequacy of the SUD benefit coverage and the utilization of SUD care by service members and their dependents are presented in Chapter 7. This section describes whether and how the policies and programs reviewed in this chapter and Appendix D specifically target military dependents.

DODI 1010.6, which addresses rehabilitation and referral of alcohol and drug abusers, contains a specific clause referencing dependents: "Rehabilitative and educational services shall be provided, when feasible, to the family members of DoD personnel and other eligible beneficiaries." While this policy grants permission to extend SUD services to family members, the committee found that in practice, this is beyond the capacity of most programs given the decade of involvement in overseas conflicts and the need to devote resources to the highest-priority issues affecting force readiness. As discussed in Chapter 7, only a fraction of family members have made use of SUD treatment services in the direct care system. Table 6-1 lists the DoD and branch programs that make specific mention of targeting military family members, according to the *Comprehensive Plan* (DoD, 2011).

TABLE 6-1 Military Programs Mentioning Dependents

Program	Clinical Focus	Target Population
DoD National Red Ribbon Campaign	Prevention	Active duty, dependents
DoD Military Pathways Program	Prevention, screening	Active duty, Reserves, National Guard, dependents
DoD Real Warriors Campaign	Prevention	Active duty, dependents
Adolescent Substance Abuse Counseling (ASAC) Program	Prevention, screening, diagnosis, treatment	Dependents
Military OneSource	Referral	Active duty, Reserves, National Guard, dependents
Air Force Culture of Responsible Choices (CoRC)	Prevention, screening, diagnosis, treatment	Active duty, dependents
Air Force, Navy, and Marines Drug Education for Youth (DEFY)	Prevention	Dependents
Air Force Enforcing Underage Drinking Laws (EUDL)	Prevention	Active duty, dependents
Army Employee Assistance Program (EAP)	Prevention, screening	Dependents, civilian employees
Navy Drug and Alcohol Advisory Council (NDAAC)	Prevention	Active duty, Reserves, dependents

Appendix D contains a description of these programs, which are assessed only briefly below.

Prevention

While some prevention resources target military spouses and children, no single uniform DoD program provides comprehensive prevention programming for dependents, and the committee found no reports on the effectiveness of prevention resources for this population. A number of programs targeting primarily service members, however, do include services for military family members.

The Red Ribbon campaign is a universal prevention campaign aimed at addressing peer pressure and prosocial bonding in youth, as well as parental monitoring. Thus, it is most developmentally appropriate for young military members with families. Red Ribbon Week is an annual campaign that is conducted nationwide in the United States every October both at the community level and on military bases. There is no evidence on this program's effectiveness, and both military bases and communities vary widely in the activities they sponsor under the auspices of the campaign. There is presently no published information on Red Ribbon's theoretical basis or on its outcomes.

Military Pathways is described as inclusive of universal and selective prevention approaches. The private contractor has developed family resiliency materials designed to help educate and support military families in coping with deployment stress, recognizing signs and symptoms of mental health problems, and building resiliency, and to help service members reconnect with their children.

The Real Warriors Campaign is an initiative launched by the Defense Centers of Excellence for Psychological Health and Traumatic Brain Injury (DCoE). Its goal is to "promote the processes of building resilience, facilitating recovery and supporting reintegration of returning service members, veterans and their families" (DCoE, 2012, p. 1); it is not aimed specifically at the prevention of SUDs. Further, as suggested by its title, the program's primary emphasis is not on family members but on assisting service members returning from deployment.

The Air Force's CoRC program appears to be aimed primarily at service members. However, it includes Toolkit 4, a training and resource guide for Command, ADAPT staff, and Drug Demand Reduction staff focused on building community collaborations for prevention. This toolkit includes training in prevention concepts, screening, social norms, consulting to the community, and prevention program management. It follows evidence-based practices for community implementation processes and prevention operating systems (Hawkins and Catalano, 1992). The committee did not hear testimony on CoRC implementation or its use to reach Air Force dependents.

DEFY is a comprehensive prevention program offered by the Air Force, Navy, and Marine Corps. It is operated worldwide and consists of a summer leadership camp (Phase 1) and a school-year mentoring program (Phase 2). The program's curriculum encompasses a variety of topics, including substance abuse prevention and other vital life skills, such as conflict resolution, self-management skills, study skills, leadership, and community service.

The EUDL program was a pilot that showed significant reductions in underage drinking (Spera and Franklin, 2010). Its primary target appears to be drinking among underage airmen, although some components include environmental changes in the community that may also benefit spouses and child dependents. The committee learned that EUDL was a demonstration project and that there are currently no plans to expand it to all Air Force bases; however, some of its components will be implemented within other Air Force–wide initiatives.[5] The committee finds the EUDL program to be a promising example of an effective approach to SUD prevention in military settings.

The Army's Employee Assistance Program provides a wide variety of services addressing various adult living problems. Examples include screening, short-term counseling, and referral. The extent to which military spouses use this program is unclear.

Finally, the Navy's Drug and Alcohol Advisory Council (NDAAC) is a local and regional mechanism by which commanders can monitor and communicate achievements or lack of success in attaining prevention goals related to alcohol-related incidents. As it targets incidents resulting from alcohol misuse, it is not a primary prevention program. Furthermore, while the NDAAC is described as available to dependents, the scope of commander monitoring is most likely limited to incidents involving service members rather than family members in the community. The committee was informed that the NDAAC could provide a mechanism for establishing specific short- and long-term branch-level goals for reducing harmful alcohol use, but the means by which this might be accomplished were not described.

Screening, Diagnosis, and Treatment

The Military Pathways program includes a self-assessment/self-screening component that can serve as a secondary prevention mechanism

[5] Personal communication, Lt. Col. Mark S. Oordt, Ph.D., USAF ADAPT Program, October 25, 2011.

for military members or spouses who self-identify as being at personal risk for SUD and subsequently seek help. The committee found that these materials appear to follow evidence-based principles. A RAND report estimates that this intervention reaches more than 305,000 active duty service members and their families each year (Weinick et al., 2011).

The *Comprehensive Plan* identifies the Adolescent Substance Abuse Counseling (ASAC) program as an Army contract, but in January 2010, DoD extended a blanket purchase agreement with a value of up to $80 million so the program could serve dependents of members of the Air Force, Navy, and Marine Corps (SAIC, 2010). The focus is described as children of military families in grades 6-12 who are considered at risk for substance use and who are authorized to use military treatment facilities. Services specified in the contract include treatment, identification and referral, and prevention education in community settings (U.S. Army, 2011b). The committee did not hear testimony on this program from any branch representatives, which appears to suggest that use of an independent private contract has not led to maximum coordination of these services with Command-directed programs.

Finally, Military OneSource provides a confidential means for service members and their families to be screened for SUDs and referred to resources. The counseling provided by Military OneSource's contracted providers is nonmedical in nature (e.g., connecting people to resources; counseling on relationship issues, readjustment, and stress). The committee did not learn of the volume of referrals made through this service.

Other than the above three programs, the committee is not aware of organized, stand-alone SUD screening, diagnosis, or treatment initiatives for military spouses or children in the direct care system. Note that while this discussion has focused on policies and programs relevant to military dependents, the TRICARE benefit pays for certain SUD services, including assessment and diagnosis by SUD professionals, in specialty programs. The adequacy of the benefit and utilization of these services are discussed in Chapter 7.

SUMMARY OF KEY FINDINGS

The committee's review of SUD policies and programs within DoD, the Air Force, the Army, the Navy, and the Marine Corps revealed both strengths and limitations. Policies outline roles, responsibilities, and options for SUD prevention, screening, diagnosis, and treatment services and provide the foundation for program implementation. Variation in program implementation, however, reflects a lack of standardization and reveals inconsistency in the interpretation of policy. Increased standardization of SUD prevention, screening, diagnosis, and treatment services across the branches of the U.S. military could enhance the effectiveness and efficiency of these services and permit branches to share resources and provide more consistent and higher-quality services.

Finding 6-1: DoD and branch policies recognize the deleterious effects of alcohol and other drug use and support the need for SUD prevention, but programs fall short of meeting this need.

DoD, Army, Navy, Air Force, and Marine Corps policies on alcohol and other drug use among service members, their dependents, and civilian employees consistently address the impact and the need for services. First, all of the policies are based on recognition that alcohol and other drug use can be harmful to individuals and hamper their ability to perform their military jobs. Second, there is a need within each of the branches to address SUDs through prevention, screening, referral to proper services, diagnosis, and treatment. Current policies assign primary responsibility for identification and referral to unit commanders and health personnel. Air Force and Navy policies provide guidance on the behaviors that may indicate alcohol and other drug use problems, such as driving while intoxicated, public intoxication, and domestic violence. These policies also recognize that personnel may self-refer for help with alcohol and other drug use, and describe Command procedures for addressing self-referral.

DoD policy recognizes the need to prevent substance abuse and maintain fitness for duty among its forces. As a prevention strategy, drug testing has a presumed deterrent effect through increased awareness of the consequences of testing positive for illicit drug use (i.e., separation from the military). There is no research, however, showing that drug testing is an effective prevention strategy for service members and their dependents. Reports that cite decreasing rates of illicit drug use as evidence of the effectiveness of drug testing do not take into account causality, secular trends, or other factors that affect rates of illicit drug use. By focusing on drug testing as prevention, the branches may fail to implement more evidence-based prevention strategies with proven effectiveness. Finally, drug testing does not address risky alcohol use or prescription drug abuse, which is epidemiologically a far more prevalent problem in the military than illicit drug use. However, the committee finds that the changes recently made to the panel of tested drugs to include often abused prescription medications such as hydrocodone and benzodiazepines (U.S. Army, 2012) demonstrate DoD's attention to these problems and efforts to deter the abuse of prescription medications.

As discussed in Chapter 5, ample opportunities exist for the military to implement systems-level environmental strategies to curb alcohol and prescription drug problems. However, the committee's site visits and other information gathering activities revealed inconsistencies in actual adoption and implementation of these strategies. The first major environmental alcohol abuse prevention strategy outlined in Chapter 5 is controlling affordability through pricing and taxation. The committee finds that while the U.S. military cannot control the prices or taxation of alcohol sold in communities around bases, it does have control over the prices of alcohol sold at stores located on bases, which are often discounted.

The second environmental strategy is restricting the availability of alcohol for purchase. The very existence of liquor stores on bases is in direct conflict with this approach. The committee heard during its site visits that in addition to military bases allowing alcohol use on base, revenues from the sale of alcohol support recreational and morale programs. Ironically, curbing the sale of alcohol would affect the amount of non-alcohol-related recreational activities available on base. In addition, below-market prices on alcohol (i.e., no state taxes) likely encourage elevated rates of unhealthy alcohol use. During visits to bases and from presentations during its information gathering meetings, the committee learned that while there is some military cooperation with the local communities surrounding bases, the extent of this cooperation varies site to site. Commanders may or may not elect to pursue it as part of an overall policy to prevent alcohol and illicit drug use by military personnel.

The third strategy is altering the context in which alcohol is consumed. In particular, bases that sell alcohol only for off-base consumption and those without liquor stores can work with the community, especially local bar owners, in the implementation of the server interventions described in Chapter 5. However, the committee's review of policies and programs revealed that such partnerships with local authorities and hospitality-related businesses (e.g., bars, hotels, casinos) are not mandated by policy and therefore are inconsistent.

The fourth strategy is prevention of impaired driving. Sobriety checkpoints and random breath testing can be applied to driving on military bases. However, the effectiveness of these measures is contingent on consistency of enforcement. Among the various military bases the committee visited, Keesler Air Force Base was the only one that administered random breath testing for those returning from leave and driving back onto the base.

The committee did find some examples of promising environmental prevention and deterrence strategies to address alcohol abuse. One was the Air Force's EUDL program (discussed briefly above and in detail in Appendix D). The committee determined that this program incorporates many of the best-practice environmental strategies reviewed in Chapter 5. A recent evaluation demonstrated declines in arrest rates for minors in possession of alcohol and for driving under the influence at sites that implemented the program (Spera et al., 2012). The committee found another example of a promising strategy for addressing alcohol abuse in the Navy's plan to institute a random breath testing program on board its ships during 2012. Those who test positive will be referred to the SARP for further screening and possible treatment. While the committee finds these efforts by the Air Force and Navy to be promising, similar efforts in the Army and Marine Corps (where prevalence rates for alcohol abuse are higher) may be needed.

To deter prescription drug abuse, DoD instituted stricter limits on the length of prescriptions for controlled drugs in May 2012. Previously, if a service member tested positive for a prescription drug but had a valid prescription on file within the past 6 months, the medical review of the positive test would likely determine that the use was legal. If a service member does not have a valid prescription, a positive test is determined to indicate illicit use, just as with any other illicit drug, with possible personnel consequences. Under the new policy, service members who need ongoing treatment with controlled substances will have greater contact with their prescribing physician, and those who need these medications only on a short-term basis will not be allowed to continue using them beyond their 30-day prescription without risking the personnel consequences of a positive drug test. By limiting prescriptions for controlled substances to 30 days, DoD is tightening the controls of these medications—a clear example of an environmental prevention strategy. The committee finds this policy change to be a promising effort to deter prescription drug abuse; however, it remains to be seen whether the change will be effective in accomplishing this goal.

Finding 6-2: DoD and branch screening policies and programs fall short of identifying all service members who have or are at risk for developing SUDs.

Current policy and screening practices tend to rely on random urine tests to detect the use of illicit drugs and on alcohol-related incidents to detect problematic alcohol use. These practices are relatively inefficient and identify only a portion of drug users at risk for developing severe SUDs and individuals with unhealthy alcohol use. Systematic screening in health care settings could be a more efficient strategy for identifying those with unhealthy alcohol use. The *VA/DoD Clinical Practice Guideline for Management of Substance Use Disorders* (VA and DoD, 2009) specifies that patients seen in general medical and general mental health settings should be screened for unhealthy alcohol use. Routine annual screening using validated tools has the potential to identify at-risk substance users before use becomes problematic and more severe. DoD and branch policies and programs, however, do not explicitly reference the VA/DoD guidance (VA and DoD, 2009), and the *Comprehensive Plan* notes that evidence-based screening tools are not consistently utilized in settings outside of deployment health assessments (DoD, 2011b). Rigorous screening of those newly entering the military for any current SUDs or a history of such disorders is also important to identify those who have SUDs or may be at risk for relapse.

Requirements for Command notification when an SUD is diagnosed may be inhibiting routine medical screening for at-risk alcohol use. Therefore, DoD's clarification that health care providers may not notify Command when they offer substance abuse education services (DoD, 2011a) provides an opportunity for enhanced screening and brief intervention. The public health goal of screening is early identification to prevent the development of more severe problems. DoD support for substance abuse screening and brief intervention in health care settings should encourage the Military Health System to implement the VA/DoD guidance on routine annual screening for unhealthy alcohol use.

With regard to identifying those individuals who are misusing and/or abusing prescription medications, DoD's PEC has developed tools that can be used by health care providers and commanders to review pharmacy data. Overall, the committee finds the activities of PEC to be comprehensive, yet it did not learn whether providers are fully using the available tools to monitor prescriptions received by patients from other physicians. Efforts should be made to encourage the use of these tools and to improve them to make them as comprehensive and as physician-friendly as possible. The committee also finds that the inability of pharmacy systems to track all prescription medications dispensed in theater is a major barrier to identifying misuse and abuse of these drugs.

Finding 6-3: Military policies reflect different attitudes toward alcohol and other drug use.

Military policies treat alcohol and other drug use differently because alcohol use is legal for those aged 21 and older, whereas other drug use is not legal. The differences appear in at least three areas. First, as stated in the discussion of **Finding 6-1**, drug testing is regarded as the main emphasis in prevention of substance abuse across all branches of the military, but currently focuses primarily on illicit drugs, not alcohol. Second, military bases allow alcohol use and use alcohol revenues to support recreational and morale programs. Below-market prices on alcohol probably encourage elevated rates of unhealthy alcohol use. While difficult to evaluate systematically, information derived from the committee's site visits suggests that drinking is acceptable as long as one is not caught with an infraction (e.g., driving under the influence) or does not show up for an active duty assignment incapacitated by alcohol. Third, alcohol misuse or abuse does not appear to carry the same consequences as illicit drug use with respect to military separation. If an individual receives a diagnosis of alcohol abuse or dependence, he/she receives treatment, whereas other drug abuse/dependence diagnoses result in initiation of separation proceedings and possible enrollment in treatment, although the policies on this issue vary (e.g., the Air Force policy is the strictest, whereas Army policy requires referral to treatment for drug "dependent" individuals but not drug "abusers"). The difference in perceived potential for rehabilitation and treatment between soldiers with alcohol and other drug dependence is not supported by scientific evidence. While the committee understands the desire to separate service members who violate laws against illicit drug use, a more systematic and evaluative approach might result in retaining highly skilled service members. Also, it should be noted that when the fifth edition of the DSM is released in May 2013, the distinction between "abuse" and "dependence" will be eliminated, and diagnosis will instead be classified as "mild," "moderate," or "severe." Therefore, DoD and branch policies that call for different personnel and treatment decisions based on diagnoses of "abuse" and "dependence" will need to be revised.

Finding 6-4: There is substantial variability among SUD-related policies, programs, procedures, and instruments across the military branches.

DoD policy lays out strategies and guidelines for SUD prevention, screening, diagnosis, and treatment, but the actual implementation of these strategies and guidelines varies according to specific branch-level policies. While DoD offers several SUD programs that could be utilized across the branches, it does not require or monitor their adoption by the branches. The RAND (Weinick et al., 2011) analysis of psychological health and TBI programs for U.S. military service members and their families yielded similar observations about the lack of standardization and the variability of implementation across the armed forces. With the exception of the Air Force's Substance Abuse Prevention Specialist Training and CoRC and the Navy's Alcohol and Drug Abuse for Managers and Supervisors (ADAMS) and Prevention Specialist programs, the branches do not make use of standardized training processes or protocols for implementers of prevention programs or for the leaders who oversee them. Programs for youth (e.g., DEFY) are delivered by contractors, and spouses and other family members receive prevention services through health care service agencies or programs such as Families OverComing Under Stress (FOCUS) (reviewed in Appendix D).

Lack of standardization is an issue of concern for screening and diagnosis as well. As noted in the discussion of **Finding 6-2,** DoD and branch policies acknowledge and emphasize screening as a key strategy in combating SUDs, but do not specify standardized screening procedures or instruments. Air Force policy and the *VA/DoD Clinical Practice Guideline for Management of Substance Use Disorders* identify specific instruments to be used in screening (e.g., AUDIT-C). These policies, as well as DODD 1010.4, also recognize that there are standardized criteria for SUD diagnoses in DSM-IV-TR. Aside from these examples, however, policies do not identify specific screening instruments or the health care professions authorized to screen and diagnose (e.g., nurses, physician assistants, licensed counselors, physicians). Standardized psychiatric interviews are not identified for diagnostic assessments.

Current governance policies are high-level and have gaps that allow for variation among the branches in such key areas as SUD program evaluations and the influence of Command on treatment plans. Expansion of the "umbrella structure" of governance discussed earlier in this chapter could promote increased coordination of resources and services and enhance consistency across the armed forces for measurement of system/program effectiveness and performance and efficiency. The *Comprehensive Plan* (DoD, 2011b) notes that utilization of the *VA/DoD Clinical Practice Guideline for Management of Substance Use Disorders* is inconsistent across DoD facilities. DoD does not systematically monitor compliance with its policies or with the VA/DoD Clinical Practice Guideline, and the branches do not routinely monitor compliance with policy across installations. Consequently, the sophisticated planning and design that go into the development of SUD prevention and treatment policies can be lost in translation as principles filter through the branches to local installations. Further, the committee would be remiss not to acknowledge that each military branch's distinctive history and culture undoubtedly play a role in the variation that exists from branch to branch in policy and program design, adoption, and delivery. The additional cultural and contextual differences that exist between the active duty population and members of the National Guard and Reserves further complicate the situation and cannot be ignored in addressing the needs of all service members across all branches of the military.

Finding 6-5: DoD and the branches do not evaluate programs and initiatives consistently and systematically.

The committee found little evidence of systematic evaluation of cognitive, affective, or behavioral change resulting from prevention programs or treatment interventions using single- or multiple-group design evaluations. The *Comprehensive Plan* (DoD, 2011b) and the RAND report (Weinick et al., 2011) also identify program evaluation as an area for improvement.

Current research projects (see Box 6-3) may yield benchmarks, such as voluntary participation rates and change in risky behaviors related to SUD development and relapse, which could be used for systematic evaluation processes and metrics. These studies are testing the extension of programs

BOX 6-3
Military Studies of the National Institute on Drug Abuse and National Institute on Alcohol Abuse and Alcoholism

National Institute on Drug Abuse

- *Use and Abuse of Prescription Opioids among Operation Enduring Freedom/Operation Iraqi Freedom Veterans*
  University of Arkansas for Medical Sciences at Little Rock
- *Integrated Treatment of Operation Enduring Freedom/Operation Iraqi Freedom Veterans with Post Traumatic Stress Disorder and Substance Use Disorders*
  Medical University of South Carolina
- *First Longitudinal Study of Missed Treatment Opportunities Using DoD and VA Data*
  Brandeis University
- *Integrated Cognitive Behavioral Therapy for Co-Occurring Post Traumatic Stress Disorder and Substance Use Disorders*
  Dartmouth College
- *Effectiveness of a Web-Enhanced Parenting Program for Military Families*
  University of Minnesota, Twin Cities

National Institute on Alcohol Abuse and Alcoholism

- *Stress-Induced Drinking in Operation Enduring Freedom/Operation Iraqi Freedom Veterans: The Role of Combat History and PTSD*
  Medical University of South Carolina
- *Veteran Reintegration, Mental Health and Substance Use in the Inner-City*
  National Development and Research Institutes, Inc., in New York City
- *Web-Based Cognitive Behavioral Therapy for Substance Misusing and Post Traumatic Stress Disorder Symptomatic Operation Enduring Freedom/Operation Iraqi Freedom Veterans*
  National Development and Research Institutes, Inc., in New York City and Syracuse University
- *Personalized Drinking Feedback Interventions for Operation Enduring Freedom*
  Operation Iraqi Freedom Veterans/University of Missouri–Columbia

effective with civilian populations to service members and their families. NORTH STAR, for example, uses community-based prevention research from Communities That Care (Hawkins et al., 1992), the Midwestern Prevention Project (Riggs et al., 2009), and Steps Toward Effective Prevention (STEP) (Valente et al., 2007). The Comprehensive Soldier Fitness program is based on the Penn resiliency program (Seligman, 1998) for preventing and reducing depression. ADAPT (After Deployment: Adaptive Parenting Tools, differentiated from the overall ADAPT program used by the Air Force) is based on the Parent Management Training Model-Oregon (Forgatch and Patterson, 2010; Gewirtz et al., 2011), used with parents whose children are exhibiting behavioral problems. And FOCUS is based on resiliency and coping training for families experiencing stress (Forgatch and Patterson, 2010; Gewirtz et al., 2011).

Finding 6-6: DoD and branch policies support the use of evidence-based prevention and treatment but do not identify specific practices.

This finding is overarching and applies to both policies and programs for prevention, screening, diagnosis, and treatment. It is also highlighted in both the *Comprehensive Plan* (DoD, 2011b) and the RAND (Weinick et al., 2011) analysis. Current policies have been ineffective in preventing alcohol abuse and prescription drug misuse. These policies could make better use of scientific evidence on the nature of alcohol and other drug use behaviors and the best prevention and treatment efforts for the full range of SUDs. As stated in **Finding 6-3,** DoD and branch policies treat alcohol and other drugs very differently. They place differential emphasis on the implementation of screening for alcohol and other drugs (e.g., testing for drugs but not alcohol) and have very different repercussions for alcohol versus other drug use (e.g., zero tolerance policies for other drugs but not alcohol; CATEP is for alcohol only).

While several of the prevention programs noted in the *Comprehensive Plan* (DoD, 2011b) assert a foundation in evidence-based principles, few specify what those principles actually are. Based on the results of this committee's review, many of the programs appear to meet prevention needs in that they are appropriate to the populations served, are theory based, address multiple risk factors, and have evaluated behavioral outcomes. Examples include Military Pathways (DoD), DEFY (Navy, Air Force), EUDL (Air Force), CoRC (Air Force), FOCUS (selected Navy, Marine, Air Force, and Army installations), and NORTH STAR (multiple Air Force Commands and bases). However, these programs (with the exception of NORTH STAR, EUDL, and FOCUS) adapted materials and concepts from civilian prevention programs and have not been tested with military populations. Further, many of the prevention efforts appear to be focused on campaigns, Internet games, and camps or events (e.g., That Guy, DEFY camp, Real Warrior, Red Ribbon), with no research evidence that they affect substance use. DoD and the various branches are not making strong enough use of evidence-based environmental policies and programs (e.g., reducing availability and/or raising the price of alcohol on bases).

The committee's analysis revealed an underutilization of evidence-based pharmacological therapies, as well as insufficient continuing care. Effective treatment of substance abuse includes both pharmacological and behavioral therapies. In the military, the pharmacotherapies for acute medical withdrawal treatment focus on alcohol, sedatives, and opioids. The most effective treatment plans entail withdrawal treatment followed by relapse prevention therapy, which is frequently a combination of both medication and behavioral therapy (Kosten and McQueen, 2008). On the issue of follow-up care, the committee finds the Navy MORE program to be an innovative and promising model for the provision of ongoing recovery support and encourages the other branches to consider adopting similar approaches to improve posttreatment care for active duty service members.

Finding 6-7: Integration of SUD care with other behavioral health and medical care is lacking.

The Military Health System has clear evidence that the current operating tempo and environment are associated with increased risk of mental health disorders and SUDs and that these disorders often co-occur (U.S. Army, 2012). Separate and distinct services for mental health disorders and SUDs are neither desirable nor feasible. The committee agrees with the need to facilitate access to both types of services and provide integrated care. Integration of care can occur at two levels: (1) integration of care for mental health disorders and SUDs, and (2) integration of behavioral health care with primary care. Integration of behavioral health services with primary care may be particularly challenging in the military, whose population is often mobile and frequently changing location. The Air Force's BHOP demonstrates the feasibility and advantages of integrating behavioral health into primary care services. Integration of services for SUDs should proceed as well to reduce stigma and enhance the development of medication-assisted treatment for alcohol and other drug use disorders. The committee supports routine screening and brief intervention for alcohol misuse within primary care settings. Screening and brief intervention are evidence-based practices, and when implemented systematically can reduce the risk of alcohol-related problems within communities and populations (Babor et al., 2007). The U.S. Preventive Services Task Force also recommends routine use of screening and brief intervention in primary care settings (O'Connor et al., 2009). DODI 6490.08 clarifies that health care providers can provide substance abuse education and should assume that providing educational interventions does not require Command notification.

Integrated care is likely to be more difficult in the Army and Marine Corps because their programs for treatment of SUDs are located within the human resources organization rather than a Medical Command. Specific strategies will be required to facilitate interaction between Commands and full access to medical records. In the Navy and Air Force, SUD treatment programs are located within the Medical Command, but remain separate and distinct settings of care that often are not fully integrated within general health care settings. Treatment for SUDs in the 21st century will require the elimination of divisions between health care and specialty addiction treatment.

Finding 6-8: DoD and branch policies are largely silent on comprehensive programs and services for SUD prevention, screening and brief intervention, diagnosis, and treatment for military dependents.

While DoD policy permits the provision of SUD services to military dependents, the branches do not have the capacity to extend such services beyond reaching service members. Furthermore, based on best practices, the specialty SUD treatment services operated by the branches for military members are not appropriate for youth and adolescents, who require developmentally appropriate treatment. While some DoD prevention programming identifies spouse and child dependents as a target population, most of these initiatives, based on their descriptions, emphasize the ways in which service members are reached and the role of commanders. Some prevention initiatives are selective or indicated, taking place with at-risk individuals or after an incident occurs. The committee found no evaluation literature associated with most of these initiatives, particularly on their reach or effectiveness with military dependents (see also **Finding 6-5**).

Finding 6-9: DoD and the branches rarely use technology to enhance the delivery of screening, diagnosis, and treatment services.

The committee found few examples of technology being used to deliver SUD services in new and innovative ways. Given identified counselor shortages and challenges to staffing SUD clinics with experienced and licensed clinicians (see Chapter 8 for further discussion), as well as concern over the lack of standardized delivery of evidence-based care, DoD might consider the increased use of technology to address some of these issues. The committee identified as promising the following approaches to addressing SUD care with the use of technology.

The Navy's MORE aftercare program represents an innovative use of technology to provide recovery support for sailors deployed internationally and at sea (see Appendix D for further description of this service). MORE illustrates the use of technology to extend the counselor workforce and provide ongoing support to active duty service members when they return to their military assignment. The Navy also is currently pilot testing a new version of the MORE program that is delivered via smartphone technology. The other branches appear not to be using this type of treatment and aftercare technology. Additional research on the effectiveness of the MORE program with military populations and other innovative models for delivering treatment services by means of telephone, video conferencing, and web-based formats might provide DoD with some alternative methods for extending its counseling workforce.

Additionally, the Air Force's use of the SUAT computerized assessment tool is an example of the utilization of technology to standardize clinical processes and improve efficiency within SUD programs. The committee finds the SUAT tool to be a promising model for DoD to evaluate and consider for dissemination to the other branches.

Finally, the committee found value in the approach taken by Military Pathways of using web-based video doctor technology to reach service members and their families who might otherwise not receive screening and referral to services for mental health conditions, including alcohol abuse. A rigorous evaluation of this program and its effectiveness would provide DoD with guidance on whether this is a beneficial use of resources and whether the approach should be considered for other uses.

REFERENCES

APA (American Psychiatric Association). 2000. *Diagnostic and statistical manual of mental disorders, fourth edition, text revision (DSM-IV-TR).* Washington, DC: American Psychiatric Association.

Babor, T. F., B. G. McRee, P. A. Kassebaum, P. L. Grimaldi, K. Ahmed, and J. Bray. 2007. Screening, Brief Intervention, and Referral to Treatment (SBIRT): Toward a public health approach to the management of substance abuse. *Substance Abuse* 28(3):7-30.

Berwick, D. M. 2002. A user's manual for the IOM's "quality chasm" report. *Health Affairs* 21(3):80-90.

Chou, R., G. J. Fanciullo, P. G. Fine, J. A. Adler, J. C. Ballantyne, P. Davies, M. I. Donovan, D. A. Fishbain, K. M. Foley, J. Fudin, A. M. Gilson, A. Kelter, A. Mauskop, P. G. O'Connor, S. D. Passik, G. W. Pasternak, R. K. Portenoy, B. A. Rich, R. G. Roberts, K. H. Todd, and C. Miaskowski. 2009. Clinical guidelines for the use of chronic opioid therapy in chronic noncancer pain. *Journal of Pain* 10(2):113-130.

Compton, W. M., and N. D. Volkow. 2006. Major increases in opioid analgesic abuse in the United States: Concerns and strategies. *Drug and Alcohol Dependence* 81(2):103-107.

Crano, W. D., and M. Burgoon. 2002. *Mass media and drug prevention: Classic and contemporary theories and research.* Mahwah, NJ: Lawrence Erlbaum Associates.

DCoE (Defense Centers of Excellence for Psychological Health and Traumatic Brain Injury). 2011. *DCoE pilot project evaluation report A401: Fort Hood Intensive Outpatient Program (IOP).* Arlington, VA: DCoE.

DCoE. 2012. *The real warriors campaign.* http://www.realwarriors.net/aboutus (accessed May 29, 2012).

Defense Health Board. 2011. *Psychotropic medication prescription practices and use and complementary and alternative medicine use.* Falls Church, VA: Defense Health Board.

DoD (Department of Defense). 1985. *Instruction 1010.6: Rehabilitation and referral services for alcohol and drug abusers.* Washington, DC: DoD.

DoD. 1994. *Directive 1010.1: Health promotion.* Washington, DC: DoD.

DoD. 1997. *Directive 1010.4: Drug and alcohol abuse by DoD personnel.* Washington, DC: DoD.

DoD. 2011a. *Instruction 6490.08: Command notification requirements to dispel stigma in providing mental health care to service members.* Washington, DC: DoD.

DoD. 2011b. *Comprehensive plan on prevention, diagnosis, and treatment of substance use disorders and disposition of substance use offenders in the armed forces.* Washington, DC: Office of the Under Secretary of Defense.

DoD. 2012. *The Department of Defense pharmacoeconomic center.* http://www.pec.ha.osd.mil/ (accessed August 07, 2012).

Forgatch, M. S., and G. R. Patterson. 2010. Parent management training—Oregon model: An intervention for antisocial behavior in children and adolescents. In *Evidence-based psychotherapies for children and adolescents* (2nd ed.), edited by J. R. Weisz and A. E. Kazdin. New York: Guilford Press. Pp. 159-178.

GAO (Government Accountability Office). 2011. *Prescription drug control: DEA has enhanced efforts to combat diversion, but could better assess and report program results.* Washington, DC: GAO.

Gewirtz, A. H., C. R. Erbes, M. A. Polusny, M. S. Forgatch, and D. S. DeGarmo. 2011. Helping military families through the deployment process: Strategies to support parenting. *Professional Psychology: Research and Practice* 42(1):56-62.

Hawkins, J. D., and R. F. J. Catalano. 1992. *Communities that care.* San Francisco, CA: Jossey-Bass.

Heyman, R. E., and A. M. Smith Slep. 2001. Risk factors for family violence: Special issue. *Aggression and Violent Behavior* 6(2-3):115-356.

Heyman, R. E., A. M. Smith Slep, and J. P. Nelson. 2011. Empirically guided community intervention for partner abuse, child maltreatment, suicidality, and substance misuse. In *Risk and resilience in U.S. military families*, edited by S. M. M. Wadsworth and D. Riggs. New York: Springer. Pp. 85-110.

Humphreys, J., J. Y. Tsoh, M. A. Kohn, and B. Gerbert. 2011. Increasing discussions of intimate partner violence in prenatal care using Video Doctor plus provider cueing: A randomized, controlled trial. *Women's Health Issues* 21(2):136-144.

Jackson, R. A., N. E. Stotland, A. B. Caughey, and B. Gerbert. 2011. Improving diet and exercise in pregnancy with Video Doctor counseling: A randomized trial. *Patient Education and Counseling* 83(2):203-209.

Kosten, T. R., and K. McQueen. 2008. General approaches to substance and polydrug use disorders. In *Psychiatry*, edited by A. Tasman, J. Kay, and J. R. Lieberman. London, England: John Wiley & Sons. Pp. 922-935.

O'Connor, E. A., E. P. Whitlock, B. Gaynes, and T. L. Beil. 2009. *Screening for depression in adults and older adults in primary care: An updated systematic review.* http://www.ncbi.nlm.nih.gov/pubmed/20722174 (accessed June 14, 2012).

Office of National Drug Control Policy. 2001. *Evidence-based principles for substance abuse prevention.* Washington, DC: Office of National Drug Control Policy.

Office of National Drug Control Policy. 2011. *Epidemic: Responding to America's prescription drug abuse crisis.* Washington, DC: Office of National Drug Control Policy.

Pentz, M. A. 2003. Evidence-based prevention: Characteristics, impact, and future direction. *Journal of Psychoactive Drugs* 35(Suppl.):143-152.

Riggs, N. R., C. P. Chou, and M. A. Pentz. 2009. Preventing growth in amphetamine use: Long-term effects of the Midwestern Prevention Project (MPP) from early adolescence to early adulthood. *Addiction* 104(10):1691-1699.

Runyan, C. N., V. P. Fonseca, and C. Hunter. 2003. Integrating consultative behavioral healthcare into the Air Force medical system. In *Behavioral health as primary care: Beyond efficacy to effectiveness*, edited by W. T. O'Donohue, K. E. Ferguson, and N. A. Cummings. Reno, NV: Context Press. Pp. 145-163.

SAIC (Science Applications International Corporation). 2010. *Department of Defense awards adolescent substance abuse counseling services contract to SAIC.* http://www.militarymentalhealth.org/ (accessed August 8, 2012).

Screening for Mental Health, Inc. 2012. *Military Mental Health Screening Program.* http://www.militarymentalhealth.org (accessed August 3, 2012).

Seligman, M. E. P. 1998. *Learned optimism.* New York: Pocket Books (Simon and Schuster).

Spera, C., and K. Franklin. 2010. Reducing drinking among junior enlisted Air Force members in five communities: Early findings of the EUDL program's influence on self-reported drinking behaviors. *Journal of Studies on Alcohol and Drugs* 71(3):373-383.

Spera, C., F. Barlas, R. Z. Szoc, J. Prabhakaran, and M. H. Cambridge. 2012. Examining the influence of the Enforcing Underage Drinking Laws (EUDL) program on alcohol-related outcomes in five communities surrounding Air Force bases. *Addictive Behaviors* 37(4):513-516.

Tsoh, J. Y., M. A. Kohn, and B. Gerbert. 2010. Promoting smoking cessation in pregnancy with Video Doctor plus provider cueing: A randomized trial. *Acta Obstetricia et Gynecologica Scandinavica* 89(4):515-523.

U.S. Air Force. 2011. *Instruction 44-121: Alcohol and Drug Abuse Prevention and Treatment (ADAPT) program.* Washington, DC: Department of the Air Force.

U.S. Army. 2009. *Army regulation 600-85: The Army substance abuse program.* http://www.apd.army.mil/pdffiles/r600_85.pdf (accessed October 11, 2011).

U.S. Army. 2010. *Pain Management Task Force final report.* Washington, DC: Office of the Army Surgeon General.

U.S. Army. 2011a. *ALARACT 062/2011: Changes to length of authorized duration of controlled substance prescriptions in MEDCOM regulation 40-51.* Washington, DC: Office of the Army Surgeon General.

U.S. Army. 2011b. *ASAC standard operating procedures (revised).* Cedar Rapids, IA: Area Substance Abuse Council.

U.S. Army. 2012. *Policy Guidance on the assessment and treatment of post-traumatic stress disorder (PTSD).* Fort Sam Houston, TX: Department of the Army.

U.S. Marine Corps. 2011. *Order 5300.17: Marine Corps substance abuse program.* Washington, DC: Department of the Navy.

U.S. Navy. 1990. *BUMED Instruction 5353.3: Use of disulfiram (Antabuse).* Washington, DC: Department of the Navy.

U.S. Navy. 1999. *BUMEDINST 5353.4A: Standards for provision of substance related disorder treatment services.* Washington, DC: Bureau of Medicine, Department of the Navy.

U.S. Navy. 2009. *Operation Navy Instruction 5350.4D: Navy alcohol and drug abuse prevention and control.* Washington, DC: Department of the Navy.

U.S. Navy. 2011. *SECNAVINST 5300.28E: Military substance abuse prevention and control.* Washington, DC: Department of the Navy.

U.S. Navy. 2012a. *NAVADMIN 082/12: Implementation of urinalysis testing for synthetic compounds.* Washington, DC: Department of the Navy.

U.S. Navy. 2012b. *21st century sailor and marine*. http://www.21stcentury.navy.mil/faqs.aspx (accessed June 4, 2012).

VA (Department of Veterans Affairs) and DoD. 2009. *VA/DoD clinical practice guideline for management of substance use disorders*. Washington, DC: VA and DoD.

VA and DoD. 2010. *VA/DoD clinical practice guideline for management of opioid therapy for chronic pain*. Washington, DC: VA and DoD.

Valente, T. W., C. P. Chou, and M. A. Pentz. 2007. Community coalitions as a system: Effects of network change on adoption of evidence-based substance abuse prevention. *American Journal of Public Health* 97(5):880-886.

Weinick, R. M., E. B. Beckjord, C. M. Farmer, L. T. Martin, E. M. Gillen, J. D. Acosta, M. P. Fisher, J. Garnett, G. C. Gonzalez, T. C. Helmus, L. H. Jaycox, K. A. Reynolds, N. Salcedo, and D. M. Scharf. 2011. *Programs addressing psychological health and traumatic brain injury among U.S. military servicemembers and their families*. Santa Monica, CA: RAND Corporation.

7

Access to Care for Substance Use Disorders

A review of access to care for substance use disorders (SUDs) was a central component of two tasks in the committee's charge:

- a comparison of the adequacy of the availability of and access to care for SUDs for members of the active duty and reserve components of the armed forces; and
- an assessment of the adequacy of the availability of and access to care for SUDs for dependents of members of the armed forces, whether such dependents suffer from their own SUD or because of the SUD of a member of the armed forces.

To address these tasks, this chapter begins by defining access to care for SUDs and providing a framework for the ensuing analysis. Subsequent sections examine the availability of care, policies and other factors that affect access to care, and data on utilization of care. The chapter concludes with findings based on this analysis. The committee's analysis considers the direct care system (military treatment facilities), the Veterans Health Administration (VHA), and the system for purchase of care (TRICARE). It reviews access to SUD care for active duty personnel; military dependents; and, to the extent data were available, members of the National Guard and Reserves. The assessment examines each branch of the military where sufficient detail was available.

FRAMEWORK FOR ACCESS TO CARE

The armed forces focus on maintaining warrior fitness and promoting resilience among service members and military families. Active duty personnel experience frequent mobilizations, difficult transitions, combat situations, and an operational tempo with long and multiple periods away from their families and supports. The physical and emotional stressors experienced by many military women and men may contribute to an increase in their use of alcohol and other drugs. Access to substance use services—from prevention to a wide spectrum of interventions for substance misuse and abuse—can help military personnel and their families maintain psychological resilience and fitness. Access to routine screening, confidential brief education, brief counseling, brief interventions for those with emerging substance use problems, and more intensive treatment for those with SUDs promotes good health and may reduce the current high rates of alcohol and prescription drug misuse. If these services are delivered without sanctions or stigma, they promote an effective response to emerging alcohol and other drug use problems, and foster a system in which individuals seek help rather than hide problems.

The committee's framework for assessing access to SUD care is based on its view that alcohol and other drug use behaviors exist on a continuum, and that certain patterns of alcohol and other drug use place some individuals at high risk of developing medical and social problems and possibly abuse or dependence. The discussion here focuses on the use of legal substances (i.e., alcohol, controlled substances prescribed by a clinician) since the use of illicit substances (when detected) prompts separation proceedings.

Addressing access to brief intervention and treatment for alcohol and other drug use is a complex undertaking. Access includes both the *availability* of services and the use of *appropriate* modalities and types of services at the appropriate times. As described in Chapter 5, contemporary substance use treatment systems include frequent screening, brief counseling, brief interventions in primary care settings, a focus on client-centered motivational interviewing, multiple entry points to treatment, pharmacotherapies that reduce cravings and maintain functioning, outpatient counseling, intensive outpatient programs, residential treatment when needed, and continuous contact with counseling professionals after an intense period of treatment. Modalities of care utilize evidence-based environmental, psychosocial, and medication interventions. The standard of practice in modern SUD treatment no longer relies on inpatient hospital services, except for the most medically complex patients. Continuity and duration of ambulatory services are more important than the provision of care in residential settings (IOM, 2006).

Aday and Andersen (1974) developed a health services framework with which to examine access to medical treatment. Subsequent investigators modified this framework to assess access to services for alcohol and other drug use disorders (Hser et al., 1997; Weisner and Matzger, 2002; Weisner and Schmidt, 2001). The Aday and Andersen (1974) model addresses barriers and facilitators to access using three domains: (1) predisposing, (2) enabling, and (3) need. The *predisposing* domain consists of individual and social facilitators and barriers. Individual factors are intrinsic characteristics that describe the propensity of individuals to use health services. Social factors include marital status, family, and social networks; these are the social contextual characteristics that influence treatment seeking. In the substance abuse field, social networks are distinguished by whether they include individuals who are influences for not using versus using substances, as well as treatment seeking versus nonseeking. The *enabling* domain consists of structural/financial and environmental factors. Structural/financial facilitators are similar to those for general health care and include the supply and availability of treatment and the types of treatment and medications available. The *need* domain includes the severity of alcohol and other drug use and comorbid mental health or medical problems.

Barriers to Access in the Military

Barriers to accessing care for SUDs can be environmental, structural, social, and/or cultural. Environmental factors, such as pressure or mandates to enter treatment, sanctions, perceptions about the effectiveness of treatment, and stigma, are unique to the behavioral health field, particularly the addiction field, and more apparent in the military than the civilian sector. Civilian individuals frequently enter SUD treatment as a result of legal, welfare, employment, or family pressures or even mandates (Weisner, 1990). The same is true in the military; most service members are assessed for the need for treatment only after receiving sanctions for a substance-related incident (e.g., driving under the influence [DUI], assault) or other drug-related infraction (e.g., possession of an illegal substance) or upon having their substance use discovered through random drug testing. Thus, the most important structural factors in the military are (1) policies that treat alcohol misuse and other drug use as a discipline problem, (2) heavy reliance on deterrence (i.e., random drug testing) as the prevention approach, and (3) the lack of a standard medical protocol for early identification and brief intervention before a disciplinary infraction occurs.

While many predisposing and need-related facilitators of and barriers to treatment in the military are similar to those in the civilian sector, some structural and environmental barriers are unique to the military—notably, policies and practices that result in random drug testing as a primary pathway to obtaining substance use services. First, random drug testing technology is not applicable to alcohol or to designer drugs not yet classified as illicit (e.g., Spice, bath salts). Second, civilian best practice addresses unhealthy substance use as a preventable and treatable health problem with known risk factors and offers screening and interventions as part of primary care services early and confidentially. Military practices, however, focus on abuse and dependence and view alcohol and other drug misuse as violations of the code of conduct and/or as criminal activities (e.g., DUI, drug possession). The emergence of unhealthy use before a negative incident occurs generally goes unnoticed or is ignored by medical programs, and while policy describes the need for prevention programs (see Chapter 6), the vast majority of resources are used for random drug testing.

The lack of distinction between unbecoming conduct and a medical problem creates an environment in which engaging in substance use treatment has counterproductive implications. Receiving treatment, even when treatment causes the desired change in behavior, is perceived as resulting in a negative career trajectory. Consequently, active duty service members (ADSMs) are not highly motivated to enter treatment. This can have the unanticipated effect on public safety of having service members continue to perform critical tasks without having had their problems treated. Indeed, during its information gathering meetings and site visits, the committee heard from military treatment professionals that many service members perceive alcohol treatment as a threat to their military career and consequently avoid it.[1] The vignette in Box 7-1 describes an extreme, but not isolated, case in which early intervention with a soldier could have occurred. A random drug test in 2007 identified cocaine use, but 15 subsequent tests were negative. In 2011, the soldier self-enrolled in an Army Substance Abuse Program (ASAP), fully 8 years after a problem was first indicated.

In keeping with the military's occupational health model, policy DODI 1010.6 requires that a service member's commander be notified of and involved in treatment for an SUD (DoD, 1985, 5.2.2.2.3) (see also Chapter 6). This policy applies whether the soldier self-refers, is referred by a medical provider, or is referred by the commander, and regardless of whether an alcohol-related incident or positive drug test is involved. Branch policies impose similar requirements. For example, the Army policy for self-referral states:

> The ASAP counselor will contact the unit commander and coordinate the Soldier's formal referral using DA Form 8003, which will be signed by the

[1]Personal communication, Vladimir Nacev, Ph.D., Resilience and Prevention Directorate Defense Centers of Excellence, and Col. John J. Stasinos, M.D., Department of the Army, Office of the Surgeon General, May 4, 2011.

BOX 7-1
A Soldier's Untreated Substance Abuse

A soldier tested positive for cocaine use in March 2007. He was not required to enroll in an Army Substance Abuse Program (ASAP), and a Department of the Army (DA) Form 4833 was never completed. Despite 15 negative urinalyses from October 2008 to January 2011, the soldier self-enrolled in ASAP during the latter month for cocaine abuse and marijuana and alcohol dependence. He was apprehended in July 2011 for assault consummated by a battery (domestic violence). A review of law enforcement databases revealed that these offenses were not the beginning of the soldier's high-risk behavior; he had been arrested for criminal trespass, marijuana possession, and evading arrest in 2003—3 years prior to his delayed-entry report date of August 2006. While driving on an interstate highway in November 2011, the soldier collided with another vehicle, killing himself and two others instantly and injuring two others. He had been driving the wrong way on the highway for 2 miles at the time of the accident. While drug and toxicology results are unknown at this time, packets of Spice were found in the soldier's vehicle.

SOURCE: U.S. Army, 2012a, p. 30.

> unit commander and be annotated as a self referral. The commander will be a part of the rehabilitation program and, as a member of the Rehabilitation Team, will be directly involved in the decision of whether rehabilitation is required. (U.S. Army, 2009, p. 49)

These policies are necessary to ensure that service members are medically ready for deployment. Yet in current practice, the lack of confidential treatment even for problems that do not meet symptom criteria for substance abuse or dependence has the perverse effect of leaving many treatable problems undetected and unaddressed. As a consequence, several Army reviews have identified a high proportion of suicides, other deaths, and other negative consequences associated with untreated SUDs (U.S. Army, 2010, 2012a).

Historically, military policy has not addressed unhealthy alcohol use or reliance on prescribed medications that places service members at high risk for SUDs and later disciplinary problems. The military now has programs that provide screening and early intervention for depression and posttraumatic stress disorder (PTSD) within primary care settings to reduce the stigma associated with seeking treatment for these conditions, but it has not adopted similar early-intervention, best-practice models for discussion of emerging alcohol and other drug use problems. In civilian model programs, early intervention for problem alcohol and other drug use is available in medical care settings such as primary care and emergency rooms. A new DoD policy, DODI 64990.08, may permit further development of brief interventions in military health care settings for service members at risk of alcohol use problems.

Military culture also creates unique environmental barriers to accessing care for SUDs. First, there are few to no public health interventions targeting the medical consequences of heavy drinking. Military personnel are warned of the severe sanctions for alcohol or other substance use that results in a formal consequence (e.g., DUI); the message conveyed, however, is that heavy drinking is acceptable, while getting into trouble because of the behavior is not (Burnett-Zeigler et al., 2011; Gibbs et al., 2011; Skidmore and Roy, 2011). Second, alcohol and other drugs often are misused as coping mechanisms for combat and other stress and hence recognized on a continuum of medical problems (Stokes et al., 2003), yet many service members are treated for long periods of time with opioid pain medications and with controlled drugs to treat anxiety and sleep disorders. These high prescribing rates introduce opportunities for abuse and addiction. The epidemiological data reviewed in Chapter 2 suggest that abuse of prescribed medications used to treat pain and/or sleep disorders is growing.

While tracking of medications dispensed to individuals in theater is problematic (Defense Health Board, 2011), recent changes have been made to prescribing practices for certain controlled medications. For instance, ALARACT (All Army Activities) 062/2011 (U.S. Army Surgeon General, 2011) requires an expiration date on prescribed opioid medications. However, the U.S. Central Command (CENTCOM) Formulary still permits the dispensing of 180 days of certain controlled substances for personnel who are deployed to war zones (DoD, 2012). These prescribing practices are intended to address the potential lack of access to medications currently being taken by the service member in a deployed environment. Yet these practices may contribute to physical dependence on such medications in several ways—being given for a longer duration than is clinically prudent, given without close medical supervision, and given to service members who have alcohol or other substance use problems. The Army has made recent policy changes aimed at reducing the prescribing of medications with the potential for abuse and addiction (U.S. Army, 2012b; U.S. Army Surgeon General, 2011). As discussed in Chapter 6, DoD instated stricter limits on the length of prescription for controlled drugs in May 2012 (see **Finding 6-1**).

In both civilian and military populations, a frequently cited barrier to seeking treatment for SUDs is denial of the need for treatment among those who need it (SAMHSA, 2011). Respondents to the National Survey on Drug Use and Health described their problem as not severe enough to require treatment and said that drug use helped them cope with difficult emotional stimuli. Among military personnel returning from Iraq and Afghanistan stigma was the most frequently cited reason for not seeking treatment for combat-related mental health conditions, including substance use (Dickstein et al., 2010; Hoge et al., 2004; Stecker et al., 2007). Self-stigma was particularly poignant; it is difficult for military personnel to identify themselves as being in need. In the civilian sector, one role for brief advice from a clinician to patients is to address their perception of their need for treatment and the value of the available treatment, but this function currently does not exist in the military.

Role of Primary Care and Medical Treatment

The military's medical care model for first-line treatment of behavioral health problems that are commonly comorbid with SUDs (e.g., PTSD, depression, suicidal ideation and attempts) now relies heavily on detection and treatment in primary care. Screening for behavioral health conditions, including hazardous alcohol use, occurs routinely in primary care. As discussed in Chapter 5, evidence-based approaches of brief advice, early intervention, and referral to treatment when needed through models commonly known as screening, brief intervention, and referral to treatment (SBIRT) should be a focus of the full continuum of care. Medical protocols for SBIRT, however, have not been implemented in military primary care programs. The Department of Veterans Affairs (VA) health care system, in contrast, routinely screens for alcohol use problems and offers brief intervention and referral to further treatment if needed. As discussed in Chapter 6, the screening and brief intervention elements of the *VA/DoD Clinical Practice Guideline for Management of Substance Use Disorders* (VA and DoD, 2009) have not been implemented in the Military Health System. Primary care also is the setting in which pharmaceutical therapy for SUDs often takes place in the commercial sector. The lack of primary care protocols in the military (and policy restrictions on the use of some of these effective medication therapies) is an additional barrier to accessing SUD care and is inconsistent with the *VA/DoD Clinical Practice Guideline* (VA and DoD, 2009). Consequently, primary care is the single largest missed opportunity in the military for early and confidential identification of alcohol and other drug misuse. DoD and branch policies and practices currently do not provide for early and confidential interventions for alcohol and other drug misuse. The committee perceives this to be a tremendous barrier to service members' accessing SUD care.

CARE AVAILABILITY, ACCESS, AND UTILIZATION IN THE DIRECT CARE SYSTEM

DoD policy requires the armed services to provide alcohol and drug abuse prevention and treatment services for active duty personnel as part of medical readiness and risk reduction programs (DoD, 1997). The committee's analysis of access to and utilization of SUD care is organized by branch and includes a review of the size of the population addressed, the number of SUD programs available, and the data on utilization of services. The content of these programs is described in Chapter 6 and Appendix D, and the SUD workforce is described in Chapter 8. This section concludes with a brief review of DoD-wide programs that may enhance access to SUD care.

There is no uniform DoD reporting system for monitoring the number of detected alcohol incidents or drug-positive events, the number of referrals for assessment or treatment, or the number enrolled in direct care treatment programs. In response to queries from the committee, each branch provided data using its own definitions, formats, and level of detail. In its site visits, the committee learned that program directors at installations can query their own systems, but do not have access to system-wide data for judging overall trends or monitoring the transfer of patients from one military installation to another. The committee does not know how any methodological differences in data reporting among branches or components affected the information provided for this study.

One major challenge confronting all branches with respect to access to SUD care is that troops are dispersed across the United States, abroad in permanent stations on U.S. territories (e.g., Guam), and in foreign nations (e.g., Japan, Germany). Family members also reside with troops where there are permanent stations. Thus, access to SUD care for these troops and family members may require travel to obtain the appropriate level of clinical care. The capacity for integrated behavioral health services in areas outside the continental United States may be particularly important when SUD programs are not available.

Air Force

The Air Force provides SUD services through 75 Alcohol and Drug Abuse Prevention and Treatment (ADAPT) programs, one at each military treatment facility, with nearly 400 counselors. None of these programs offer inpatient, medically supervised treatment or residential, medically monitored treatment. The Air Force has one ADAPT program that provides intensive outpatient care at Andrews Air Force Base. The Air Force Medical Operations Agency reported to the committee that during fiscal year (FY) 2010, 736 service members self-referred to ADAPT, and 4,644 members

TABLE 7-1 Utilization of Alcohol and Drug Abuse Prevention and Treatment (ADAPT) Services by Active Duty Air Force Personnel*

FY 2006	FY 2007	FY 2008	FY 2009	FY 2010
1,559	1,429	1,532	1,565	1,454

*Includes 11-26 persons treated annually who were activated National Guard/Reserve members.
SOURCE: Personal communication, Lt. Col. Mark Oordt, Air Force Medical Operations Agency, October 25, 2011.

were referred by Command.[2] Beyond self-referrals and Command referrals, individuals can be referred to ADAPT by medical providers, but these represent the smallest proportion of referrals. Table 7-1 displays the number of active duty patients enrolled in treatment at ADAPT clinics from FY 2006 to FY 2010. Comparing the number of self- and Command referrals in FY 2010 (5,380) with the number of patients enrolled in treatment in the same period (1,454) suggests that most referrals do not lead to enrollment in treatment. As described in Chapter 6, most individuals receiving services through ADAPT do not meet diagnostic criteria for enrollment in formal treatment and instead are enrolled in alcohol brief counseling as an indicated prevention measure. The number treated has not increased over time and was lower in FY 2010 than in 3 of the 4 prior years.

Army

ASAPs are located within the Army Installation Management Command (IMCOM) as part of the human resources program (see also Chapter 6). The Army has 38 ASAPs, which typically offer American Society of Addiction Medicine (ASAM) Level I (outpatient service) care to military personnel and have insufficient capacity to serve family members with SUDs.[3] Army regulations require all ASAP counselors to have a master's or doctoral degree in psychology or social work. The ASAP counselors may be uniquely positioned to provide integrated care for service members with SUDs and comorbid mental health problems, but are credentialed only to treat SUDs and are not authorized to treat mental health problems. Military personnel who require partial hospitalization or inpatient care or have a dual diagnosis often are referred by Command to the civilian provider network. The extent to which ASAP programs are available to Army per-

[2]Personal communication, Lt. Col. Mark Oordt, Air Force Medical Operations Agency, October 25, 2011.

[3]Personal communication, Les McFarling, Ph.D., Army Center for Substance Abuse Programs, March 30, 2011.

sonnel and family members permanently stationed abroad or in states and territories outside the continental United States is unclear.

The TRICARE Management Activity (TMA) Section 596 report indicated that the Army operates only one inpatient (around-the-clock), medically monitored treatment program, which has 20 inpatient beds (DoD, 2011b, p. 30). During a site visit to Fort Belvoir Community Hospital (see Appendix A for the committee's site visit agenda), the committee learned of a newly opened residential treatment center (ASAM Level III rehabilitation program for SUDs under the Army's Medical Command). This medical service will provide care for ADSMs from all branches of the military and eligible retirees. When referred by Command, personnel may be treated in any SUD facility under a budget agreement with the military treatment facility commander; that is, commanders are not restricted to the use of TRICARE network Substance Use Disorder Rehabilitation Facilities (SUDRFs) (SUDRFs are discussed later in the purchased care section).[4]

With regard to in-theater care, a report of the Army Inspector General concludes that there is a lack of compliance with Army alcohol and other drug use policy when units are in a combat operation environment (U.S. Army, 2008). CENTCOM General Order #1 states that alcohol consumption and possession and drug use are illegal in the combat environment (United States Central Command, 2006). AR 600-85 requires that deployed commanders maintain a drug deterrence program. However, the Inspector General's report finds little compliance with these directives and notes that DoD provides no guidance on how to implement the policies and no professional staff to implement them and monitor compliance, and that the rotation of personnel in and out of the combat environment inhibits enforcement. In efforts to deter drug use during deployment, the Army updated AR 600-85 in 2009 to include new language meant to increase random drug testing in theater. To increase access to screening and treatment in theater, the Army is in the first phase of rolling out an Expeditionary Substance Abuse Program to provide SUD services during deployment, primarily through telephone contact with in-theater providers.[5]

Table 7-2 shows data on initial referrals of Army ADSMs to ASAP for FY 2006-2010. The Army Center for Substance Abuse Programs (ACSAP) reported to the committee that for FY 2010, 3,401 distinct active duty individuals enrolled in treatment as self-referrals, and 10,968 enrolled because of Command referral.[6] ACSAP provided detailed information on

[4] Personal communication, John Sparks, TRICARE Regional Office-West, March 18, 2012.

[5] Personal communication, Col. John J. Stasinos, M.D., Department of the Army, Office of the Surgeon General, March 15, 2012.

[6] Personal communication, Les McFarling, Ph.D., Army Center for Substance Abuse Programs, January 13, 2012.

TABLE 7-2 Army Active Duty Initial Referrals to the Army Substance Abuse Program (ASAP)

	FY 2006	FY 2007	FY 2008	FY 2009	FY 2010
Initial Referrals	16,826	18,164	20,316	23,044	23,093

SOURCE: Personal communication, Les McFarling, Ph.D., Army Center for Substance Abuse Programs, January 13, 2012.

gender, rank, and substance of initial referral (not treatment enrollment) for 23,093 individuals in FY 2010. According to a recent Army analysis (U.S. Army, 2012a), 52 percent of soldiers referred to treatment for either alcohol or other drug problems enrolled in outpatient treatment. Many who are referred to ASAP for assessment fail to meet diagnostic criteria for SUDs and are enrolled in the Army's indicated prevention course Prime for Life (described in Appendix D). When soldiers are enrolled in treatment at ASAP, they do not always complete the program for various reasons (e.g., deployments). The rates of successful completion of rehabilitation from FY 2001 to FY 2010 averaged 66 percent for alcohol and 47 percent for other drugs (U.S. Army, 2012a).

The committee also received data on treatment enrollment in ASAP. Figure 7-1 shows the data received on the distribution of enrollment ranked

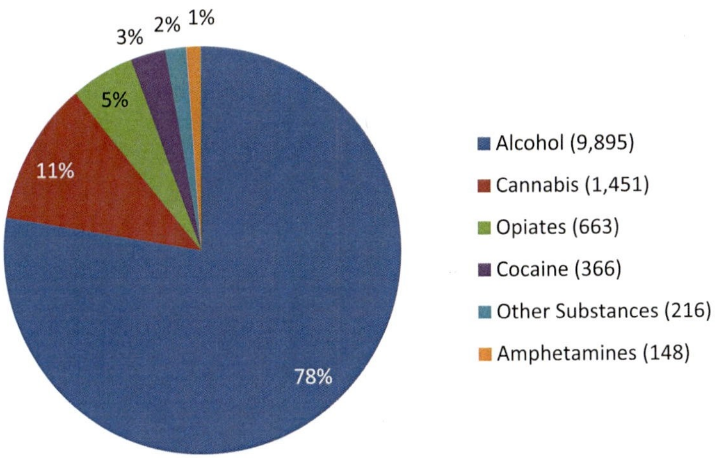

FIGURE 7-1 Number of Army Substance Abuse Program (ASAP) treatment enrollments by substance of abuse for fiscal year 2010. Enrollments for the following substances were small in number and not included in the above chart: inhalants (52), sedatives (41), hallucinogens (41), and PCP (3).
SOURCE: Personal communication, Les McFarling, Ph.D., Army Center for Substance Abuse Programs, March 30, 2011.

by type of substance in FY 2010. Alcohol misuse is the single largest reason for enrollment, followed by use of cannabis and opiates.

According to data for FY 2006-2010, women averaged about 10 percent of initial referrals to ASAP, but this proportion declined during the period from 11.2 percent to 9.8 percent. Officers represented only 2.5 percent of total initial referrals in FY 2010, but the number of officer referrals increased by 63 percent between FY 2006 and FY 2010. In FY 2010, alcohol accounted for 75 percent of initial ASAP referrals (n = 17,343/23,093), cannabis for 12.5 percent, opioids for 4.3 percent, cocaine for 3.0 percent, and all other substances for under 2 percent each. Opioid referrals grew from 238 in FY 2006 to 992 in 2010, an increase of more than 300 percent, while alcohol referrals and total referrals grew by around 36 percent. The total number of referrals to ASAP in FY 2008-2010 was about 37 percent higher than in FY 2006-2007.

ACSAP also provided counts of drug positives and alcohol violations as indicators of the need for SUD care for FY 2010. The number of persons testing positive for nonprescription illicit drugs was 6,597 (7.7 percent women), for prescription drugs was 1,363 (8.1 percent women), with a DUI charge was 4,609 (5.4 percent women), and with another alcohol-related charge was 3,439 (8.0 percent women).[7] If these counts represented distinct individuals, the sum would be 16,008 Army men and women with detected alcohol or other drug use, a number smaller than the total number of ASAP referrals (23,093). Undoubtedly, however, some individuals are double counted across classes of drug positives and alcohol violations, so the detected need would sum to fewer than 16,008 distinct individuals. Nonetheless, the number of persons with detected alcohol violations and other drug use is undoubtedly much smaller than the total need for care.

Military personnel assigned to Warrior Transition Units (WTUs) have an elevated risk for SUDs, making access to SUD care an important priority for this population. The Department of the Army established the Warrior Transition Command, which manages care for 18,000 soldiers and veterans annually. Army staff includes nearly 4,000 squad leaders, platoon sergeants, nurse case managers, and other support staff who coordinate care in WTUs and community-based WTUs (U.S. Army, 2011). On a site visit to Dewitt Army Hospital, the committee learned of a newly opened comorbid disorders program located within the Warrior Transition Brigade at Fort Belvoir. This program was designed to provide treatment for soldiers with complex mental health needs. For the committee's review and assessment of this program, see Appendix D.

[7] Personal communication, Les McFarling, Ph.D., Army Center for Substance Abuse Programs, January 13, 2012.

Navy

The Navy operates 38 Substance Abuse Rehabilitation Programs (SARPs), including 35 outpatient-only programs (in Bahrain, Guam, Italy, Japan, and Spain) and 3 U.S.-based SARPs that provide intensive inpatient care (34 days of around-the-clock counseling and rehabilitation services) (DoD, 2011b, p. 30). The largest SARPs are based at San Diego, California, and Norfolk, Virginia. The three SARPs that provide outpatient, intensive outpatient/partial hospitalization, and residential/inpatient care treat patients with comorbid disorders. All SARP patients participate in continuing care following discharge through the Navy's My Ongoing Recovery Experience (MORE) program, a Web-based and telephone program contracted through Hazelden that provides continuing care and support services to patients leaving treatment at a SARP. Marines treated at Navy SARPs may also enroll in the Navy MORE program.

The Navy Alcohol and Drug Abuse Program Office reported to the committee that 4,566 Navy patients and 5,535 Marines were treated at Navy SARPs in 2010, and 625 of the Navy patients were self-referrals.[8] Table 7-3 displays the number of active duty Navy and Marine personnel who were enrolled in treatment at SARPs for FY 2006 through FY 2010 (Marines also are treated in the Service Academy Career Conference [SACC] program, described in the next section). The number of Navy service members treated declined by 2 percent over the period (Marine utilization statistics are discussed in the next section). Nearly all Navy members were treated for alcohol use disorders, as indicated by the substance recorded at initial referral (data not shown). No other drug (opiates, cocaine, amphetamines, cannabis) was responsible for more than 17 treatment admissions in 2010, and "other drugs" accounted for a total of 71 treatment admissions. The number of Navy members receiving services for alcohol and cocaine use declined over the period, while the number for other drug types increased. Women increased as a percentage of Navy members with alcohol use disorders from 8 percent to 11 percent in the period FY 2006 to FY 2010, and Navy officers represented 3 percent of those receiving alcohol services in FY 2010.

The Navy also provided counts of drug positives and alcohol violations as indicators of the need for SUD care for FY 2010. The number of persons testing positive for nonprescription illicit drugs was 1,492 (11.1 percent women), for prescription drugs was 292 (11.3 percent women), with a DUI charge was 1,416 (women 6.9 percent), and with another alcohol-related charge was 2,489 (8.2 percent women). In contrast with the Army,

[8] Personal communication, George Aukerman, Navy Alcohol and Drug Abuse Prevention Office, February 15, 2012.

TABLE 7-3 Utilization of Substance Abuse and Rehabilitation Program (SARP) Treatment by Active Duty Navy and Marine Corps Members

	FY 2006	FY 2007	FY 2008	FY 2009	FY 2010
Navy	4,677	4,482	4,076	4,617	4,566
Marines	3,033	2,781	3,402	4,683	5,535
Total SARP	7,710	7,263	7,478	9,300	10,101
% Marines	39.3	38.3	45.5	50.4	54.8

SOURCE: Personal communication, George Aukerman, Navy Alcohol and Drug Abuse Prevention Office, February 15, 2012.

the number of Navy service members needing services for drugs other than alcohol appears to be much smaller than the number identified through drug-positive tests. The number needing services for alcohol appears to be slightly higher than the number with alcohol violations, even if no individuals were counted with both DUI and other alcohol-related charges.

Marine Corps

SACCs are located at 15 Marine installations and are under the direction and authority of the Personnel Command. Of the 15 SACCs, 14 provide outpatient treatment, and 12 provide intensive outpatient treatment. The Marine Corps reported that it attempts to have one counselor for every 2,500 active duty Marines.[9] The Marine and Family Programs Division reported utilization statistics to the committee from the Alcohol and Drug Management Information Tracking System (ADMITS). Of those Marines admitted into substance abuse treatment in FY 2011, 354 self-referred to a SACC, and 2,463 were referred by Command.[9] Table 7-4 displays the total number of active duty Marines who were screened at a SACC, the number that completed the early intervention program (Impact, which is described in Appendix D), and the number that completed outpatient or intensive outpatient treatment provided at a SACC. It is unclear whether the number completing treatment represents the total utilization of SACCs or only those who completed the full treatment course. In the past 5 years, no dependents have been treated at SACCs. Based on information for 2010, the SACCS provided services to 67 percent of persons assessed for treatment need, assuming that the number receiving early intervention does not duplicate any of those completing outpatient or inpatient treatment (Table 7-3). Most of the SACCS have the capacity to provide intensive outpatient services; the service counts provided by the Marine Corps combine intensive and regular outpatient services.

[9]Personal communication, Eric Hollins, Marine and Family Programs Division, October 25, 2011.

TABLE 7-4 Numbers of Active Duty Marines Receiving Substance Abuse Counseling Center (SACC) Screening and Completing Treatment

	FY 2006	FY 2007	FY 2008	FY 2009	FY 2010
Number of Marines screened	7,710	5,794	6,965	6,709	7,201
Completed early intervention	2,714	3,289	3,255	2,974	2,677
Completed outpatient or intensive outpatient treatment	2,144	2,873	2,224	1,974	2,204

SOURCE: Personal communication, Eric Hollins, Marine and Family Programs Division, October 25, 2011.

As discussed earlier, Marines also access care at Navy SARPs if they need higher levels of care than the SACCs offer or if a SACC program is not available at their duty location; Marines' utilization of services at SARPs was presented previously in Table 7-3. In 2010, 5,535 Marines were served by SARPs, a number that increased by 82 percent between FY 2006 and FY 2010. For fully 84 percent of those who accessed services at SARPs, alcohol was reported as the drug of initial referral in 2010. In contrast with the Navy, a substantial number of Marines were treated for use of cannabis (n = 305), opiates (82), cocaine (80), amphetamines (113), and other drugs (312), and admissions for all drugs including alcohol, except cocaine, increased substantially from FY 2006 to FY 2010 (data not shown). When Marines receive services at Navy SARPs, they often are stepping up or down from care provided at their local SACC; therefore, the numbers of Marines receiving services at SACCs and SARPs do not represent distinct individuals.

SUD Care Accessed by Dependents at Military Treatment Facilities

To understand the extent to which family members of ADSMs access SUD care at military treatment facilities, the committee reviewed data provided by TMA. Table 7-5 presents the numbers and rates[10] of dependents of ADSMs receiving SUD care at military treatment facilities. The utilization data are based on diagnosis (excluding nicotine) and may include stays for detoxification only. These data demonstrate that it is rare for dependents of ADSMs to receive SUD care in military treatment facilities. Utilization of SUD care in the purchased care sector by dependents of ADSMs is discussed later in this chapter.

The committee also received information on direct care services for all ADSMs and active duty family members (ADFMs) with an SUD diagno-

[10] See Table 7-8 for the total average number of beneficiaries by region, which was used to calculate rates.

TABLE 7-5 Numbers of Dependent Beneficiaries Receiving SUD Care in Military Treatment Facilities by TRICARE Region (FY 2010)

	West (N per 1,000)	North (N per 1,000)	South (N per 1,000)
Active Duty Family Member (ADFM) Adult Dependent Beneficiaries (ages 18 and over)			
Alcohol diagnoses	317 (1.0)	249 (0.8)	483 (1.7)
Other drug diagnoses	325 (1.0)	267 (0.8)	508 (1.8)
Both alcohol and other drug diagnoses	23 (0.1)	9 (0.0)	30 (0.1)
ADFM Child Dependent Beneficiaries (ages 14-17)			
Alcohol diagnoses	11 (0.2)	9 (0.1)	35 (0.5)
Other drug diagnoses	70 (1.2)	39 (0.6)	78 (1.2)
Both alcohol and other drug diagnoses	3 (0.1)	1 (0.0)	3 (0.0)

SOURCE: Personal communication, Frank Lee, TRICARE Management Activity, March 2, 2012.

sis, combined across branches. These data for FY 2010 show the relative reliance on different service modalities (detoxification, emergency, inpatient, and outpatient) at military treatment facilities and are summarized in Table 7-6. It should be noted that some portion of the outpatient services was not for SUD treatment but for ancillary services associated with the other three categories, as evidenced by the settings of care listed in the footnote to the table. In other words, it would be incorrect to assume that 54,043 ADSMs received outpatient counseling for SUDs, as some of the

TABLE 7-6 Number of Active Duty Service Members (ADSMs) and Active Duty Family Members (ADFMs) Who Accessed Care at Military Treatment Facilities for an SUD Diagnosis by Type of Service (FY 2010)

Type of Care	ADSM (N per 1,000)	ADFM (18 and over) (N per 1,000)	ADFM (14-17) (N per 1,000)
Detoxification	661 (0.4)	16 (0.0)	0 (0.0)
Emergency	2,815 (1.9)	677 (0.7)	83 (0.4)
Inpatient	1,845 (1.2)	192 (0.2)	9 (0.0)
Outpatient*	54,043 (35.5)	2,347 (2.6)	207 (1.1)

*Outpatient care includes care provided in any of the following settings: emergency room-hospital, hospital-outpatient, office, ambulance-land, independent laboratory, psychiatric facility (partial hospitalization), community mental health center, nonresidential substance abuse treatment facility, other unlisted facility, urgent care facility, home, public health clinic, rural health clinic, ambulatory surgical center, nursing facility, comprehensive outpatient rehabilitation facility, federally qualified health center, group home, ambulance-air or water, Indian Health Service freestanding facility, prison/correctional facility, assisted living facility, military treatment facility, independent clinic.

SOURCE: Personal communication, Greg Woskow, TRICARE Management Activity, June 8, 2012.

outpatient services counted may have been associated with and already counted under detoxification, emergency department, and inpatient care.

DoD-Wide Programs

DoD contracts for programs to expand ready access to behavioral health services and encourage help seeking among military personnel and their dependents. Some of these programs, such as Military OneSource and the Yellow Ribbon Campaign, are described in Appendix D. These programs generally provide nonmedical support services and are considered an important pathway to SUD care and other services. Box 7-2 describes these programs. The committee did not receive data on the volume of calls, consultations, or referrals provided. A recent RAND report found that many of these programs do not track outcome data and have largely not been evaluated (Weinick et al., 2011).

Summary of Access in the Direct Care System

The Air Force and Navy reported serving fewer individuals in their SUD programs in FY 2010 than in most prior years. In contrast, the Army and Marine Corps reported increased treatment admissions. No branch had high rates of self-referral to treatment, a finding consistent with the literature reviewed and reports provided to the committee regarding the perceived stigma of receiving treatment. The Army reported the highest proportion of self-referrals, which likely is due to the Confidential Alcohol Treatment and Education Pilot (CATEP) program (described in Appendix D) and contributed to higher than average utilization rates.

The committee identified a number of aspects of the organization of care, policies on and barriers to care, and other differences in how service members gain access to care that appear to contribute to some of this variation. The branches are remarkably diverse in the types of SUD programs they offer and the pathways to care they provide. Despite a far greater number of troops relative to other branches, the Army operates ASAPs at only 38 locations and acknowledges it has been trying to expand its numbers of licensed social workers and psychologists. Many Army installations have no ASAP, and the Army operates only one 20-bed medically monitored inpatient unit for SUD care. In contrast, the Navy operates 38 SARP outpatient programs, including 5 programs in foreign countries and 3 SARP inpatient/outpatient hospital units. SARPs actually provide services to more Marine Corps than Navy patients even though the number of Navy service members far exceeds the number of Marines. The Navy's SARP integrates care for comorbid mental health issues and is managed by Medical Command. The Marine SACCs are at 15 installations, and nearly

BOX 7-2
DoD-Wide Programs to Increase Access to Behavioral Health Care Services and Encourage Help Seeking

Military OneSource	Offers nonclinical counseling free of charge to active duty, Reserve, and National Guard service members and their families. Does not report to military commanders.
Military Pathways	Provides free and anonymous self-assessments online and over the telephone, with the goal of reducing stigma, raising awareness, and encouraging referrals to DoD or VA services.
Military Family Life Consultants	Invited by commanders to specific military installations with impending deployment or return of troops. The contractor provides licensed mental health professionals who offer confidential nonclinical counseling outside of the health care system, with no documentation in the medical record being required.
Defense Center of Excellence Outreach Center	Provides 24/7 behavioral health support for a range of psychological health needs and traumatic brain injury.
Yellow Ribbon Program	Offers reintegration events hosted by National Guard units at 30, 60, and 90 days after return. Guard members, Reservists, and family members receive information on, among other things, accessing services for medical, mental health, and substance abuse problems. Military family life consultants may be invited as a resource.

all offer both intensive and regular outpatient services, unlike the facilities of the other branches. The worldwide geographic distribution of service members may also explain some of the variation in SUD care. All branches cannot feasibly operate and staff specialty SUD programs in all locations. In the United States, the military can supplement its direct care SUD programs with purchased services offered by local VHA programs or TRICARE providers (discussed below). These options do not exist, by and large, for the numerous service members and family members who are stationed overseas or on ships or submarines or are deployed.

The committee's ability to make direct comparisons across branches or even within branches across years was hampered because of variations in the way data on SUD care are maintained and reported. These variations were magnified when the committee attempted to integrate direct care information with data from the TRICARE regional offices and purchased care programs. This exercise illustrated the complex nature of obtaining and reviewing data on the scope of the SUD problem DoD-wide and understanding the full extent of services offered to address alcohol and other drug problems, both emerging and chronic. The lack of consistent reporting of data DoD-wide appears to hamper monitoring of how well current programs meet the needs of the armed forces. At its various site visits, the committee learned that different systems store different types of data. Program managers must therefore consult multiple systems (typically at least one managed by Installation Command and one managed by Medical Command, and sometimes more) either weekly or daily to monitor the progress from positive drug tests to Command referrals to substance use assessment.

CARE AVAILABILITY, ACCESS, AND UTILIZATION IN THE VETERANS HEALTH ADMINISTRATION

The VHA also provides SUD services for ADSMs, and the committee reviewed the access standards for SUD care specified in *Uniform Mental Health Services in VA Medical Centers and Clinics* (VHA Handbook 1160.01) (VA, 2008). These standards are consistent with the National Voluntary Consensus Standards for Treatment of Substance Use Conditions endorsed by the National Quality Forum (NQF, 2007) and with the *VA/DoD Clinical Practice Guideline for Management of Substance Use Disorders* (VA and DoD, 2009). Box 7-3 lists the services that must be readily available, according to the access standards, to all patients when clinically indicated.

Currently, the VA provides care for SUDs in 108 intensive outpatient clinics, 237 residential rehabilitation treatment programs (8,443 operational beds), and 63 programs with specialty SUD bed sections (1,658 beds). The Opioid Treatment Program includes 32 in-house and 22 contracted off-site formally approved and regulated opioid treatment clinics using methadone or buprenorphine as agonist medications. Office-based buprenorphine treatment is offered by "waivered" physicians in nonspecialty settings (e.g., primary care), including 132 medical centers and 109 community clinics. The VA provides an SUD-PTSD specialist funded at each facility to promote integrated care. These specialists provide treatment based on the *VA/DoD Clinical Practice Guideline for Management of Substance Use Disorders* (VA and DoD, 2009) and its counterpart for PTSD

BOX 7-3
Access Standards of the Veterans Health Administration for SUD Care

Treatment Modalities

- Pharmacotherapy and psychosocial interventions are important treatment options for veterans with SUDs.
- Regardless of the particular intervention chosen, motivational interviewing style must be used during therapeutic encounters with patients, and the common elements of effective interventions must be emphasized.

Screening and Brief Intervention

- At least annual screening must be provided across settings for alcohol misuse and tobacco use.
- Targeted case finding must be conducted for use of illicit drugs or misuse of prescription or over-the-counter agents.
- Further assessments must be performed to determine the level of misuse and to establish a diagnosis.
- Referral to treatment must be offered for those with dependence.
- All providers must systematically promote the initiation of treatment and ongoing engagement in care for patients with SUDs.

Other Program Standards

- Appointments for follow-up treatment must be provided within 1 week of completion of medically supervised withdrawal management.

(VA and DoD, 2010).[11] A recent Government Accountability Office (GAO) (2011b) study concluded that in general, the VA service delivery system is comprehensive, but the actual provision of specialty services varies among VA facilities. Starting in 2004, VA medical facilities became authorized TRICARE providers and expanded the SUD continuum of care available to certain ADSMs living near one of these facilities (DoD, 2011b). TMA reported to the committee, however, that few ADSMs accessed VA treatment through TRICARE during 2011 (West Region = 15, North Region = 77, and South Region = 18).[12]

As members of the National Guard and Reserves are not eligible for direct care unless activated (i.e., placed on federal orders for deployment

[11] Personal communication, Daniel Kivlahan, Department of Veterans Affairs, November 16, 2011.

[12] Personal communication, Frank Lee, TRICARE Management Activity, March 2, 2012.

- Intensive substance use treatment programs must be available for all veterans who require them to establish early remission from an SUD.
- Multiple (at least two) empirically validated psychosocial interventions must be available for all patients with SUDs who need them, whether psychosocial intervention is the primary treatment or an adjunctive component of a coordinated program that includes pharmacotherapy.
- Pharmacotherapy with approved, appropriately regulated opioid agonists (e.g., buprenorphine or methadone) must be available to all patients diagnosed with opioid dependence for whom it is indicated and for whom there are no medical contraindications in addition to, and directly linked with, psychosocial treatment and support.
- If agonist treatment is contraindicated or not acceptable, antagonist medication (e.g., naltrexone) must be available and considered for use when needed.
- Patients with an SUD must be offered long-term management for that disorder and any other coexisting psychiatric and general medical conditions. The patient's condition must be monitored in an ongoing manner, and care must be modified, as appropriate, in response to changes in the patient's clinical status.

SOURCE: VHA Handbook 1160.01 (VA, 2008).

or another contingency order), VA health care is a relatively new source of care for these personnel returning from deployments to Operation Enduring Freedom (OEF) and Operation Iraqi Freedom (OIF) (38 U.S.C. § 1710[a], 38 CFR §§ 17.36, 17.38 [2009]). ADSMs discharged from service also have new eligibility. Specifically, this recent policy change states that

> any veteran who has served in a combat theater after November 11, 1998, including OEF/OIF veterans, and who was discharged or released from active service on or after January 28, 2003, has up to 5 years from the date of the veteran's most recent discharge or release from active duty service to enroll in VA's health care system and receive VA health care services.[13]

[13] National Defense Authorization Act of 2008, Public Law 110-181, 110th Congress (January 28, 2008).

The nature of the need and demand for SUD treatment may differ for reserve and active duty component service members, although their role in the recent conflicts has been equally prominent. Reserve component citizen soldiers may transition repeatedly throughout their military career from active duty to civilian status. The Guard and Reserve forces are recognized as indispensable and integral parts of the nation's defense. In the Army, in particular, the total size of the reserve component was approximately equal to that of the active duty component in FY 2010-2011, and in recent history, its size exceeded that of the active duty component (see Chapter 2).

A GAO (2011b) analysis examined mental health services in the VHA system and utilization of the services among OEF/OIF veterans. GAO estimated that there are 2.6 million living veterans from the OEF/OIF era (12 percent of all living veterans). OIF/OEF veterans accounted for 12 percent (n = 139,167) of veterans who received mental health services in FY 2010 and 10 percent (n = 36,797) of veterans treated for an SUD.[14] Thus, among VA recipients of SUD services, OIF/OEF veterans' use of mental health services is high; OEF/OIF veterans receive mental health care at a higher rate (38 percent) than all other veterans (28 percent) (GAO, 2011b).

The VHA provided the utilization data presented in Table 7-7. VA SUD services are offered in both specialty and primary care settings. The patient numbers shown in Table 7-7 are for veterans, including members of the National Guard and Reserves who have been demobilized from active duty but not released from service; in other words, they may be called to another deployment and return to active duty status. The percent change in diagnosed individuals over the last four quarters shows a clear increase in incidence. Table 7-8 presents data on VA SUD services provided to OEF/OIF/Operation New Dawn (OND) veterans, separating out care provided to those who were ADSMs and those who were members of the National Guard and Reserves in FY 2006-2010. The 4.6-fold increase in numbers treated for SUDs during the 5-year reporting period suggests that the VA has become an important source of SUD treatment services for the armed forces.

CARE AVAILABILITY, ACCESS, AND UTILIZATION IN THE PURCHASED CARE SYSTEM

Under the TRICARE insurance plans, network and non-network providers deliver services for SUD care in civilian-operated settings (purchased

[14] A veteran was counted as having a mental health condition if, at any point in the fiscal year, his or her medical record indicated at least two outpatient encounters with any mental health diagnosis (with at least one encounter having a primary mental health diagnosis) or an inpatient stay in which the veteran had any mental health diagnosis.

TABLE 7-7 Substance Use Disorders of Operation Iraqi Freedom (OIF)/ Operation Enduring Freedom (OEF)/Operation New Dawn (OND) Veterans in Department of Veterans Affairs Programs, 2002-2012

	Number (Cumulative from 1st Quarter FY 2002)	% Change Over Most Recent 4 Quarters for Which Data Are Available
Total OIF/OEF/OND patients with behavioral health disorder	404,060	
Alcohol abuse (ICD 305.0)	49,793	26.6
Alcohol dependence syndrome (ICD 303)	46,753	29.8
Nonalcohol abuse of drugs (ICD 305.2-9)	32,908	33.7
Drug dependence (ICD 304)	24,550	34.7

NOTE: ICD = International Classification of Diseases.
SOURCE: Personal communication, Daniel Kivlahan, Department of Veterans Affairs, July 3, 2012.

TABLE 7-8 Number of Operation Iraqi Freedom (OIF)/Operation Enduring Freedom (OEF)/Operation New Dawn (OND) Veterans Treated in Department of Veterans Affairs Programs for an SUD Diagnosis*

	2006	2007	2008	2009	2010
Active duty	4,696	8,272	13,249	19,950	26,440
Guard/Reserves	4,423	6,594	9,576	12,860	16,058
Total	9,119	14,866	22,825	32,810	42,498

*Analysis includes OEF/OIF/OND veterans who accessed the VHA for an inpatient stay or outpatient encounter and had a primary and/or secondary SUD diagnosis.
SOURCE: Personal communication, Barbara Swailes, Department of Veterans Affairs, March 9, 2012.

care) (see Chapter 3). These purchased care settings extend the capability of the Military Health System to treat ADSMs with SUDs and also are reimbursed under the TRICARE benefit for services to ADFMs, retirees and their family members, and certain other civilians.

TRICARE Benefits and Access Standards

The *Code of Federal Regulations* (CFR) 32 199.4 specifies the required TRICARE benefits for SUD care, including emergency and inpatient hospital care for complications of alcohol and drug dependency.[15] In contrast

[15] Title 32: National Defense. Part 199: Civilian Health and Medical Program of the Uniformed Services (CHAMPUS): Basic Program Benefits. 32 C.F.R. § 199.4 (June 27, 2012).

with commercial managed care contracts, TRICARE contractors are not required to have specific SUD care capabilities within their networks.[16] The level of care within a network generally includes detoxification, hospitalization, and partial rehabilitation, and regulations permit detoxification and rehabilitation care with limits. In contrast with the commercial sector, intensive outpatient programs are not a designated level of care in the TRICARE SUD benefit, although commanders have the discretion to purchase such care on a case-by-case basis (TMA, 2008). Also unlike the commercial sector, TRICARE does not reimburse for office-based individual counseling for an SUD unless it is comorbid with a mental health disorder that is the primary diagnosis. TRICARE benefit limits for SUD care are summarized in Box 7-4. These benefit limits are inconsistent both with current standards of care for SUDs based on recent legislation requiring parity of mental health and substance abuse care and other medical services and with requirements in the Patient Protection and Affordable Care Act of 2010 (as discussed in Chapter 4). The benefit coverage for pharmaceutical therapy for SUDs is limited to anticonvulsants, benzodiazepines, and naltrexone during alcohol detoxification and rehabilitation. While opioid detoxification may employ buprenorphine or naloxone, the medications are not covered as maintenance therapies.

The policies that govern access to SUD care (Box 7-4) are described in Chapter 7 of the *TRICARE Operations Manual* (TMA, 2008). Regulations require that all SUD services, including outpatient services, be delivered by an SUDRF. An SUDRF is defined as a Joint Commission–accredited hospital that offers an SUD program or a freestanding Joint Commission–accredited facility. To obtain the designation of an SUDRF, these facilities must be certified as such by KePRO, the quality monitoring contractor for TRICARE (KePRO, 2011). KePRO publishes a monthly listing of all certified mental health facilities on its website; as of June 2012, the listing included just 20 freestanding SUDRFs across the United States with current certification. According to a 2007 report of the DoD Task Force on Mental Health, "38 states have no approved substance abuse residential facility including heavily populous states (e.g., New York, Ohio, Illinois) and states with a large military presence (e.g., Washington, Maryland, Virginia, and Washington, DC)" (DoD, 2007, p. 51). On KePRO's June 2012 mental health facility listing, the only state to have gained an SUDRF since that report was released is Virginia, which now has two such facilities. As a result of the restriction of care to such facilities, SUD services for TRICARE beneficiaries are available neither through most community-based addiction treatment centers nor through licensed independent practitioners who are not affiliated with an SUDRF.

---

[16] Personal communication, John Sparks, TRICARE Regional Office-West, July 19, 2011.

BOX 7-4
TRICARE Policies Governing Access to SUD Care

- Must be obtained in an authorized Substance Use Disorder Rehabilitation Facility (SUDRF).
- For outpatient care in an SUDRF, up to 60 visits are allowed per benefit period; however, office-based individual counseling is limited to cases in which the primary diagnosis is a mental disorder and the SUD a comorbidity.
- Alcohol/chemical dependency counselors are the only category of providers specifically licensed for substance abuse treatment. Alcohol/chemical dependency counselors are not among the "qualified mental health providers" reimbursed by TRICARE.
- Residential (inpatient or partial day)—up to 21 days and 7 days for detoxification.
- Family therapy—up to 15 visits per benefit period.
- Restricted to three treatment benefit episodes in a lifetime (defined as 365 days after the first service regardless of the care used). Emergency department or hospital care is not counted as the start of an episode.
- Coverage is specifically allowed for antabuse, but not for the use of certain medically assisted treatments, including methadone and buprenorphine, as a maintenance program.

SOURCE: *TRICARE Operations Manual* (TMA, 2008, Chapter 7).

The *TRICARE Operations Manual* (TMA, 2008, Chapter 7, section 3) describes the reimbursement and cost sharing for TRICARE beneficiaries (these policies govern medical and behavioral health care generally and are not specific to SUDs). Reimbursement rates can become a barrier to access when they are out of line with rates paid by the majority of health plans. The committee heard testimony that the TRICARE rate-setting method leads to unacceptably low rates for some SUDRFs, diminishing access to care.[17] The TRICARE maximum allowable payment to providers is set equal to the Medicare payment rate. A 2009 reimbursement rate study, not specific to SUDRFs, examined 13 medical specialties, including psychiatry and psychology. Commercial rates were found to be higher than TRICARE reimbursement rates for these specialties in almost all of the geographic market areas analyzed, implying that a facility would be less willing to take

[17] Personal communication, John Sparks, TRICARE Regional Office-West, February 2, 2012.

a new TRICARE patient than a commercially insured patient when space was available (Kennell et al., 2009).

Population at Risk and Utilization of SUD Care

Table 7-9 shows the mean number of beneficiaries by region eligible for care through the TRICARE network. These numbers provide a basis for estimating the total population of beneficiaries eligible for care. Table 7-10 presents the number and rate per 1,000 of beneficiaries receiving SUD care in the purchased care sector (based on diagnosis rather than setting of

TABLE 7-9 Average Number of Beneficiaries by TRICARE Region for Fiscal Year 2010*

	West	North	South
Active duty service members	548,086	532,163	440,337
Active duty family members (ADFMs), aged 18 and over	320,446	318,528	278,445
ADFMs, aged 14 to 17	59,634	68,854	64,573

*Computed as monthly average enrollment in TRICARE Prime across FY 2010.
SOURCE: Personal communication, Frank Lee, TRICARE Management Activity, March 2, 2012.

TABLE 7-10 Number and Rate per 1,000 Beneficiaries Utilizing the Purchased Care Sector for SUD Care, by TRICARE Region (FY 2010)

	West (N per 1,000)	North (N per 1,000)	South (N per 1,000)
Active Duty Service Member Beneficiaries[a]			
Alcohol diagnoses	2,443 (4.5)	1,924 (3.6)	1,808 (4.1)
Other drug diagnoses	676 (1.2)	875 (1.6)	715 (1.6)
Both alcohol and other drug diagnoses	137 (0.2)	160 (0.3)	154 (0.3)
Active Duty Family Member (ADFM) Adult Dependent Beneficiaries[b] **(aged 18 and over)**			
Alcohol diagnoses	1,075 (3.3)	1,252 (3.9)	924 (3.3)
Other drug diagnoses	980 (3.0)	1,640 (5.1)	1,135 (4.0)
Both alcohol and other drug diagnoses	133 (0.4)	158 (0.5)	117 (0.4)
ADFM Child Dependent Beneficiaries[b] **(aged 14-17)**			
Alcohol diagnoses	177 (2.9)	153 (2.2)	79 (1.2)
Other drug diagnoses	283 (4.7)	312 (4.4)	220 (3.3)
Both alcohol and other drug diagnoses	39 (0.6)	20 (0.3)	5 (0.1)

[a]May include a small number of reserve component members enrolled in TRICARE Reserve Select or with transitional benefits.
[b]May include a small number of dependents of reserve component members enrolled in TRICARE Reserve Select or with transitional benefits.
SOURCE: Personal communication, Greg Woskow, TRICARE Management Activity, May 7, 2012.

care) in each region. The utilization data are based on diagnosis (excluding nicotine) and may include stays for detoxification only. In Table 7-9, the total served includes detoxification services, counseling, and rehabilitation in SUDRFs and outside of SUDRFs in network and non-network purchased care facilities. The overall rate of receiving SUD care per 1,000 beneficiaries for adult ADFMs is small in each region when summed across alcohol and other drugs, ranging from 6.7 per 1,000 beneficiaries in the West Region to 9.5 in the North. In the North and South Regions, the number of adults treated for other drug diagnoses exceeds the number treated for alcohol diagnoses. In contrast with adult ADFMs, the utilization rate for ADFM children in the West Region (7.6 per 1,000 beneficiaries) is higher than that in the other regions; all regions had more child beneficiaries receiving services for other drugs than for alcohol.

In all regions, the greatest number of ADSMs received services for an alcohol diagnosis. The rate ranges from 3.6 to 4.5 per 1,000 ADSM beneficiaries. The rate of purchased care services for other drug disorders is very low (1.2-1.6 per 1,000 ADSM beneficiaries). Note that these services are in addition to those of direct care providers; however, it is unknown whether these ADSM individuals were also served by the military program (e.g., for outpatient care or aftercare) and already counted under direct care, or are distinct individuals. Branch policies permit commanders to refer their ADSMs to SUD services that cannot be provided in the direct care system. The TRICARE regional offices assist military commanders in finding the care that is needed. It is unknown whether the ADSMs who received SUD services in these purchased care settings received any coordination of their treatment plan or aftercare by a branch military program as well. It is possible that some of these individuals were at installations without SUD programs.

Table 7-11 presents TRICARE data for FY 2010 on the total days' supply and total number of users of pharmacological SUD treatments for adult ADSMs and ADFMs being treated for alcohol or other drug use disorders. Chapter 5 describes the evidence for use of these medications as best practice for addiction care, and the use of pharmacological treatment is also recommended by the *VA/DoD Clinical Practice Guideline for Management of Substance Use Disorders* (VA and DoD, 2009). In Table 7-11, each medication category includes the total number of individuals who received the medications from military treatment facility, retail, and mail order pharmacies; there may be some duplication across those three categories if an individual filled prescriptions for these medications via multiple pharmacy systems. Additionally, the number of individuals who received pharmacological treatment are not distinct across the medication categories, so some individuals who received multiple medications throughout the course of treatment would be represented multiple times. Therefore,

TABLE 7-11 Medications for Addiction Treatment Given to Active Duty Service Members and Active Duty Family Member Adult Dependent Beneficiaries (aged 18 and over), All Systems of Care (FY 2010)

	Active Duty Service Members		Active Duty Family Members	
Medication	Sum of Days' Supply	No. of Users	Sum of Days' Supply	No. of Users
Antabuse	35,560	605	14,127	214
Buprenorphine	35,966	405	60,718	668
Campral	30,024	619	21,736	343
Methadone	250	6	1,405	20
Naltrexone	54,057	1,034	26,518	371
Vivitrol	956	14	270	3

SOURCE: Personal communication, Greg Woskow, TRICARE Management Activity, May 7, 2012.

the actual number of distinct individuals who received pharmacological treatment is lower than the counts shown.

As the table shows, the single most common medication prescribed for SUD care was naltrexone, with 1,034 ADSM users and 371 ADFM users. The long-acting form of naltrexone (vivitrol) was rarely prescribed, and medications for treatment of opioid addiction (buprenorphine, methadone) were prescribed for only a small number of users, presumably for detoxification as maintenance on these medications is not a covered benefit. When one compares the number of ADSMs diagnosed with alcohol use disorders in Table 7-10 (6,175) with the number who received either naltrexone (1,034, some of which would have been prescribed for alcohol dependence, but some for opioid dependence), antabuse (605), and camparal (619), it is clear that many individuals with alcohol use disorders did not receive medication therapy. Among those diagnosed with drug use disorders (2,900), only 400 were prescribed buprenorphine. It is apparent that the use of these medications is not an integral part of SUD treatment for most individuals despite the evidence for their effectiveness.

Tables 7-12 through 7-15 summarize SUD services by type of facility for the TRICARE North, West, and South Regions. These data were provided by each regional office and thus provide different levels of detail. The committee requested data that were based on analyses of primary SUD diagnoses (excluding nicotine-only diagnoses). Thus, settings that delivered detoxification services or emergency department services associated with alcohol or other drug intoxication would be counted.

Table 7-12 presents the total number of ADSM and ADFM users of SUD care in the purchased care North Region by type of facility and whether the facilities participated in the TRICARE network. These data show that an equal number of ADSMs were treated in network and non-

TABLE 7-12 Number of Beneficiaries Receiving SUD Care by Type of Purchased Care Facility, North Region (FY 2010)

Setting	Active Duty Service Members	Active Duty Family Members (Adult and Child)
Network freestanding SUDRF	688	359
Network hospital-based SUDRF	552	234
SUDRF Total	**1,240 (50%)**	**593 (36%)**
Non-network provider	557	494
Other network provider	685	574
Non-SUDRF Total	**1,242 (50%)**	**1,068 (64%)**

NOTE: SUDRF = Substance Use Disorder Rehabilitation Facility.
SOURCE: Personal communication, Marie L. Mentor, TRICARE Management Activity, February 27, 2012.

network SUD facilities, and that many more ADFMs were treated in non-network than in network facilities. From these data, it is clear that ADSM beneficiaries were equally likely to receive some alcohol or other drug care in non-SUDRF facilities and SUDRFs, and that ADFM beneficiaries were more likely to receive care in non-SUDRF facilities. Non-SUDRF facilities include hospitals that offer SUD care but do not have certification from KePRO as an SUDRF. Of beneficiaries who received care from a SUDRF, 40 percent or more received it in a hospital-based rather than a freestanding facility.

Table 7-13 presents the total numbers of ADSMs, ADFM spouses, and ADFM children receiving inpatient and outpatient SUD care in the West Region in both network and non-network facilities. These data demonstrate that among all beneficiary groups, the vast majority received inpatient rather than outpatient services. The West Region had a different pattern from the North Region in that the majority of SUD care was provided in network facilities.

Table 7-14 presents the number of ADSM, ADFM adult, and ADFM child beneficiaries receiving SUD care in freestanding or hospital SUDRFs. The South Region data suggest there is some capacity to treat child dependents for SUD care in that network. The majority of care again was provided in hospital-based rather than freestanding SUDRFs.

To examine further what types of care are being provided in different settings, the committee reviewed additional data from TMA on the numbers of beneficiaries whose claims were selected based on diagnosis and classified by setting as detoxification, emergency, inpatient, and outpatient service for SUDs. Table 7-15 displays the services associated with an SUD diagnosis provided in purchased care settings, along with the rates of use

TABLE 7-13 Number of Beneficiaries Receiving SUD Care by Type of Purchased Care Facility, West Region (FY 2010)

Setting	Active Duty Service Members	Active Duty Family Members (Aged 18 and Over)	Active Duty Family Members (Aged 14-17)
Inpatient: non-network	238	148	15
Inpatient: network	852	465	55
Total Inpatient	**1,090 (80%)**	**613 (90.5%)**	**70 (98.6%)**
Outpatient: non-network	59	8	0
Outpatient: network	214	56	1
Total Outpatient	**273 (20%)**	**64 (9.5%)**	**1 (1.4%)**
Totals	1,363	677	71
Network total	1,066 (78.2%)	156 (23.0%)	56 (78.9%)[a]
Non-network total	297 (21.8%)	521 (77.0%)	15 (21.1%)[b]

[a]All but one are inpatient.
[b]All are inpatient.
SOURCE: Personal communication, Frank Lee, TRICARE Management Activity, March 2, 2012.

TABLE 7-14 Number of Beneficiaries Receiving SUD Care by Type of Purchased Care Facility, South Region (FY 2010)

Setting	Active Duty Service Members	Active Duty Family Members (Aged 18 and Over)	Active Duty Family Members (Aged 14-17)
Freestanding SUDRF	283 (20.4%)	186 (30.8%)	53 (36.6%)
Inpatient other network	1,102 (79.6%)	417 (69.2%)	92 (63.4%)
Total	1,385	603	145

NOTE: SUDRF = Substance Use Disorder Rehabilitation Facility.
SOURCE: Personal communication, Frank Lee, TRICARE Management Activity, March 2, 2012.

per 1,000 beneficiaries. Note that Table 7-6 presented earlier in the section on direct care and Table 7-15 may include some duplication if beneficiaries had claims for care in both military treatment facilities and purchased care settings during the year. Table 7-6 also shows that the rate of use of direct care for ADFMs was very low—well under 1 per 1,000 beneficiaries—in all settings but outpatient care and for both adult and child dependents. Furthermore, the outpatient setting includes, to an unknown extent, ancillary services associated with detoxification, emergency, or inpatient care (as indicated by the footnote to Table 7-6); thus the 2,347 adults and 207 youth may not all have received outpatient counseling services. It is clear that military treatment facilities have limited capacity to provide SUD ser-

TABLE 7-15 Number of Beneficiaries with Claims in Purchased Care Settings, by Type of SUD Care (FY 2010)

Type of Care	Active Duty Service Members (n per 1,000)	Active Duty Family Members (Aged 18 and Over) (n per 1,000)	Active Duty Family Members (Aged 14-17) (n per 1,000)
Detoxification			
Institutional SUDRF	229 (0.2)	192 (0.2)	4 (0.02)
Professional SUDRF	293 (0.2)	313 (0.3)	0 (0.0)
Other setting	1,269 (0.8)	897 (1.0)	21 (0.1)
Emergency			
Institutional SUDRF	0 (0.0)	0 (0.0)	0 (0.0)
Professional SUDRF	34 (0.02)	49 (0.05)	5 (0.02)
Other setting	2,752 (1.8)	2,796 (3.0)	411 (2.1)
Inpatient			
Institutional SUDRF	413 (0.3)	260 (0.3)	7 (0.03)
Professional SUDRF	52 (0.03)	62 (0.1)	3 (0.02)
Other setting	3,235 (2.1)	1,834 (2.0)	212 (1.1)
Outpatient*			
Institutional SUDRF	0 (0.0)	0 (0.0)	0 (0.0)
Professional SUDRF	1,208 (0.8)	563 (0.6)	68 (0.4)
Other setting	7,716 (5.1)	6,160 (6.7)	1,025 (5.3)

NOTE: SUDRF = substance use disorder rehabilitation facility.
*Outpatient care includes care provided in any of the following settings: emergency room-hospital, hospital-outpatient, office, ambulance-land, independent laboratory, psychiatric facility (partial hospitalization), community mental health center, nonresidential substance abuse treatment facility, other unlisted facility, urgent care facility, home, public health clinic, rural health clinic, ambulatory surgical center, nursing facility, comprehensive outpatient rehabilitation facility, federally qualified health center, group home, ambulance-air or water, Indian Health Service freestanding facility, prison/correctional facility, assisted living facility, military treatment facility, independent clinic.
SOURCE: Personal communication, Greg Woskow, TRICARE Management Activity, June 8, 2012.

vices for ADFMs—hence the importance of the TRICARE purchased care program. This implies that family members who receive the bulk of their primary care at a military treatment facility may experience some challenges in having their SUD care integrated with the rest of the care they receive.

The committee received information that the institutional SUDRFs represented in Table 7-15 included hospital-based programs only. The definition of a professional SUDRF the committee received was that it represented a professional service claim emanating from an SUDRF; the committee presumed this denoted outpatient counseling or services within the hospital-based setting for an individual not admitted for overnight care. The committee was told the data system did not permit separate identification of SUDRF overnight or professional services in freestanding facilities.

While the definition of these settings is unclear, the table supports the finding that few individuals received SUD care in the purchased care system. This finding is not surprising for ADSMs given that in most circumstances, they have access to outpatient services at their military treatment facility and potentially to other levels of care if transferred to inpatient programs offered by the larger installations. As noted in Table 7-6, however, typically fewer than 1 per 1,000 ADFMs received SUD care at military treatment facilities. Combined with the low utilization rates in Table 7-15, these data are evidence that ADFMs face strong barriers to gaining access to SUD care in the military treatment facility and purchased care systems combined.

Data in Table 7-15 on the treatment of SUDs in purchased care facilities further demonstrate that network facilities do not provide all the SUD care received by ADFMs. In part, this reflects the finding that non-SUDRF hospitals are used for emergency detoxification and withdrawal from substances. Nevertheless, these data also show that the majority of inpatient SUD care was delivered outside of SUDRFs. The majority of outpatient services were received from settings other than professional SUDRFs. However, some of these outpatient services may represent not counseling services but claims for ancillary services associated with other types of care.

The data in Table 7-15 indicate a substantial underutilization of care but do not directly identify the full range of barriers that contribute to this pattern. It is apparent that there is a lack of capacity in network SUDRFs; in some states there are no SUDRFS, and in most regions the SUDRFs serve only some geographic areas and are too distant to accommodate many military families. Further, all SUDRF care is facility rather than office based as prescribed by regulation, and a substantial or majority portion is in inpatient hospital facilities. This implies a reliance on the highest-cost setting for SUD care, an approach not supported by the evidence (see Chapter 5) and no longer practiced in the commercial insurance sector. According to practice guidelines, most individuals can be treated with outpatient SUD protocols.

Taken together, these data imply an extreme shortage of outpatient settings for SUD care for ADFM adults and children. There may also be a shortage of outpatient services for ADSMs who lack access to SUD programs at their military treatment facility. Outpatient settings are the appropriate setting of care for most individuals with SUD needs, and they are also the setting in which aftercare services should be provided for those individuals who have undergone an inpatient episode of care.

SUMMARY OF KEY FINDINGS

The committee's review of access to SUD care suggests that while services are available for ADSMs through military treatment facilities, the number of patients treated is below epidemiological expectations. Many barriers to care apparently inhibit ADSMs' use of these services. These barriers include the structure and location of the services, a reliance on residential care, and stigma that substantially inhibits help-seeking behavior in a system in which regulation requires the "employer" (i.e., commander) to be informed about any use of services for SUDs. Further, many policies (e.g., drug testing and Command involvement) may actually inhibit rather than enhance access (as intended) to early SUD treatment and discourage screening and brief intervention in medical settings for alcohol use disorders. Additionally, access to care for ADFMs is extremely limited in TRICARE's purchased care system. The barriers to care in the purchased care system appear to be associated with the limitations of benefit coverage (far different from the standard of coverage in the commercial sector) and the requirements for SUDRF certification (again different from the standards used in the commercial sector). The restriction of services to SUDRFs leads to an expensive reliance on geographically distant hospital-based treatment services, a lack of access to existing community-based outpatient and intensive outpatient services, and poor transition from SUDRF care to primary care and from inpatient to outpatient services. Thus, access to prevention and treatment services that incorporate the latest scientific evidence and predominate in the commercial sector (pharmaceutical therapy, individual therapy, intensive outpatient programs), as well as care in individual practitioners' offices and outpatient clinics, is limited in the military largely by an outdated benefit structure, outdated benefit limits, and other unique policy restrictions that appear to be inconsistent with the military's goal of providing the best possible SUD care to those who need it.

Finding 7-1: There is a significant unmet need for SUD care among service members in the U.S. armed forces.

DoD policy mandates a postdeployment assessment and screening interview to identify emerging health problems, and each branch has its own procedures for ensuring the medical fitness or readiness of its personnel for future deployments. These surveillance programs generate data on the impact of deployment and combat on mental health, including concerns about drinking, depression, and stress-related symptoms. Unfortunately, the identification of problems does not lead to referral for treatment. A recent study showed that of 6,669 Army soldiers self-reporting levels of drinking categorized as alcohol misuse, only 0.2 percent received a referral for alcohol services, and only 29 of these were seen within 90 days (Milliken et al., 2007). Figure 2-3 and Table 2-3 in Chapter 2 provide anonymous survey data illustrating high rates of heavy drinking. Given the epidemiological data showing high rates of weekly binge drinking among military personnel (Bray et al., 2009), it is apparent that only a fraction of those needing brief intervention and advice to change their alcohol-related behavior are being reached.

This low level of access is potentially attributable to the lack of a clear public health message and vision within DoD with respect to its characterization of SUDs. A full range of SUD service modalities is not available to ADSMs and their dependents in the direct and purchased care sectors. Particularly lacking are any medical services for prevention and early intervention for emerging problems that could be identified through confidential medical discussions about behaviors that increase the risk of developing alcohol use disorders. While the civilian world has protocols for routine standardized medical screening, brief advice, brief counseling, and brief treatment, the armed forces lack these protocols and practices. Although medical protocols for brief intervention for those individuals who have unhealthy alcohol use are recommended in the *VA/DoD Clinical Practice Guideline for Substance Use Disorders* (VA and DoD, 2009), the committee found little evidence of their actual use. While the estimated unmet need for SUD care is significant, it is of note that DoD is not consistently tracking measures of need for care across service branches. The committee found that DoD has no uniform reporting system for monitoring the number of detected alcohol incidents or drug-positive events, the number of referrals for assessment or treatment, and the number enrolled in direct care treatment programs. While individual service branches have their own databases for collecting this information, it is challenging to understand the extent of the unmet need for care without more consistent data that are incorporated into the medical record.

Finding 7-2: Access to care is restricted by the TRICARE SUD benefit's lack of coverage of intensive outpatient services, office-based outpatient services, and certain evidence-based pharmacotherapies.

The committee concurs with the assessment in DoD's *Comprehensive Plan on Prevention, Diagnosis, and Treatment of Substance Use Disorders and Disposition of Substance Abuse Offenders in the Armed Forces* (*Comprehensive Plan*) that additional inpatient and residential capacity for SUD care is not needed. However, the committee disagrees with that report's conclusion that the full range of SUD services is sufficient. As discussed above, current policies that limit outpatient services to SUDRFs inhibit access to care and require the use of expensive and increasingly antiquated inpatient facilities. In reviewing data provided by TMA, the committee found that much of the SUD care that is claimed under the TRICARE benefit is provided in inpatient settings. A comparison of TRICARE utilization data with commercial practices suggests that TRICARE overemphasizes inpatient settings and underutilizes outpatient care. According to contemporary standards, however, systems of care for SUDs should rely on outpatient services and ongoing management of a potentially chronic disorder, particularly after episodes of inpatient and residential treatment. Both the direct care and TRICARE systems lack the necessary capacity for providing intensive outpatient and outpatient services.

The implication of the current SUDRF regulations is that many SUD services delivered through community-based addiction treatment centers or through licensed independent practitioners are not available to TRICARE beneficiaries. This particularly affects access to SUD care for dependents of service members, who generally are unable to receive care at military treatment facilities since programs give priority to providing care to service members. Continued reliance on a small number of hospital-based and free-standing SUDRFs and limits on the settings and levels of care contribute to overall low utilization rates and to a lack of continuity in care. According to a draft update to the *Comprehensive Plan*, DoD is aware of this issue and is currently drafting policy language for internal review and coordination that would expand the authorized providers of SUD treatment services beyond SUDRFs.[18] While it was outside the charge for this study to investigate total expenditures on SUD services, the committee notes that the current configuration of capacity and the current TRICARE benefit structure promote use of the most expensive settings of care and limit access to lower-cost modalities that are evidence based (outpatient counseling, intensive outpatient, and partial hospitalization modalities). The restriction of care to SUDRFs appears to be unwarranted in the current health care environment, in which the quality of services and the need for different levels of care can be determined using managed care technologies. In reviewing claims data from TMA, the committee also found limited use of pharmacological therapies for alcohol and other drug use disorders, presumably due in part to the TRICARE benefit's limit on the use of maintenance pharmacotherapy for the treatment of SUDs. The committee finds that underutilization of effective treatment modalities such as outpatient therapy and maintenance medications inhibits service members and their dependents from accessing effective and quality care for the treatment of SUDs.

Finding 7-3: Low rates of ADSM self-referral to treatment corroborate reports provided to the committee regarding the perceived stigma of receiving treatment.

When the numbers of self-referrals to treatment are compared with the numbers of Command referrals, it is clear that, across the different

[18] Personal communication, Alfred J. Ozanian, Ph.D., TRICARE Management Activity, June 6, 2012.

branches, the numbers of self-referrals remain very low. The Army had a higher proportion of self-referrals than the other branches in FY 2010, a differential that presumably is due to the Army Confidential Alcohol Treatment and Education Pilot (CATEP) program (described in Chapter 6), which offers confidential treatment. The committee finds that policies requiring Command notification for the treatment of SUDs encourage ADSMs and their families to avoid rather than seek care and therefore contribute to low numbers of self-referrals. These policies also inhibit medical professionals from conducting routine screening for alcohol misuse and identifying those at risk and in need of intervention.

> **Finding 7-4: Access to SUD care is inhibited by various structural, social, and cultural barriers that are specific to military procedures, programs, and policies.**

A primary barrier to access to the full continuum of SUD care for military populations is the body of DoD and branch policies that rely first and foremost on the detection and adjudication of alcohol and other drug misuse as a disciplinary problem. These policies have the effect of attaching negative consequences and stigma to seeking help for alcohol and other drug use disorders (Gibbs et al., 2011). Studies have shown that negative attitudes and beliefs about treatment can inhibit help seeking among service members as well (Kim et al., 2011; Stecker et al., 2007). The mistaken belief that seeking help and receiving treatment are a sign of weakness, coupled with policies that tie negative career consequences to alcohol and other drug misuse, creates a climate that hampers military leaders who wish to help service members, inhibits accurate screening and diagnosis by medical professionals who care for service members, and leads to very low self-referral rates for SUD treatment.

In addition to this inhibition of care seeking, there are key structural barriers to SUD care in the armed forces. Specifically, military treatment facilities lack the full continuum of SUD services. In the smaller installations of some branches, there are no specialty treatment programs. In no branch did the committee learn of early, primary care-based indicated prevention for substance use problems that do not meet clear diagnostic criteria. Furthermore, there are severe practice restrictions on prescribing some pharmaceutical therapies known to support patients who wish to cut down on or abstain from alcohol and other drug use, and utilization data indicate a much lower than anticipated use of pharmaceutical therapies that are approved and known to be efficacious. One explanation for the low use of approved medications is the lack of SUD service delivery through primary care settings. Overall, the committee found a lack of adherence in practice to the *VA/DoD Clinical Practice Guideline* for SUD care (VA and DoD, 2009) that has been acknowledged as the military's standard of care.

The committee's findings are in line with earlier findings of the DoD Task Force on Mental Health (DoD, 2007). That task force observed that the stigma of mental health disorders inhibits military members and their families from seeking care. The task force recommended that DoD (1) develop public education campaigns to dispel this stigma; (2) embed mental health professionals in primary care to improve access and reduce stigma; (3) train officers, families, and medical professionals to value and promote psychological health and services; and (4) recognize that DoD regulations often inhibit seeking care (DoD, 2007). Recommendation 5.1.4.1 specifically addresses the effects of policy on care for alcohol use disorders and suggests policy changes to promote access to care:

> The Department of Defense should promote earlier recognition of alcohol problems to enhance early and appropriate self-referral. If, in the clinician's judgment, alcohol use does not warrant a diagnosis, mechanisms should exist to ensure that service members receive appropriate and non-prejudicial education and preventive services, without a requirement for command notification. Evaluations resulting in a diagnosis of substance abuse or dependence or entry into a formal outpatient or inpatient treatment program should continue to require command notification, as should reporting of alcohol-related incidents. (DoD, 2007, p. 21)

Lack of confidentiality is a persistent barrier to SUD care and appears as well to influence the lack of preventive and early intervention services that may prevent the development of an SUD. To reduce the stigma associated with seeking help for mental health and substance abuse problems, a recent DoD policy (DODI 6490.08) gives health care providers more latitude in responding to requirements for notifying Command of mental health and substance abuse disorders. The policy clarifies that if a service member voluntarily seeks drug and alcohol abuse education and does not meet diagnostic criteria, brief intervention services can be provided without Command notification (DoD, 2011a). The instruction also creates an opportunity for health care providers in primary care or other medical settings to screen for alcohol and other drug misuse and provide patient education. The committee suggests that policies such as DODI 64990.08 are a step toward creating confidential systems of intervention and may encourage help-seeking behavior. If DoD and branch policies do not provide for early and confidential treatment of alcohol and other drug misuse, the committee believes that stigma will remain a significant barrier to SUD services. While these subclinical behaviors are not detected or treated, they may still have a tremendous impact on force health and readiness.

The committee finds that the structure of SUD services in the armed forces also inhibits access to care. For example, DoD's *Comprehensive Plan* acknowledges that "gender-specific programs to treat SUDs in women are not available at MTFs [military treatment facilities]" (DoD, 2011b, p. 26). With increased enrollment of women in the military and their greater exposure to combat deployments, the need for gender-specific services is apparent. Additionally, the availability of SUD treatment at the time it is sought is an important principle in the commercial sector. On-base substance abuse programs typically offer care during duty hours, so participation in treatment programs often necessitates notifying Command to arrange adjustments to one's work schedule. If SUD services were available at times that did not conflict with work duties (perhaps through increased use of telemental health technologies, which could provide care outside of duty hours delivered remotely by a provider in another time zone), ADSMs would have greater opportunities to enter care before the severity of an SUD required leave from their duty assignment. While this conflict with work duties is one rationale for commander involvement on the treatment team, it also is a perceived barrier to seeking care, particularly for career-minded service members who see daytime therapy appointments as often conflicting with job demands (Kim et al., 2011).

Similarly, while waiting to enter treatment or in the middle of treatment, a service member may leave on deployment. Upon return, he or she may receive a different permanent station, which again disrupts continuity of care. The DoD Task Force on Mental Health reached similar findings and recommended that DoD support a full continuum of services for service members and their families, and develop policies that would ensure continuity of care during deployment transitions and transitions between civilian and military providers (DoD, 2007). The task force encouraged DoD to develop strategies for recruiting and retaining mental health professionals, including social workers. The task force's findings raised concern about access to mental health services within TRICARE and led to recommendations for policy revisions to require access to care within 7 days, competitive reimbursement rates, the use of intensive outpatient services and other new approaches to care, and the use of qualified professionals not affiliated with hospitals to provide outpatient services (DoD, 2007).

Finding 7-5: Members of the National Guard and Reserves have no or limited access to SUD care within the Military Health System.

The large numbers of National Guard and Reserve personnel who have been activated and deployed to Iraq and Afghanistan raise concern about specific barriers to SUD care that they confront. Reserve component personnel often are dispersed within the civilian community and often live in rural areas a great distance from a VA medical center. Outreach efforts are challenged by this geographic dispersion, and must rely on innovative delivery methods such as Web-based outreach, telephone counseling, and telemedicine consultation. Additionally, members of the National Guard and Reserves and their families may not qualify for the same services as active duty personnel, who receive comprehensive care through the military's direct care system. Discharge status also can present barriers to accessing care. Reserve component and discharged military personnel must have an honorable or general discharge to be eligible for the special combat veteran medical care at VA health centers. Combat veterans with SUDs are more likely to receive a less than honorable discharge because of disciplinary infractions. Consequently, those in need of care may be ineligible. Furthermore, while family members may be involved in a veteran's care, VA clinics do not provide individual therapy for family members.

An additional system-level barrier is the lack of a "warm hand-off" from the Military Health System to the VA health system (GAO, 2011a). Service members who have substance use or mental health problems must navigate the complex transition from one system to the other on their own. In contrast with physical injuries (which may result in medical treatment within the military, visible impairment, and a disability rating from the VA), the fact that many military personnel do not receive needed substance abuse care while in the military also means they do not receive a formal referral to VA care. Further, the GAO noted that demobilized members of the National Guard and Reserves may be concerned about a perceived lack of confidentiality of their VA medical record with regard to their current military service. The GAO's 2011 report identifies key barriers gleaned from a literature review and corroborates those findings through interviews. The barriers identified in that report included stigma, a lack of understanding or awareness of mental health care, logistical challenges to accessing mental health care, and concerns about the quality or appropriateness of the care provided by the VA (GAO, 2011b).

REFERENCES

Aday, L. A., and R. Andersen. 1974. A framework for the study of access to medical care. *Health Services Research* 9(3):208-220.

Bray, R. M., M. R. Pemberton, L. L. Hourani, M. Witt, K. L. Olmsted, J. M. Brown, B. Weimer, M. E. Lance, M. E. Marsden, and S. Scheffler. 2009. *Department of Defense survey of health related behaviors among active duty military personnel.* Research Triangle Park, NC: RTI International.

Burnett-Zeigler, I., M. Ilgen, M. Valenstein, K. Zivin, L. Gorman, A. Blow, S. Duffy, and S. Chermack. 2011. Prevalence and correlates of alcohol misuse among returning Afghanistan and Iraq veterans. *Addictive Behaviors* 36(8):801-806.

Defense Health Board. 2011. *Psychotropic medication prescription practices and use and complementary and alternative medicine use.* Falls Church, VA: Defense Health Board.

Dickstein, B. D., D. S. Vogt, S. Handa, and B. T. Litz. 2010. Targeting self-stigma in returning military personnel and veterans: A review of intervention strategies. *Military Psychology* 22(2):224-236.

DoD (Department of Defense). 1985. *Instruction 1010.6: Rehabilitation and referral services for alcohol and drug abusers*. Washington, DC: DoD.

DoD. 1997. *Directive 1010.4: Drug and alcohol abuse by DoD personnel*. Washington, DC: DoD.

DoD. 2007. *An achievable vision: Report of the Department of Defense Task Force on Mental Health*. Washington, DC: DoD Task Force on Mental Health.

DoD. 2011a. *Instruction 6490.08: Command notification requirements to dispel stigma in providing mental health care to service members*. Washington, DC: DoD.

DoD. 2011b. *Comprehensive plan on prevention, diagnosis, and treatment of substance use disorders and disposition of substance use offenders in the armed forces*. Washington, DC: Office of the Under Secretary of Defense.

DoD. 2012. *Deployment medication information resource page*. http://pec.ha.osd.mil/pmart/deployment.php (accessed July 11, 2012).

GAO (Government Accountability Office). 2011a. *DoD and VA health care: Action needed to strengthen integration across care coordination and case management programs*. Washington, DC: GAO.

GAO. 2011b. *VA mental health number of veterans receiving care, barriers faced, and efforts to increase access: Report to the ranking member, Committee on Veterans Affairs, House of Representatives*. Washington, DC: GAO.

Gibbs, D. A., K. L. Rae Olmsted, J. M. Brown, and A. M. Clinton-Sherrod. 2011. Dynamics of stigma for alcohol and mental health treatment among Army soldiers. *Military Psychology* 23(1):36-51.

Hoge, C. W., C. A. Castro, S. C. Messer, D. McGurk, D. I. Cotting, and R. L. Koffman. 2004. Combat duty in Iraq and Afghanistan, mental health problems, and barriers to care. *New England Journal of Medicine* 351(1):13-22.

Hser, Y. I., M. D. Anglin, C. Grella, D. Longshore, and M. L. Prendergast. 1997. Drug treatment careers: A conceptual framework and existing research findings. *Journal of Substance Abuse Treatment* 14(6):543-558.

IOM (Institute of Medicine). 2006. *Improving the quality of health care for mental and substance-use conditions: Quality chasm series*. Washington, DC: The National Academies Press.

Kennell, D., A. Brooks, C. Witsberger, L. Cottrell, and K. Caney. 2009. *Comparison of commercial, Medicaid, and TRICARE reimbursement rates for physicians*. Falls Church, VA: Kennell and Associates, Inc.

KePRO. 2011. *TRICARE Quality Monitoring Contractor (TQMC)*. http://tricare.kepro.com (accessed June 13, 2012).

Kim, P. Y., T. W. Britt, R. P. Klocko, L. A. Riviere, and A. B. Adler. 2011. Stigma, negative attitudes about treatment, and utilization of mental health care among soldiers. *Military Psychology* 23(1):65-81.

Milliken, C. S., J. L. Auchterlonie, and C. W. Hoge. 2007. Longitudinal assessment of mental health problems among active and reserve component soldiers returning from the Iraq war. *Journal of the American Medical Association* 298(18):2141-2148.

NQF (National Quality Forum). 2007. *National voluntary consensus standards for the treatment of substance use conditions: Evidence-based treatment practices*. Washington, DC: NQF.

SAMHSA (Substance Abuse and Mental Health Services Administration). 2011. *Results from the 2010 National Survey on Drug Use and Health: Summary of national findings, national survey on drug use and health series*. Rockville, MD: U.S. Department of Health and Human Services, SAMHSA, Center for Behaviorial Health Statistics and Quality.

Skidmore, W. C., and M. Roy. 2011. Practical considerations for addressing substance use disorders in veterans and service members. *Social Work in Health Care* 50(1):85-107.

Stecker, T., J. C. Fortney, F. Hamilton, and I. Ajzen. 2007. An assessment of beliefs about mental health care among veterans who served in Iraq. *Psychiatric Services* 58(10):1358-1361.

Stokes, J. W., H. Greer, and P. S. Hammer. 2003. Combat stress control and force health protection. In *Military preventive medicine: Mobilization and deployment*. Vol. 1, edited by P. W. Kelley. Washington, DC: Office of The Surgeon General, Department of the Army.

TMA (TRICARE Management Activity). 2008. *TRICARE policy manual 6010.57-M*. Falls Church, VA: TMA.

United States Central Command. 2006. *General order number 1B: Prohibited activities for U.S. Department of Defense personnel present within the United States Central Command area of responsibility*. Macdill Air Force Base, FL: Office of the Commander, United States Central Command.

U.S. Army. 2008. *Inspection of the Army's substance abuse program during unit deployments*. Washington, DC: Department of the Army.

U.S. Army. 2009. *Army regulation 600-85: The Army substance abuse program*. http://www.apd.army.mil/pdffiles/r600_85.pdf (accessed July 11, 2012).

U.S. Army. 2010. *Health promotion, risk reduction, and suicide prevention report*. Washington, DC: Army's Suicide Prevention Task Force.

U.S. Army. 2011. *America's Army: At a strategic crossroads*. Washington, DC: Department of the Army.

U.S. Army. 2012a. *Army 2020: Generating health & discipline in the force*. Washington, DC: Department of the Army.

U.S. Army. 2012b. *Policy guidance on the assessment and treatment of post-traumatic stress disorder (PTSD)*. Fort Sam Houston, TX: Department of the Army.

U.S. Army Surgeon General. 2011. *ALARACT 062/2011: Changes to length of authorized duration of controlled substance prescriptions in MEDCOM regulation 40-51*. Washington, DC: Department of the Army.

VA (Department of Veterans Affairs). 2008. *Uniform mental health services in VA medical centers and clinics: VHA handbook 1160.01*. Washington, DC: VA.

VA and DoD. 2009. *VA/DoD clinical practice guideline for management of substance use disorders*. Washington, DC: VA and DoD.

VA and DoD. 2010. *VA/DoD clinical practice guideline for management of post-traumatic stress disorder and acute stress reaction*. Washington, DC: VA and DoD.

Weinick, R. M., E. B. Beckjord, C. M. Farmer, L. T. Martin, E. M. Gillen, J. D. Acosta, M. P. Fisher, J. Garnett, G. C. Gonzalez, T. C. Helmus, L. H. Jaycox, K. A. Reynolds, N. Salcedo, and D. M. Scharf. 2011. *Programs addressing psychological health and traumatic brain injury among U.S. military service members and their families*. Santa Monica, CA: RAND Corporation.

Weisner, C. 1990. Coercion in alcohol treatment. In *Broadening the base of treatment for alcohol problems*. Washington, DC: National Academy Press. Pp. 579-607.

Weisner, C., and H. Matzger. 2002. A prospective study of the factors influencing entry to alcohol and drug treatment. *Journal of Behavioral Health Services and Research* 29(2):126-137.

Weisner, C., and L. A. Schmidt. 2001. Rethinking access to alcohol treatment. In *Recent developments in alcoholism*. Vol. 15, edited by M. Galanter. New York: Kluwer Academic/Plenham. Pp. 107-136.

8

Substance Use Disorder Workforce

The committee's charge included two tasks that required an analysis of the credentials and numbers of physicians and nonphysician health care professionals treating alcohol and other drug use disorders in members of the armed forces:

- analyze the adequacy and appropriateness of current credentials and other requirements for physician and nonphysician health care professionals treating members of the armed forces with substance use disorders (SUDs); and
- address and offer recommendations on evidence-based methodology(ies) for determining the advisable ratio of physician and nonphysician health care providers of care for SUDs to members of the armed forces.

This chapter reviews the regulations and instructions governing addiction counselors and licensed practitioners in each branch of the U.S. armed forces. In response to the committee's queries, the Air Force, Army, Navy, and Marine Corps provided counts of the current counseling and physician workforce credentialed to treat alcohol and other drug use disorders. The committee also examined the Psychological Health Risk-Adjusted Model for Staffing (PHRAMS) to understand the current ratios of physicians and nonphysician health care professionals assigned to treat alcohol and other drug use disorders. The sections that follow describe and critique the addiction workforce in each branch of the U.S. armed forces. The chapter ends with a summary of key findings.

AIR FORCE WORKFORCE

The Air Force's 75 Alcohol and Drug Abuse Prevention and Treatment (ADAPT) programs provide services to prevent and treat SUDs. Located organizationally in the Mental Health Flight, three types of providers staff ADAPT clinics: (1) licensed clinical social workers with master's or doctoral training; (2) licensed clinical psychologists with doctoral training; and (3) certified Air Force alcohol and drug counselors (Oordt, 2011). The certified alcohol and drug counselors make up the primary staffing for the ADAPT programs. They work under the supervision of an ADAPT program manager (a licensed psychologist or social worker). Licensed mental health counselors (military and civilian) assigned to the behavioral health clinic may also work with ADAPT patients, diagnosing, developing and amending treatment plans, and terminating treatment within the scope of their licenses. The number of privileged providers assigned specifically to each ADAPT clinic depends on the local need for services. The Air Force identified two physicians (one civilian internal medicine provider and one civilian anesthesiologist) certified in addiction medicine. In addition, the Air Force reported 144 active duty psychiatrists and 12 civilian psychiatrists; although none was certified in addiction medicine, it was reported that psychiatrists frequently provide treatment services in the ADAPT clinics. Table 8-1 shows the numbers of ADAPT providers by job title.

Air Force Instruction 44-121, section 3.13, indicates that the primary objective of the treatment team for an individual ADAPT client is "to guide the clinical course of treatment of the client after examining all the facts" (U.S. Air Force, 2011b, p. 21). The treatment team meets within 14 days of the initial assessment. It includes (1) the client's unit commander or first sergeant, (2) the client's immediate supervisor, (3) the ADAPT program manager (treatment team leader), (4) alcohol and drug counselors and mental health technicians involved in the case, (5) medical providers if needed, (6) other individuals as needed, and (7) the client (unless deemed clinically inappropriate).

Air Force Instruction 44-121 (U.S. Air Force, 2011b) also establishes guidance for the ADAPT program and implements Air Force Policy Directive 44-172, *Medical Operations for Behavioral Health Flight* (U.S. Air Force, 2011c). The instruction applies to all active duty Air Force members and to members of the Air Force Reserve Command and Air National Guard. Air Force policy requires health care personnel to complete annual training on substance misuse and abuse. According to information provided to the committee by the Air Force, the training begins with a review of the mandate that all suspected or diagnosed cases of substance abuse be referred to mental health services for assessment. The training reviews standardized screening tools (Alcohol Use Disorders Identification Test

TABLE 8-1 Alcohol and Drug Abuse Prevention and Treatment (ADAPT) Workforce

Position	Active Duty	Civilian
Physicians		
Nonpsychiatrist M.D.s certified in addiction medicine	0	2
Psychiatrists certified in addiction medicine	None (144 total psychiatrists)	None (12 total psychiatrists)
Licensed Independent Practitioners		
Licensed clinical psychologists (Ph.D.)	218[a]	117[a]
Licensed clinical social workers	206[a]	216[a]
Counselors		
Certified alcohol and drug counselors (ADCs) II	289[b]	96[b]

[a] The numbers in the table reflect the numbers of providers in each specialty area who are qualified to provide SUD treatment. Providers are authorized and assigned to the Mental Health Flight at each military treatment facility; they are not necessarily assigned to the ADAPT clinic but may provide treatment for SUDs when needed. Some of these providers may currently be assigned outside the military treatment facility setting (e.g., staff jobs, operational roles). At a minimum, each of the 75 Air Force military treatment facilities has one ADAPT program manager and one mental health technician working in the ADAPT program.

[b] Noncertified mental health technicians work in ADAPT while in training for their ADC certification. These individuals are not reflected in the numbers shown.

SOURCE: Personal communication, Lt. Col. Mark Oordt, Air Force Medical Operations Agency, October 25, 2011.

[AUDIT] and Post-Deployment Health Reassessment [PDHRA]) and signs of commonly abused drugs and encompasses diagnosis, intervention, and the mandatory notification of ADAPT (U.S. Air Force, 2011a).

The Air Force Substance Abuse Counselor Certification Board establishes standards for counselor certification. The Air Force is a member of the International Certification and Reciprocity Consortium (IC&RC), which sets standards globally for certified substance abuse counselors (IC&RC, 2012), and adheres to its certification standards. The Air Force Substance Abuse Counselor Certification Board encourages mental health technicians, mental health providers, and nurses providing substance abuse treatment in a military treatment facility to seek certification as a substance abuse counselor (U.S. Air Force, 2010). Licensed practitioners (physicians, psychologists, social workers) are not required to obtain certification but may apply.

The ADAPT program manager in each clinic reviews and approves applicants for certification. Certification applicants must sign the USAF Alcohol and Drug Counselor Code of Ethics and obtain 6 hours of training in counselor ethics provided by the program manager (U.S. Air Force, 2010). Applicants complete formal education, supervised/practical training, and work experience prior to certification (U.S. Air Force, 2010):

- Formal education
  - 270 hours of training in domains for alcohol and other drug counseling
  - required reading (Chapters 1-5 of the *Alcoholics Anonymous Big Book* [Alcoholics Anonymous World Services, 1939])
- Supervised/practical training
  - 300 hours of documented supervision and 10 hours of supervision in each of eight core functions
  - attendance at a minimum of five support groups and five aftercare sessions during a 3-year internship
- Work experience
  - 6,000 hours of supervised work experience (3 years)
  - 1 year of work in the ADAPT program
  - following of one diagnosed patient from the beginning to the end of treatment

The required hours of work experience can be reduced based on education: a 1,000-hour reduction for an associate's degree, 2,000 hours for a bachelor's degree, and 4,000 hours for a master's degree. Certified counselors must complete 60 hours of continuing education every 3 years to maintain certification.

Mental health technicians who are not certified alcohol and drug counselors must have written training plans to develop competence in working with patients with alcohol and other drug use disorders. The training plan must include completion of Qualification Training Package 1, which includes the Twelve Core Functions of Substance Abuse Counselors identified by IC&RC (U.S. Air Force, 2010) (see Box 8-1). Training continues until the technician has the education and field experience required to qualify for certification and pass the oral and written certification exams.

ADAPT program managers are licensed psychologists or social workers who in many cases function as the sole licensed independent practitioner for the ADAPT clinic. There are no formal requirements for the ADAPT program manager to have specialty training in providing care for SUDs. The ADAPT program manager "coordinates clinic resources to provide effective education, identification, assessment and treatment programs as well as coordinates with the Resiliency Element (RE) to provide prevention programs" (U.S. Air Force, 2011b, p. 7). He/she is also responsible for budget management, workload reporting, coordination with off-base resources, development and implementation of education programs, assistance in the

BOX 8-1
12 Core Functions of Substance Abuse Counselors

- Screening
- Intake
- Orientation
- Assessment
- Treatment planning
- Counseling (individual, group, and significant others)
- Case management
- Crisis intervention
- Patient education
- Referral
- Reports and record keeping
- Consultation with other professionals with regard to patient treatment/services

SOURCE: U.S. Air Force, 2010.

identification and referral of individuals needing ADAPT services, supervision of nonprivileged personnel, development and tracking of quality improvement metrics, and chairing of treatment team meetings. Additional responsibilities relate to HIV testing requirements; coordination with the Resiliency Element on community referral guidelines; coordination with Air Force Reserve and National Guard members, including ensuring that they receive appropriate services; and provision of monthly status reports on all ADAPT program clients and fitness-for-duty or status recommendations.

ARMY WORKFORCE

AR 600-85 specifies staffing requirements for the Army Substance Abuse Programs (ASAPs). ASAPs operate under the direction of alcohol and drug control officers (ADCOs), who are responsible for staff management and supervision, management of the drug and alcohol testing program, coordination of all risk reduction and prevention services, coordination of and assistance with Command referrals, development of an ASAP staff training plan, evaluation of prevention activities, and preparation and approval of all reports. A prevention coordinator, an employee assistance program coordinator, a drug testing coordinator, a risk reduction program coordinator, a suicide program manager, a clinical director, counselors, clinical consultants, and substance abuse professionals support the ADCO and the delivery of ASAP services. As of February 2012, 63 ADCOs supervised 349 ASAP prevention staff. Table 8-2 shows the number of individuals in nonclinical positions, who generally provide support for prevention and drug testing efforts.

TABLE 8-2 Army Substance Abuse Program (ASAP) Prevention Workforce

Position	Civilian
Alcohol and drug control officers (ADCOs)	63
Risk reduction program coordinators	55
Drug testing coordinators	132
Suicide program managers	34
Prevention coordinators	81
Employee assistance program coordinators	47
Total	412

SOURCE: Personal communication, Les McFarling, Ph.D., Army Center for Substance Abuse Program, February 22, 2012.

Clinical providers must have a master's or doctoral degree in social work, psychology, counseling, or marriage and family therapy from an accredited university and a state-issued independent license. Counselors not licensed as independent practitioners must have a master's degree and a national recognized certification in substance abuse rehabilitation. ASAP requires a minimum of 2 years of sobriety or postrehabilitation experience for counselors in recovery from an SUD. Department of Defense (DoD) regulations require Medical Command (MEDCOM) to continue to credential ASAP clinicians despite the recent relocation of ASAP's clinical services to the Installation Management Command (IMCOM). The credentialing process follows regulations specified in AR 40-68 (*Medical Services: Clinical Quality Management*). Table 8-3 shows the numbers of clinical providers currently assigned to ASAP. As the table indicates, ASAP staffing does not include physicians. Military treatment facilities provide physician support when needed for SUD patients with comorbid conditions, including suicidality, posttraumatic stress disorder (PTSD), and traumatic brain injury, and those requiring medication assistance. The committee heard testimony that as of May 2011, the staffing rate for the ASAP clinics was just 66 percent.[1] During 2011, the Army made substantial efforts to recruit and retain ASAP practitioners, but there were too few applicants who met the Army's counselor requirements, and ASAPs continue to be understaffed.

NAVY WORKFORCE

Navy Instruction 5350-4D (U.S. Navy, 2009) specifies the operation of the Navy's alcohol and drug abuse prevention and control programs. Bureau of Medicine (BUMED) Instruction 5353.4A operationalizes the

[1]Personal communication, Col. John Stasinos, M.D., Addiction Medicine Consultant for the Army Office of the Surgeon General, May 3, 2011.

TABLE 8-3 Army Substance Abuse Program (ASAP) Clinical Workforce as of December 2011

Position	Civilian
Physicians	
Nonpsychiatrist M.D.s certified in addiction medicine	None authorized for ASAP
Psychiatrists certified in addiction medicine	None authorized for ASAP
Licensed Independent Practitioners	
Licensed clinical psychologists (Ph.D.)	17
Licensed clinical social workers	219
Licensed professional counselors	165
Licensed marriage and family therapists	70
Counselors (not licensed independent practitioners)	
Master's-level substance abuse certification	406
Other	
Social workers (not licensed clinical social workers)	24

SOURCE: Personal communication, Les McFarling, Ph.D., Army Center for Substance Abuse Program, February 22, 2012.

standards for provision of SUD-related treatment services (U.S. Navy, 1999). Substance Abuse Rehabilitation Program (SARP) site directors are usually psychiatrists or doctoral-level psychologists licensed as independent practitioners. Licensed clinical social workers also are available to see patients. Civilian counselors are certified or licensed. Active duty alcohol and drug counselors must be certified or seeking certification. The Navy Certification Board is a member of IC&RC.

Navy instructions are silent on the credentials and training required for alcohol and drug abuse counselors. The Navy School of Health Sciences hosts the Navy Drug and Alcohol Counselor School (NDACS), which provides training to meet certification standards for alcohol and drug counselor I (nonreciprocal), alcohol and drug counselor II, and certified clinical supervisor. NDACS holds five 10-week classes per year. Three weeks of clinical rotation are included in the 10-week course. Course work, based on the Substance Abuse and Mental Health Services Administration (SAMHSA) Center for Substance Abuse Treatment's Treatment Assistance Protocol 21 (SAMHSA, 1998), emphasizes counseling skills, group counseling skills, integration of 12-step programs with treatment, and biopsychosocial and spiritual aspects of substance abuse and dependence. The 1,172-page *Student Guide for Navy Drug and Alcohol Counselor School* (U.S. Navy, 2011) includes a lesson on the pharmacology of alcohol and other drug use and the effects on the brain. The discussion of pharmacological therapy, however, is limited to psychiatric medications and the need to continue taking those medications even when there is peer pressure to stop their use. There is no discussion of medications with Food and Drug Administration approval for treatment of alcohol and opioid use disorders.

In addition, NDACS offers a prevention specialist course to provide education and training on designing and implementing evidence-based SUD prevention programs at the local Command level. The prevention specialists are trained to use the strategies of SAMHSA's Center for Substance Abuse Prevention and to use the National Registry of Evidence-Based Programs and Practices to select prevention programs for their local community (DoD, 2011, Appendix C). Intern counselors must complete 270 hours of alcohol and other drug abuse education (including 3 hours of ethics training) during 7 weeks of the NADCS curriculum and 120 hours (3 weeks) of supervised practical experience to complete the 10-week curriculum. Certified alcohol and drug counselors I must complete 195 hours of supervised practical experience plus 2,000 hours (1 year) of supervised work experience and must pass the alcohol and drug counselor I certification exam. Alcohol and drug counselors II must complete 6 hours of ethics training, 300 hours of supervised practical experience, and 6,000 hours of supervised work experience and must pass the IC&RC alcohol and drug counselor certification exam. Certified clinical supervisors must have alcohol and drug counselor II certification plus 30 hours of clinical supervision training, 10,000 hours of work experience, and 4,000 hours of supervision experience and must pass the IC&RC certified clinical supervision certification exam. All counselors must have a minimum of 50 hours of supervision per year (1 hour per week). See Table 8-4 for numbers of SARP providers by job title.

TABLE 8-4 Substance Abuse Rehabilitation Program (SARP) Workforce

Position	Active Duty	Civilian	Contractor
Licensed Independent Practitioners			
Licensed clinical social workers		16	1
Licensed clinical psychologists		18	2
Psychiatrists		5	
Counselors			
Substance abuse counselors (alcohol and drug counselors I)	87	11	2
Substance abuse counselors (alcohol and drug counselors II)	39	43	3
Certified prevention specialists		8	

SOURCE: Personal communication, Charles Gould, Naval Bureau of Medicine, March 1, 2012.

The San Diego SARP is the Navy's largest and most intensive SARP, providing both residential and outpatient services.[2] Eleven interdisciplinary teams (substance abuse counselors, senior addiction counselors, licensed providers) can access medical support, a psychiatrist, and specialized mental health providers. A family counselor, recreation therapists, a creative art therapist, case managers, and chaplain support also are available. The residential staff includes 13.5 licensed providers (2 active duty), 2.5 recreation therapists, 36 alcohol and drug counselors (13 active duty), 14 administrative staff, and 14 medical staff. The outpatient staff includes 4 licensed providers (1 active duty), 16 alcohol and drug counselors (8 active duty), and 3 administrative staff. During a site visit, the committee learned that the San Diego SARP was evolving its services to fully address comorbid mental health disorders. The program now meets criteria for a dual-diagnosis enhanced program and has trained its providers in the treatment of comorbid disorders accordingly.

MARINE CORPS WORKFORCE

The Marine Corps operates 15 Substance Abuse Counseling Centers (SACCs), 14 of which have the capability to provide outpatient services. SACCs that do not provide outpatient group therapy are located at smaller installations and generally provide one-on-one counseling or refer to an outside agency. The Marine Corps transitioned to a civilian workforce for its SACCs to improve service delivery and allow for uniformity and stability while returning Marines to their primary military occupational specialty. The SACCs include both treatment and prevention staff. Counselors, directors, and medical officers implement and coordinate screening, assessment, and treatment services. Alcohol abuse prevention specialists and drug demand reduction coordinators have lead responsibility for prevention activities. Substance abuse control officers (SACOs), discussed further below, work closely with SACCs to facilitate Command referrals for screening and to supervise and implement annual drug screening. Alcohol abuse prevention specialists must complete certification as a prevention specialist within 180 days of assignment. They conduct annual assessments of alcohol abuse prevention needs, including a risk assessment, and develop annual alcohol abuse prevention plans. They also provide a monthly train-the-trainers course—Building Alcohol Skills Intervention Curriculum (BASIC)—to support alcohol abuse prevention (see Appendix D for further review of BASIC). Drug demand reduction coordinators assess needs for drug abuse prevention (which includes performing a risk assess-

[2]Personal communication, CAPT Mary K. Rusher, M.D., Substance Abuse Rehabilitation Program Department Head, Naval Medical Center San Diego, March 1, 2012.

ment) and develop an annual prevention plan with measurable objectives. They also provide education on illicit and prescription drugs.

Civilian certified substance abuse counselors screen, assess, and counsel patients and draft treatment plans under the supervision of the SACC director and SACC medical officer. Counselors enter patient data into the Alcohol and Drug Management Information Tracking System (ADMITS). The SACC director is responsible for the overall SACC operation and the accuracy of data entered into the ADMITS database, consistent with Marine Corps Order 5300.17. Directors are certified as clinical supervisors and as alcohol and drug counselors. Directors provide individual and group counseling when counselors are unavailable. SACC directors report to the director of behavioral health programs. A medical officer (physician or clinical psychologist credentialed and privileged through the Naval hospital) assigned to a local military treatment facility makes formal diagnoses, approves individualized treatment plans, authorizes changes in treatment plans, and makes discharge decisions. Each Command has an assigned SACO who provides technical assistance to that commander and education to the Marines on prevention of substance abuse and the related Marine Corps policies. SACOs also are responsible for urinalysis screening and act as the liaison between the Command and the SACC. As part of their training, SACOs attend a mandatory 40-hour course that provides an overview of their duties and responsibilities.

Staffing ratios for each SACC are determined by installation commanders based on need and other factors. The ratio is typically 1 counselor per 2,500 active duty Marines. Table 8-5 shows the numbers of providers by job title that the Marine Corps reported to the committee. The Marine Corps is assessing the feasibility of amending credentialing requirements to include licensed professional counselors and licensed clinical social workers as licensed independent practitioners.

Marine Corps Order 5300.17 requires that certified counselors staff SACCs but is otherwise silent on training and qualification. Because the Marine Corps hires certified or licensed practitioners, it no longer uses

TABLE 8-5 Substance Abuse Counseling Center (SACC) Workforce

Position	Civilian
Substance abuse counseling directors	10
Substance abuse counselors (alcohol and drug counselor I)	7
Substance abuse counselors (alcohol and drug counselor II)	56
Drug demand reduction coordinators	23
Certified prevention specialists	8

SOURCE: Personal communication, Charles Gould, Naval Bureau of Medicine, March 1, 2012, and Eric Hollins, Marine and Family Programs Division, October 25, 2011.

NDACS for counselor certification. The school continues to provide training for certified clinical supervisor and prevention certifications.

DoD EFFORTS TO REVIEW STAFFING REQUIREMENTS

The committee determined early on in its deliberations that while its statement of task called for providing "recommendations on evidence-based methodology(ies) for determining the advisable ratio of physician and nonphysician health care providers of care for SUDs to members of the armed forces," doing so would require information and use of DoD's data systems that were unavailable to the committee. The committee determined that appropriate staffing ratios can be determined only with a thorough understanding and knowledge of the health needs of the population in question and access to health data records. Because DoD recently developed and implemented a model that takes into account the psychological health needs of its population and estimates psychological staffing requirements, the committee deemed it most helpful to review this existing model and examine whether the ratios related to SUDs are adequate.

The impetus for the development of a staffing model began when DoD's Mental Health Task Force reviewed the resources available to support psychological health among service members and their families. The task force concluded that funding and personnel were insufficient "to adequately support the psychological health of service members and their families in times of peace and conflict" (DoD, 2007, p. 41). In response to the task force's recommendations for increased staffing for a full continuum of psychological care within the Military Health System and the TRICARE purchased care system, the Office of the Assistant Secretary of Defense for Health Affairs contracted for the development of a risk-adjusted population-based model for psychological health staff. The resulting PHRAMS model defines psychological health services and needs broadly to include prevention services, diagnosis and treatment of mental health conditions, and behavioral and psychological health issues not defined as mental health conditions (Harris and Marr, 2011).

PHRAMS forecasts staffing requirements to meet the estimated annual need by type of provider. Need is estimated on the basis of longitudinal trends in service utilization by condition type and adjusted for underutilization. The model includes a risk adjustment for recent deployment history; need varies by the number, length, and recency of deployments based on service utilization data. "PHRAMS includes all encounters reported in the direct care professional encounters or purchased care non-institutional MDR [Military Health System Data Repository] files regardless of what type of provider it was with, what clinical setting (inpatient or outpatient) it occurred in, or what sector (direct or purchased care) it was delivered in—as long as the encounter was psychological health in nature" (Harris and Marr, 2011, p. 17). More specifically, the total staffing requirement is the sum of encounter-based plus non-encounter-based staffing requirements. The encounter-based staffing requirement is based on the estimated number of encounters divided by the productivity expectation. The encounter estimate reflects the population covered in the Defense Health Plan, multiplied by the prevalence rate of the specific psychological health needs, multiplied by the encounter rate. Separate estimates are generated for each risk group and 12 diagnostic groups (see Box 8-2 for details). Non-encounter-based staffing requirements are the sum of enrollee-based requirements, plus structural unit requirements, plus support staff requirements and reflect work requirements in addition to clinical productivity (encounters).

PHRAMS Version 3.0 software is available as a compact disc-based user application plus user's guide. The databases can be updated annually to reflect changing service needs. Soft parameters allow users to modify the proportion of direct versus purchased care at the primary planning unit level, adjust the productivity metrics, change the estimates for underutilization, and alter the distribution of service members projected to fall into the deployment experience categories.

For 2012, PHRAMS estimates that the DoD direct care system requires 146.1 full-time equivalents (FTEs) of counselor time to provide treatment for SUDs. The estimate for the purchased care system is 151.5 FTEs (Harris and Marr, 2011). The estimates increase to 192.7 (direct care) and 227.1 (purchased care) FTEs in 2017. The 2012 staffing requirement estimates for substance abuse counselors vary by branch: Air Force = 6.6 FTEs, Army = 112.9 FTEs, and Navy = 26.6 FTEs (Harris and Marr, 2011). (Requirements for the Marine Corps are largely included in the Navy estimates because the Navy provides clinical services for the Marines.)

The committee notes that these estimates for substance use counselor staffing are far below the current staffing levels. The PHRAMS data appear to be incomplete. The PHRAMS need estimates reflect primarily services that occur in military treatment facilities and are captured in the MDR. Encounters for SUDs that occur in the specialized treatment settings for these disorders (e.g., ADAPT, ASAP, SARP) apparently are not included in the MDR. Moreover, if care occurs under the supervision of licensed practitioners, the encounters are attributed to the type of practitioner supervising the case (e.g., psychologist, social worker).

SUMMARY OF KEY FINDINGS

This chapter has reviewed the workforce standards for health care professionals providing prevention and treatment services for SUDs for

BOX 8-2
Psychological Health Risk-Adjusted Model for Staffing (PHRAMS) Diagnosis and Risk Groups

- Diagnosis Groups
  - Affective psychosis (including major depressive disorder)
  - Nonpsychotic depression
  - Other neurotic disorders
  - Adjustment disorder or acute stress reaction (excluding posttraumatic stress disorder [PTSD])
  - PTSD
  - Psychotic and nonpsychotic substance use
  - Nonpsychotic childhood disorder
  - All other psychotic disorders
  - Psychological health V-codes (excluding Post-Deployment Health Assessment/Reassessment [PDHA/PDHRA])
  - Psychological health V-codes for PDHA/PDHRA
  - Other psychological health not elsewhere classified

- Risk Groups (more than 30,000 unique risk groups)
  - Service (Army, Air Force, Navy, Marines, unknown)
  - Beneficiary category (service member, service family member, all other)
  - Gender (male, female)
  - Age group (under 18, 18-24, 25-44, 45-64, 65 and older)
  - Rank group (junior enlisted, senior enlisted, junior officer, senior officer)
  - Component (active duty, reserve, neither)
  - Enrollment (enrolled in a military treatment facility, enrolled in the purchased care network, not enrolled)
  - Deployment exposure history (never deployed, moderate–not recent deployment, moderate-recent deployment, high–not recent deployment, high-recent deployment, currently deployed)

SOURCE: Harris and Marr, 2011.

members of the armed forces. The committee's analysis of the credentialing and other requirements used by each branch led to findings on the adequacy and appropriateness of these requirements.

Finding 8-1: Credentialing and required training for SUD counselors vary among the branches.

The Air Force, Navy, and Marine Corps rely on certified alcohol and drug counselors, while the Army requires individuals to have graduate training and professional licenses as psychologists, social workers, or counselors. The committee finds that few licensed professionals (physicians, psychiatrists, psychologists, social workers, licensed professional counselors, marriage and family counselors) are available to individuals seeking treatment for SUDs in the U.S. armed forces. Currently, each branch sets requirements for the staffing of its SUD programs; DoD has set forth no overarching guidelines. The result is considerable variability from branch to branch in the size and makeup of the SUD counseling workforce.

The certified counselor specialty emerged in the 1980s because licensed professionals were not trained and had little interest in treating alcohol and other drug use disorders. In 1979, fewer than one in four counselors (22 percent) held a graduate degree (Camp and Kurtz, 1982). Counselor certification is a useful tool for setting minimum standards. Certification standards, however, have not evolved to keep pace with scientific developments and the emergence of evidence-based pharmacological and behavioral therapies for SUDs. Women and men seeking treatment for SUDs are increasingly burdened with comorbid mental health and physical health disorders. In the U.S. military, comorbid posttraumatic stress disorder (PTSD) diagnoses are common. Treatment for comorbid mental health diagnoses is outside the scope of practice for most certified alcohol and drug counselors.

The nation's SUD workforce is evolving in response to the changing needs of the patient population. A 2007 workforce analysis found that 42 percent of counselors and 58 percent of counselor supervisors working within treatment centers participating in the National Drug Abuse Treatment Clinical Trials Network held a master's or doctoral degree; in outpatient treatment settings, moreover, 53 percent of counselors held graduate degrees (McCarty et al., 2007). Nationally, health care reforms are likely to limit the use of unlicensed credentialed counselors. Payers will require independent licensure for counselors providing care for SUDs (McCarty et al., 2009).

Instead of continuing to use a 20th-century workforce to treat SUDs, DoD is challenged to structure and staff treatment services for alcohol and other drug use disorders for the 21st century. As discussed in Appendix F, the emerging model of SUD care uses multidisciplinary treatment teams to create a varied workforce with carefully articulated roles and training. Individuals in recovery provide peer support instead of serving as primary counselors. Certified counselors work under the supervision of licensed practitioners. Treatment plans include evidence-based pharmacological and behavioral therapies, as well as long-term continuing care with peer support. To increase caseloads and enhance productivity, services emphasize outpatient and intensive outpatient modalities, rely on relatively brief intensive group therapy, use computer-assisted cognitive-behavioral techniques, and include long-term support and ongoing recovery monitoring.

The U.S. military needs to begin to reconfigure the workforce providing alcohol and other drug treatment services so that active duty military personnel have the same level of professional care that is afforded to the civilian population (as discussed in Appendix F). The U.S. military also appears to have an increased need for licensed practitioners to support its members with comorbid mental health disorders and SUDs.

Finding 8-2: The SUD counselor training manuals of the Air Force and Navy are dated, do not address the use of evidence-based pharmacological and behavioral therapies, and do not reference the *VA/DoD Clinical Practice Guideline for Management of Substance Use Disorders.*

Chapter 10 of the *Air Force Alcohol and Drug Counselor Certification Handbook* (U.S. Air Force, 2010) outlines knowledge and skill requirements. The listed skills are based on the Model Professional Standards for Counselor Credentialing released in 1984 (Birch and Davis Associates, Inc., 1984). The standards developed under contract for the National Institute on Alcohol Abuse and Alcoholism were crafted to stimulate and support voluntary credentialing efforts (Birch and Davis Associates, Inc., 1984). The standards are obsolete and do not address medication-assisted treatment for alcohol and opioid use disorders, nor do they describe evidence-based behavioral therapies. The Center for Substance Abuse Treatment released an update (Technical Assistance Publication [TAP] 21, *Addiction Counseling Competencies*) in 2008, but it, too, overlooks important developments in the use of pharmacological and behavioral therapies. The next revision of Chapter 10 of the *Air Force Alcohol and Drug Counselor Certification Handbook* should be updated to address the use of evidence-based pharmacological and behavioral therapies. Similarly, NDACS bases its curriculum on the Center for Substance Abuse Treatment's TAP 21, which as noted does not address pharmacological and behavioral therapies for treatment of alcohol and other drug use disorders. An updated curriculum should more fully encompass emerging developments in evidence-based treatments for SUDs. Counselor training in both the Navy and Air Force neglects the *VA/DoD Clinical Practice Guideline for Management of Substance Use Disorders* (VA and DoD, 2009). The *Clinical Practice Guideline*, developed in collaboration between the Department of Veterans Affairs (VA) and DoD, should be a core element of counselor training.

Finding 8-3: Physicians who provide care in military treatment facilities and have received training in addiction medicine or addiction psychiatry are a rarity.

While the current SUD workforce serving the military falls short of meeting the need for SUD services generally, a particular shortfall is that few physicians have received training in addiction medicine or addiction psychiatry. General medical officers and flight surgeons receive minimal instruction in SUDs, yet often are on the front lines of diagnosis, suggesting that these providers should receive additional training to diagnosis and treat alcohol and other drug-related disorders. Beyond specialty training, one opportunity to increase background SUD training among the larger workforce of primary care physicians who provide care to military personnel is for these physicians to have a continuing medical education requirement in screening, brief intervention, and referral to treatment (SBIRT) and SUD treatment. As an example, the American Society of Addiction Medicine (ASAM) offers highly regarded state-of-the-art courses in this area and the Ruth Fox Course for Physicians (which educates doctors on addiction medicine) at its annual conferences. The committee also reviewed a webinar course on SBIRT created by the Defense Centers of Excellence that was offered in January 2012 to DoD providers. The committee finds this effort to train DoD providers in evidence-based practices such as SBIRT a promising step toward building a more knowledgeable workforce; however, the extent to which this course is widely disseminated and whether providers are implementing the practices learned through the webinar are unclear. The committee also learned of an additional effort by the Defense Centers of Excellence to further educate providers in SUDs and their treatment. A toolkit was developed for this purpose and became available for provider use in early 2012. The committee's review of this toolkit revealed that the materials are comprehensive and represent an excellent start toward training providers in best practices for treatment of SUDs. Because the toolkit was developed and released recently, however, the extent of its dissemination and of implementation of the practices at the provider level is unknown.

Finding 8-4: The PHRAMS program is a reasonable start toward determining the quantitative relationship between the need for SUD care and staffing levels.

PHRAMS appears to be a useful tool for assessing staffing needs for care for mental health disorders. The Government Accountability Office noted that the Army, Air Force, and Navy are using PHRAMS to estimate mental health staffing requirements for their budget requests (GAO, 2010). The committee finds that PHRAMS provides an underestimate of the staffing required to address alcohol and other drug use disorders. DoD's *Comprehensive Plan on Prevention, Diagnosis, and Treatment of Substance Use Disorders and Disposition of Substance Use Offenders in the Armed Forces* similarly finds that SUD treatment is in some cases not being counted in the MDR database from which PHRAMS calculates estimates for staffing. PHRAMS therefore requires modification before it can be applied to estimate staffing needs for alcohol and drug counselors (DoD, 2011).

The PHRAMS analysis, however, includes interesting data related to alcohol and drug use treatment needs. During fiscal year (FY) 2010, 10.4 percent of the psychological health encounters in the MDR database were related to "psychotic and nonpsychotic substance use," with a mean of 3.5 encounters among individuals with a substance use encounter (Harris and Marr, 2011). PHRAMS assumes that each substance use patient should receive a mean of 9 encounters. The PHRAMS database (FY 2003 through FY 2010) shows increasing use of psychological health services over the 8-year span and variations by service branch (Harris and Marr, 2011). Based on the trend of increasing encounters and adjusting for underutilization and changes in demographics, PHRAMS estimates an increasing need for services related to SUDs. It should be kept in mind, however, that the PHRAMS FTE estimate reflects only services reported in the MDR database.

The committee's charge included offering recommendations on evidence-based methods for estimating staffing needs to address SUDs. The PHRAMS software appears to include the key variables required for estimating staffing needs, including the ratio of physician and nonphysician health care providers. The underestimated need for counselors to treat SUDs, however, suggests that the parameters for making estimates need substantial modification and that the data used to generate the staffing estimates for SUD treatment may be incomplete. Refinement and complete data are required if PHRAMS is to be used to estimate staffing needs for substance use encounters.

Finding 8-5: All of the branches appear to have shortages of SUD counselors.

The branches all reported shortages of counselors in their SUD programs. The Army was actively recruiting licensed practitioners to staff ASAPs while the committee met. The Navy had unfilled authorized positions. The Air Force and Marine Corps reported minimal staffing levels in their programs as well. It is apparent that the branches have pressing needs for additional qualified counselors to staff their SUD programs.

In both civilian and military programs, recruitment and retention of practitioners skilled in addressing SUDs is an ongoing challenge because the positions have low prestige, offer low salaries, and tend to attract entry-level practitioners. The low prestige reflects the lack of professional training and licensure. Credentialed counselors who are not licensed often are seen as paraprofessionals who are not as skilled or trained as practitioners with graduate training and professional licensure. The stigma of addiction contributes to the low prestige and the view that counselors who treat only alcohol and other drug use disorders are not full professionals. Because much of the SUD workforce lacks graduate training and is unlicensed, the individuals who fill these positions accept low salaries. Low salaries in turn enhance the perception that the positions lack professional status. Staff turnover is a related issue, as industries with lower salary levels tend to have higher levels of turnover. Annual turnover rates in SUD counseling positions approach 25 percent (Eby and Rothrauff-Laschober, 2012). As a result, treatment programs are constantly recruiting and training new staff, who tend to be entry-level and to require more training investment.

The U.S. military faces similar staffing challenges for SUD counselors. While higher salaries and a focus on graduate-trained individuals with professional licensure could help address some of these staffing challenges, the stigma of addiction lingers and makes positions focused on addiction treatment less attractive. Full integration with mental health and primary care services could enhance the professional status and prestige of treating alcohol and other drug use disorders.

Finding 8-6: Each of the military branches could benefit from a better trained and staffed prevention workforce.

While the statement of task for this study did not specifically require an examination of SUD prevention providers, during the course of its review the committee learned that each branch could benefit from improved workforce standards and staffing for SUD prevention as well as treatment.

REFERENCES

Alcoholics Anonymous World Services. 1939. *Alcoholics Anonymous.* New York: Works Publishing, Inc.

Birch and Davis Associates, Inc. 1984. *Development of model professional standards for counselor credentialing* (Vol. 1). Rockville, MD: U.S. Department of Health and Human Services, Public Health Service, Alcohol, Drug Abuse, and Mental Health Administration, National Institute on Alcohol Abuse and Alcoholism.

Camp, J. M., and N. R. Kurtz. 1982. Redirecting manpower for alcoholism treatment. In *Prevention, intervention and treatment: Concerns and models.* Rockville, MD: U.S. Department of Health and Human Services, Public Health Service, Alcohol, Drug Abuse, and Mental Health Administration, National Institute on Alcohol Abuse and Alcoholism. Pp. 371-397.

DoD (Department of Defense). 2007. *An achievable vision: Report of the Department of Defense Task Force on Mental Health.* Washington, DC: DoD Task Force on Mental Health.

DoD. 2011. *Comprehensive plan on prevention, diagnosis, and treatment of substance use disorders and disposition of substance use offenders in the armed forces.* Washington, DC: Office of the Under Secretary of Defense.

Eby, L. T., and T. C. Rothrauff-Laschober. 2012. The relationship between perceptions of organizational functioning and voluntary counselor turnover: A four-wave longitudinal study. *Journal of Substance Abuse Treatment* 42(2):151-158.

GAO (Government Accountability Office). 2010. *Military personnel: Enhanced collaboration and process improvements needed for determining military treatment facility medical personnel requirements.* Washington, DC: U.S. Government Printing Office.

Harris, D. M., and L. M. Marr. 2011. *The Psychological Health Risk-Adjusted Model for Staffing (PHRAMS): Update for version 3.0.* Alexandria, VA: CNA Analysis and Solutions.

IC&RC (International Certification & Reciprocity Consortium). 2012. *Setting global standards for addiction professionals.* http://internationalcredentialing.org (accessed May 28, 2012).

McCarty, D., B. E. Fuller, C. Arfken, M. Miller, E. V. Nunes, E. Edmundson, M. Copersino, A. Floyd, R. Forman, R. Laws, K. M. Magruder, M. Oyama, K. Prather, J. Sindelar, and W. W. Wendt. 2007. Direct care workers in the National Drug Abuse Treatment Clinical Trials Network: Characteristics, opinions, and beliefs. *Psychiatric Services* 58(2):181-190.

McCarty, D., K. J. McConnell, and L. A. Schmidt. 2009. *Policies for the treatment of alcohol and drug use disorders: A research agenda for 2010-2015.* Princeton, NJ: Robert Wood Johnson Foundation.

Oordt, M. 2011. *Air Force substance abuse policies and programs.* Lackland Air Force Base, TX: Air Force Medical Operations Agency.

SAMHSA (Substance Abuse and Mental Health Services Administration). 1998. *Addiction counseling competencies the knowledge, skills, and attitudes of professional practice.* Rockville, MD: U.S. Department of Health and Human Services, Public Health Service, SAMHSA.

U.S. Air Force. 2010. *Air Force alcohol and drug counselor certification handbook.* Washington, DC: Department of the Air Force.

U.S. Air Force. 2011a. *AFMS annual training on substance misuse and abuse for healthcare personnel.* Washington, DC: Department of the Air Force.

U.S. Air Force. 2011b. *Instruction 44-121: Alcohol and Drug Abuse Prevention and Treatment (ADAPT) program.* Washington, DC: Department of the Air Force.

U.S. Air Force. 2011c. *Instruction 44-172: Mental health.* Washington, DC: Department of the Air Force.

U.S. Navy. 1999. *BUMEDINST 5353.4A: Standards for provision of substance related disorder treatment services.* Washington, DC: Bureau of Medicine, Department of the Navy.

U.S. Navy. 2009. *Operation Navy Instruction 5350.4D: Navy alcohol and drug abuse prevention and control.* Washington, DC: Department of the Navy.

U.S. Navy. 2011. *Student guide for Navy Drug and Alcohol Counselor School.* San Diego, CA: Navy Drug and Alcohol Counselor School.

VA (Department of Veterans Affairs) and DoD. 2009. *VA/DoD clinical practice guideline for management of substance use disorders.* Washington, DC: VA and DoD.

9

Conclusions and Recommendations

One of the most important lessons learned in recent years is that we cannot simply deal with health or discipline in isolation; these issues are interrelated and will require interdisciplinary solutions.
—GEN Peter W. Chiarelli, 2012 Army 2020 Report, p. 6

The charge for this study directed the committee to assess the adequacy and availability of and access to services for the prevention, diagnosis, screening, treatment, and ongoing management of substance use disorders (SUDs) for military members and their families (Chapter 1). In response, the committee examined the scope of SUD problems in the military (Chapter 2) and the Military Health System that provides services for military personnel with those problems (Chapter 3); identified modern standards of SUD care (Chapter 4) and best practices from research and practice (Chapter 5); analyzed the SUD-related Department of Defense (DoD) and branch-level SUD policies and programs and compared them with standards of care and best practices (Chapter 6); inventoried access to care for service members, members of the National Guard and Reserves, and military dependents (Chapter 7); and assessed the credentialing and adequacy of staffing for the workforce providing SUD care (Chapter 8). Based on the findings of this comprehensive review, the committee developed conclusions and recommendations designed to enable DoD and the branches to deliver to military members and their families with SUDs the best possible support and care that would be efficient, realistic, up to date, evidence-based, and in conformance with DoD policies. These conclusions and recommendations are presented in this chapter.

The committee recognizes the challenge of managing one of the nation's largest health systems, but notes that the different branches tend to operate their SUD services with minimal direction from and accountability to DoD. Consequently, DoD needs to acknowledge that the current levels of substance use and misuse among military personnel (e.g., reported binge drinking among 47 percent of active duty service members in 2008 [Bray et al., 2009]) and their dependents constitute a public health crisis; require consistent implementation of prevention, screening, and treatment services; and assume the leadership necessary to achieve this goal. This complex task will undoubtedly require changes to military culture, which is perceived by many as inhibiting case finding and discouraging self-referral for alcohol and other drug use problems. Based on the demographics of the U.S. armed forces (i.e., the majority of men and women under age 30), the results of self-report surveys on drug and alcohol use (Bray et al., 2009), and the ready access to relatively inexpensive alcohol on military bases, the committee recognizes that the need for prevention and treatment efforts and services is higher than the utilization data reported in Chapter 7 suggest. The committee believes that the foundation for SUD policy and program formulation and resource allocation should be an understanding that the levels of alcohol and other drug use constitute a public health crisis in the military. The highest leadership levels throughout the military should recognize that alcohol and other drug use problems

- are currently at unacceptably high levels and detrimental to readiness and total force fitness;
- should be addressed with an arsenal of public health strategies (e.g., universal, selective and indicated prevention programs and policies) applied to population groups, particularly those at high risk;
- require medical and behavioral interventions for individuals with emergent problems;
- can be prevented and treated when detected early and addressed with confidential interventions; and
- demand the attention of unit leaders and commanders.

The committee recognizes the need for disciplinary action when criminal behavior occurs, supports a strong surveillance program to detect the use of substances that impair performance, and applauds current efforts to enhance the quality and effectiveness of SUD prevention and treatment services. Increased routine screening for unhealthy alcohol use and mechanisms to support brief interventions and confidential treatment (each of which is discussed in the recommendations that follow) could inhibit the development of severe alcohol and other drug use disorders, promote force readiness, and prolong careers. The recommendations presented in this chapter focus on

- increasing emphasis on efforts to prevent SUDs in service members and their dependents;
- developing strategies for identifying, adopting, implementing, and disseminating evidence-based programs and best practices for SUD care (including prevention, screening, brief intervention, diagnosis, treatment, and ongoing management);
- increasing access to care for military service members and their dependents; and
- strengthening the workforce treating SUDs within the armed services.

In addition, although this issue is not addressed by a specific recommendation in this report, DoD and the branches will need to update policy and program language to reflect the forthcoming changes in SUD diagnostic labels and criteria in the *Diagnostic and Statistical Manual of Mental Disorders*, Fifth Edition (DSM-5).

INCREASING EMPHASIS ON EFFORTS TO PREVENT SUBSTANCE USE DISORDERS

Culture change will require the use of strong prevention programs that use the full range of evidence-based prevention interventions. Institute of Medicine (IOM) reports have differentiated three levels of prevention: (1) *universal* strategies that target communities to reduce the population risk for specific problems (e.g., enforcement of laws on minimum drinking age that affect everyone under age 21); (2) *selective* prevention strategies that target groups at elevated risk for specific disorders to reduce the probability of their developing those disorders (e.g., a program to prevent tobacco use among children whose parents smoke); and (3) *indicated* efforts that target individuals who have early signs of a disorder but do not meet diagnostic criteria (e.g., screening and brief intervention for service members seen in primary care) (IOM, 1994; NRC and IOM, 2009).

Recommendation 1: DoD and the individual branches should implement a comprehensive set of evidence-based prevention programs and policies that include universal, selective, and indicated interventions.

In **Finding 6-1,**[1] the committee identified the extent to which military policies and programs fall short of incorporating best practices in the field of SUD prevention. The most effective universal, population-based environmental prevention strategies increase the price of and reduce access to alcohol and other drugs. Successful environmental prevention strategies that DoD and the branches should adopt include consistent enforcement of regulations on underage drinking, a reduced number of alcohol outlets, and limited hours of operation for those outlets. Availability on bases can be reduced by controlling the types of alcohol sold, the days and hours of sale, and the amount of purchase per sale and by enforcing the minimum legal purchase age. While each of these measures is relevant, working with communities to reduce availability by enforcing the minimum legal drinking age is particularly important given that a considerable proportion of military personnel are between the ages of 18 and 20, or under the legal age for drinking. Efforts such as the Enforcing Underage Drinking Laws (EUDL) program (reviewed in Chapter 6 and Appendix D) should be expanded and investigated more broadly across military sites as part of efforts to stem underage drinking. With respect to availability off base, Commands can work actively with local authorities in surrounding communities to ensure that existing controls on availability are implemented and to develop control measures where such measures are not already in place. The committee sees partnerships with local authorities and hospitality-related businesses (e.g., bars, hotels, casinos) as critically important, and their absence is a missed prevention opportunity. Commands should undertake partnerships with local communities and businesses as a rule rather than as an exception. Commands, especially those on large bases, have considerable control over access to a large population of consumers important to the local economy. Thus, they can influence the level of enforcement of alcohol control laws, as well as help with such enforcement. Commands should also work with local authorities to make sure that driving under the influence (DUI) prevention measures are implemented and enforced consistently in communities surrounding military bases.

Similarly, as a universal prevention strategy, DoD and the individual branches should proactively prevent the misuse and abuse of prescription medications by limiting access to controlled medications. On this latter point, DoD currently participates in Drug Enforcement Administration (DEA)-approved prescription drug take-back programs, which can reduce the amount of unused medications in the community that otherwise could be diverted and abused. DoD's participation in drug take-back events should continue to be promoted at all military sites. A recent change in

[1] The findings that support the committee's conclusions and recommendations are numbered by chapter and are discussed in detail in the respective chapters (Chapters 6-8).

policy to set limits on the length of prescriptions and the quantity dispensed for controlled substances (U.S. Army Surgeon General, 2011) has the potential to decrease ready access to some of the most commonly abused medications. Monitoring of the implementation of this policy change, coupled with an enhanced prescription drug monitoring system, could identify risky use, abuse, and questionable prescribing practices.

Additionally, DoD should conduct research on the current utilization of Pharmacoeconomic Center (PEC) programs intended to support the clinicians who care for service members receiving prescriptions for long-term (i.e., more than 180 days) use of controlled substances (at a minimum, opioids and benzodiazepines) that may impair their health and combat readiness. This research should identify the extent to which clinicians make use of the Controlled Drug Management Analysis and Reporting Tool (CD-MART) and Deployment MART to identify and monitor the use of controlled substances among all individuals with long-term use, as well as the clinical response among medical personnel preparing service members for deployment. DoD should investigate how it can enhance the clinical utilization of these PEC reporting tools by disseminating additional clinical guidelines on the prescribing of controlled substances and instructions on the use of the tools for providers, or by promulgating mandates, regulations, and policy changes requiring the use of these tools in caring for service members. DoD should also investigate the extent to which individuals with high-risk alcohol use behavior or aberrant drug use behavior are receiving long-term supplies of controlled substances for use during deployment. This research should focus on determining whether additional guidance or policy changes are needed to ensure that controlled medications are given only when not clinically contraindicated for individuals at risk of developing an alcohol or other drug use disorder. While it is necessary for Army medics and Navy corpsmen to be able to dispense medications in the field that have the potential for abuse, such as opioids and benzodiazepines, enhanced training is needed on dose limitations and signs of aberrant behavior or abuse. Health care professionals at all levels (e.g., general medical officers, flight surgeons, medics) should be trained in recognizing patterns of substance abuse and misuse and provided clear guidelines for referral to specialty providers, including pain management specialists and mental health providers. Training and ongoing education should also be provided to all clinicians on effective pain management, with attention to the risks associated with prescribing pain medications, particularly short-acting opioids, which have a high potential for abuse and have not been found to be effective for treating chronic pain conditions (Martell et al., 2007).

Beyond general training and education of providers, a system is needed to monitor the implementation of the *VA/DoD Clinical Practice Guide-*

line for Management of Opioid Therapy for Chronic Pain (VA and DoD, 2010), with clear and measurable standards of practice and accountability of providers to deliver evidence-based care. DoD should move forward to implement the recommendations in the final report of the Army pain management task force, particularly those related to routinely assessing for drug abuse in patients on opioid therapy and implementing sole provider programs to prevent "doctor shopping" (U.S. Army, 2010). DoD currently does not share its pharmacy data with state-run prescription drug monitoring programs (PDMPs). Because many service members and their dependents fill prescriptions in community pharmacies, it is important for DoD to partner with community efforts to identify those individuals who are abusing prescription drugs. During its site visit to Fort Belvoir, the committee heard that physicians at the military treatment facility routinely checked the locally available state-run PDMPs before dispensing controlled substances.[2] However, the extent of this practice among military physicians is unknown. The committee therefore recommends that DoD providers routinely check any locally state-run PDMPs before dispensing prescription medications that have abuse potential. As the state-run PDMPs or other related community efforts are further developed, DoD should consider investigating the potential value of sharing its pharmacy data with those programs and efforts.

With regard to prevention programming, DoD and the branches should focus on adapting and testing efficacious developmentally focused universal, selective, and indicated prevention initiatives for children and families, including broader child development programs that do not address substance abuse specifically. Branch policy makers and commanders in charge of units should develop procedures that routinely include family members in evidence-based prevention programs at the entry, predeployment, and postdeployment stages for active duty members and at entry for members of the reserve component until they become active. The military branches, through their respective surgeon general or Command structure, should coordinate the sharing and use of evidence-based programs and models of standardized annual training of program implementers and their supervisors. Several evidence-based programs that are already being disseminated across branches (e.g., Families OverComing Under Stress [FOCUS], New Orientation to Reduce Threats to Health from Secretive Problems That Affect Readiness [NORTH STAR]) appear to have been disseminated as part of a research trial rather than DoD or branch policy. Standardized training models are included in the Alcohol and Drug Abuse Managers/Supervisors (ADAMS) and Culture of Responsible Choices (CoRC) pro-

---

[2]Personal communication, Ben Krepps, M.D., Director of the Pain Clinic at Fort Belvoir Community Hospital, November 15, 2011.

grams, which are used in the Navy and Air Force, respectively (see Appendix D for descriptions of these programs).

Finding 6-5 states that neither DoD nor the branches evaluate their programs and initiatives consistently or systematically. This finding is in line with a recent RAND report examining the psychological health programs available to service members, which also notes a lack of evaluation of program effectiveness (Weinick et al., 2011). To address this gap, the committee advises DoD and each branch to require annual evaluation of the effects of prevention programs. Benchmarks with which to determine whether programs are effective or need to be changed should be established as part of the evaluation design.

As noted in **Finding 6-1,** DoD and the individual branches use drug testing as an integral component of their prevention strategies; however, the committee notes the limitations of these drug testing programs in preventing SUDs. The committee encourages DoD to sponsor research on the cost-effectiveness of the current urinalysis programs. Considering the complexity of drug use behavior and the continuing problem it poses for the armed forces, this research should identify ways to improve the deterrence effect of these programs and provide insight into how the programs affect service members' attitudes toward the use of tested and untested illicit drugs. The research should also yield quantitative data on the cost per annual drug user deterred that can be compared with the cost-effectiveness of alternative evidence-based prevention programs, particularly those that may be implemented to deter alcohol misuse, which is far more prevalent than other drug misuse in the military. There appears to be a temporal correlation between the introduction of random urinalysis testing to detect and deter illicit drug use among military personnel and a declining trend in the prevalence of some drug use in the military. However, no other data are available on the effectiveness of drug screening in the armed forces, and this temporal association by itself does not meet the burden of proof for establishing a causal relationship. Further, the panel of tested substances is minimal and historically has not included some opioids and benzodiazepines that are frequently abused. Recently, DoD made changes to its drug testing program to expand the panel of tested substances to include hydrocodone and benzodiazepines, two of the most widely abused prescription medications. DoD should continue to revise the panel of tested substances as feasible to include the detection of emerging drugs of abuse, such as Spice and bath salts. DoD should also undertake evaluations to determine whether decreases in prevalence rates occur for substances recently added to the testing panel. The committee cautions DoD not to take hasty action by reducing funding for its drug testing programs before reviewing the results of cost-effectiveness research regarding whether decreased illicit drug use is causally related to these programs.

A public health approach to prevention of SUDs would integrate universal, selective, and indicated prevention within the medical care system. Research has found that routine screening and brief intervention in medical settings can allow health care professionals to point out the risks of high levels of alcohol use and consistently support reductions in population levels of use (Whitlock et al., 2004). As noted in **Finding 7-1,** the need for this type of early screening and intervention is high within military populations. Additionally, while the *VA/DoD Clinical Practice Guideline for Management of Substance Use Disorders* (VA and DoD, 2009) indicates the appropriateness of screening and brief intervention protocols, the committee found a lack of implementation of these protocols. Integration of screening and brief intervention for alcohol misuse into primary care settings could reduce stigma and expand access to care. DoD should explore ways to increase the use of screening and brief intervention for alcohol misuse in all medical care settings to make it possible to identify those at risk of developing alcohol use disorders and intervene before more intensive care may be needed. It may be noted that, while there is clear evidence in support of screening and brief intervention in primary care to address alcohol use (Kaner et al., 2009; Whitlock et al., 2004), the efficacy of this approach for other substances besides alcohol is less apparent (Polen et al., 2008).

Ultimately, among the most important factors to consider in selecting evidence-based policies, programs, and practices is the extent to which they fit logically into an appropriate overarching strategic plan that addresses the unique conditions found in differing environments. To inform their decision making regarding the selection and implementation of appropriate evidence-based practices, DoD and the service branches will need to adopt a reliable, consistent, yet flexible problem-solving framework. Further, no single evidence-based practice in isolation is likely to result in a significant change in substance use behavior; the optimal prevention strategy will involve the coordination of multiple, mutually reinforcing evidence-based universal, selective, and indicated efforts at both the environmental and individual levels.

DEVELOPING STRATEGIES FOR IDENTIFYING, ADOPTING, IMPLEMENTING, AND DISSEMINATING EVIDENCE-BASED PROGRAMS AND BEST PRACTICES FOR SUD CARE

The use of evidence-based practices in the care of SUDs (as well as the training of providers in these practices) is integral to ensuring that individuals receive effective, high-quality care. In **Finding 6-6,** the committee notes that while DoD and individual branches advocate for the adoption and implementation of evidence-based practices throughout their policies and program literature, scant detail is provided on the specific practices to be used. As a result, adoption and implementation are highly variable both across and within branches. In collaboration with the Department of Veterans Affairs (VA), DoD has already developed evidence-based guidelines for the treatment of SUDs (VA and DoD, 2009); however, the committee found a lack of implementation, as well as monitoring of implementation, of these guidelines (**Finding 6-4**). Recent DoD reports present similar findings about the lack of dissemination and implementation of clinical practice guidelines across branches and settings of care (Defense Health Board, 2011; DoD, 2007, 2011b).

> **Recommendation 2: DoD should assume leadership in ensuring the consistency and quality of SUD services. DoD also should require improved data collection on substance use and misuse, as well as the operation of SUD services.**

Findings 6-4, **6-5**, and **6-6** identify problems arising from the lack of standardization, monitoring, and evaluation of SUD policies and programs by DoD or the individual branches, as well as the underutilization of evidence-based practices. The committee struggled to obtain from DoD and the branches basic data on the number of prevention events and participation rates, individuals treated for SUDs, and the characteristics of the workforce treating SUDs. The committee also noted a lack of benchmarks and standards for prevention, screening, diagnosis, and treatment services. DoD and the individual branches need accurate and valid performance measures to better monitor the implementation and effectiveness of SUD prevention, screening, and treatment services. Consequently, DoD should assume responsibility for ensuring the consistency and quality of these services. Each branch organizes these services idiosyncratically, with little consistency in service implementation and data collection. DoD should monitor adherence to policies and the implementation of clinical practice guidelines, develop performance measures related to SUD prevention and treatment, and hold providers and systems accountable for their performance on these measures. Specifically, full implementation of the *VA/DoD Clinical Practice Guideline for Management of Substance Use Disorders* (VA and DoD, 2009) in general medical care and specialty care settings would facilitate implementation of the committee's recommendations for routine screening, effective prevention and treatment efforts, integration with general medical care and mental health services, greater use of technology, confidential care, and greater use of ambulatory and continuing care. Where evidence-based prevention, screening, diagnosis, and treatment practices are nationally known and accepted, they should be incorporated into the principles and structures of DoD policies as an overarching expectation for all branches as a means of driving consistency and minimizing variability. DoD operates one of the nation's largest health care systems and should use 21st-century management standards and process improvement tools to ensure the quality and effectiveness of its services.

Recommendation 3: DoD should conduct routine screening for unhealthy alcohol use, together with brief alcohol education interventions.

Finding 6-1 acknowledges that DoD and branch policies emphasize screening as a key strategy in combating SUDs in the military, but **Finding 6-2** points out that screening policies and programs fall short of identifying all service members with SUDs or those who are at risk for developing them, while **Finding 7-1** makes note of the unmet need for effective screening and brief intervention strategies. Additionally, the committee notes in **Finding 6-3** that DoD and branch policies reflect very different (and somewhat disconcerting) attitudes toward alcohol and other drugs. Annual screening for unhealthy alcohol use in all patients is recommended in the *VA/DoD Clinical Practice Guideline for Management of Substance Use Disorders* (VA and DoD, 2009) based on extensive evidence that such screening, followed by brief alcohol counseling, is efficacious in reducing drinking. Routine screening during annual medical checkups includes use of a validated screening instrument to identify individuals drinking above recommended daily and weekly limits (i.e., 4 drinks per day and 14 drinks per week for men and 3 drinks per day and 7 drinks per week for women). The screening should identify patients who are drinking despite contraindications to alcohol use (i.e., pregnant or trying to conceive; liver disease, including hepatitis C; pancreatitis; congestive heart failure; use of medications with clinically important interactions with alcohol) even if they screen negative for unhealthy alcohol use. Outside of deployment health assessments, the committee found little evidence of the actual implementation of these components of the *VA/DoD Clinical Practice Guideline* (**Finding 7-1**). Likewise, DoD's *Comprehensive Plan on Prevention, Diagnosis, and Treatment of Substance Use Disorders and Disposition of Substance Use Offenders in the Armed Forces* (*Comprehensive Plan*) finds that evidence-based screening tools are not used consistently in the military, particularly in primary care settings (DoD, 2011b). In an update to the *Comprehensive Plan*, DoD notes that policy language is currently under development to call for more consistent use of screening measures in primary care settings.[3] The committee recommends that DoD move forward with this action and specifically cite the use of validated screening tools and adherence to the screening procedures identified in the *VA/DoD Clinical Practice Guideline*.

[3] Personal communication, Alfred J. Ozanian, Ph.D., Addiction Medicine Program Manager, TRICARE Management Activity, June 6, 2012.

Further, it is imperative that screening for unhealthy alcohol use be available without stigma or disciplinary consequences so that screening responses will be truthful, and a brief intervention can be delivered clinically, either by Internet programs or in direct clinical encounters, such as in a primary care setting. Screening and brief intervention should be understood according to DoD policy to be an educational intervention akin to an indicated prevention approach. Screening is not diagnosis, and brief advice is not treatment. The applicable DoD policy supporting this approach is Instruction DODI 6490.08, *Command Notification Requirements to Dispel Stigma in Providing Mental Health Care to Service Members* (DoD, 2011a). DoD providers should be trained to follow the guidelines in DODI 6490.08, which allow for administration of a brief and confidential prevention intervention to those who are identified as at risk for SUDs but do not yet meet diagnostic criteria. Branch policies and programs should allow for the delivery of indicated prevention programming for those at risk for SUDs without the notification of commanders (within the guidelines of DODI 6490.08).

Recommendation 4: Policies of DoD and the individual branches should promote evidence-based diagnostic and treatment processes.

As discussed above, while DoD and the branches advocate for the adoption and implementation of evidence-based practices, their policies and program literature provide little detail on specific practices; the result is great variation in practices both across and within branches. Also as noted above, DoD supports implementation of the *VA/DoD Clinical Practice Guideline for Management of Substance Use Disorders* (VA and DoD, 2009), but the committee found little evidence of its implementation within the branches. The lack of routine screening, limited use of anticraving and agonist medications, minimal training in the use of psychosocial interventions, and the poor connections between specialty SUD care and general medical care suggest passive rather than active implementation of the guideline. DoD needs to review the guideline's implementation at the branch level and develop system measures with which to monitor ongoing implementation and compliance. Implementation measures might include tracking the percentage of active duty service members annually completing routine screening, the percentage of patients referred for SUD assessment who complete an assessment and engage in care, and the number of prescriptions for addiction-focused pharmacotherapy. The SUD measures tracked by the National Committee for Quality Assurance using the Healthcare Effectiveness Data and Information Set should be adapted for use in the direct and purchased care systems of the Military Health System.

Specifically, the committee found in the purchased care system underutilization of effective treatment modalities such as individual outpatient therapy provided in office-based settings and the use of maintenance medications (**Finding 7-2**). DoD should move forward to promote such evidence-based treatment modalities. All patients with SUDs should be evaluated for and provided appropriate pharmacotherapy to treat their addiction in line with current evidence-based practices, as described in Chapter 5 and recommended in the National Quality Forum's *National Voluntary Consensus Standards for the Treatment of Substance Use Conditions* (NQF, 2007). Providers should be trained to offer patients education in the benefits of such therapies and be required to provide them when clinically indicated. DoD should enforce efforts to train providers in the use of pharmacotherapy. Electronic training programs are currently available to certify medical providers to dispense buprenorphine for opioid addiction, and primary care clinicians can also be trained to administer naltrexone and extended-release naltrexone for the treatment of alcohol and opioid use disorders. While the military should be concerned with how medication therapies may affect service members' performance and safety, there are model programs in the civilian sector for highly skilled professionals whose performance affects public safety (airline pilots, physicians, nurses) in which primary care physicians and addiction specialists prescribe therapeutic medications and carefully monitor patient performance and abstinence. These programs are considered some of the most effective in the United States (McLellan et al., 2008). DoD should look to these models when developing its own treatment policies and systems of care.

SUD patients in direct and purchased care settings should also be offered individual and group outpatient counseling using evidence-based protocols when clinically indicated. To this end, DoD should expand its capacity to offer local outpatient services in both the direct and purchased care systems. In the direct care system, this may require the addition of addiction specialists to supervise clinical staff and the expansion of training and certification in addiction medicine for mental health practitioners (see Chapter 8). In the purchased care system, mechanisms will be required to certify individual licensed clinicians in an addiction specialty and to certify the TRICARE network of community-based addiction and mental health programs regardless of Substance Use Disorder Rehabilitation Facility (SUDRF) status. (See **Recommendation 7** below for the committee's guidance on how to update the TRICARE SUD benefit to reflect current evidence-based treatment modalities.)

Finally, DoD and individual branch policies will require revision following the release of the fifth edition of the *Diagnostic and Statistical Manual of Mental Disorders*, Fifth Edition (DSM-5) in May 2013. At present, the policies are based on the DSM-IV-TR SUD definition, which includes diagnoses of "abuse" and "dependence," but no such distinction will be made in the new manual. Consequently, policies that require separation following drug abuse or dependence diagnoses will no longer be applicable. In the latest iteration of the manual, SUD diagnoses will be differentiated as "mild," "moderate," or "severe" depending on the number of symptoms present. The committee recommends that DoD and the individual branches make it a consistent practice to review the language and content of their policies to reflect changes such as this, as well as future advances in field.

Recommendation 5: DoD and the individual branches should better integrate care for SUDs with care for other mental health conditions and ongoing medical care.

In **Finding 6-7**, the committee points out the lack of integration of SUD care with other behavioral health and medical care, most notably within the Army and Marine Corps. The committee also notes that this lack of integration can lead to structural and social barriers that inhibit individuals from accessing care (**Finding 7-4**). These findings are not unexpected; indeed, similar findings are presented in a report by DoD's Task Force on Mental Health (DoD, 2007). Integration of care can occur at two levels: (1) integration of care for mental health disorders and SUDs, and (2) integration of alcohol and other drug prevention with primary care. Primary care is the single largest missed opportunity in the military for early and confidential identification of and brief intervention in alcohol and other drug misuse. The Air Force's Behavioral Health Optimization Program (described in Appendix D) demonstrates the feasibility and advantages of integrating behavioral health into primary care services. Integration of services for SUDs should proceed as well to reduce stigma and enhance the use of medication-assisted treatment for alcohol and opioid use disorders. Integration will require that physicians be permitted to address misuse of alcohol without having to include Command when developing service plans for those individuals who do not meet diagnostic criteria and are in need of only brief education. This approach is supported by the new DoD Instruction DODI 6490.08, discussed under **Recommendation 3** above.

To better integrate treatment for SUDs and comorbid mental health problems, the Army Substance Abuse Program (ASAP) needs to alter provider credentialing. Currently, licensed independent practitioners working in ASAP are credentialed only to treat SUDs. Even though they are trained mental health practitioners (psychologists and social workers), they are not authorized to treat comorbid conditions such as depression and posttraumatic stress disorder (PTSD). Because the current operational environment increases the probability of comorbid disorders, the Army can no longer afford to maintain separate services for mental health disorders and SUDs. An additional strategy the committee suggests is the return of SUD services to the Medical Command.

Recommendation 6: The Military Health System should reduce its reliance on residential and inpatient care for SUDs in its direct care system and build capacity for outpatient and intensive outpatient SUD treatment using a chronic care model that permits patients to remain connected to counselors and recovery coaches for as long as needed.

The Military Health System appears to have sufficient access to inpatient beds within existing regulations. The direct care system needs to build capacity for intensive outpatient and outpatient services. Contemporary systems of care for SUDs rely on outpatient services and ongoing disease management. For many individuals, SUDs are relapsing conditions that require ongoing monitoring and periodic stabilization. Monitoring systems similar to those used by the Department of Transportation and physician assistance programs allow highly trained individuals to continue to work without jeopardizing health and safety. The military branches are well positioned to provide the most effective environment for alcohol and other drug treatment in the nation. In so doing, they can emulate the services and structure of state programs for physicians with alcohol and drug use disorders (DuPont et al., 2009; McLellan et al., 2008). The elements critical to high rates of recovery appear to be ongoing care in an outpatient setting, coupled with routine monitoring and clear consequences associated with a return to use (loss of license). A similar program in military treatment facilities would facilitate retention of trained personnel, noncommissioned leadership, and commissioned leadership while enhancing unit capacity and safety.

INCREASING ACCESS TO CARE

As described in Chapter 7, the committee's review of access to SUD services revealed substantial unmet need and policies and practices that inhibit access to care (**Findings 7-1, 7-2, 7-3, 7-4,** and **7-5**). The committee's findings on access are in agreement with findings from the report of DoD's Mental Health Task Force, which documents many barriers faced by service members and their families in accessing mental health services in both direct and purchased care settings (DoD, 2007). The following recommendations outline strategies for improving access to and enhancing utilization of SUD care.

Recommendation 7: DoD should update the TRICARE SUD treatment benefit to reflect the practices of contemporary health plans and to be consistent with the range of treatments available under the Patient Protection and Affordable Care Act.

This recommendation is based on **Finding 7-2,** which notes that access to care is restricted by the TRICARE SUD benefit's lack of coverage for intensive outpatient services, office-based outpatient services, and certain evidence-based pharmacological therapies. This recommendation is related to **Recommendation 6** regarding the expansion of intensive outpatient and office-based outpatient treatment in the direct care system. As outlined in Chapter 5 and incorporated in the *VA/DoD Clinical Practice Guideline for Management of Substance Use Disorders* (VA and DoD, 2009), contemporary SUD care includes the use of maintenance medications and a focus on outpatient rather than residential treatment. The TRICARE benefit at present does not permit use of maintenance medications in the treatment of SUDs and thus deprives many patients of therapies that could help reduce craving and support long-term recovery. Further, TRICARE coverage does not permit use of office-based individual therapy (outside of SUDRFs) to treat SUDs, although such therapy is permitted for other mental health disorders. This restriction is inconsistent with current best practices reflecting parity in coverage for SUDs and mental health disorders, as well as medical conditions. The TRICARE benefit for SUD care should provide coverage for all evidence-based forms of care, including maintenance medications. DoD recently proposed a rule to remove the prohibition on the use of maintenance medications in 32 *Code of Federal Regulation* (CFR) Part 199, and the proposed rule was published in the *Federal Register* to elicit public comment (DoD, 2011c). DoD should move forward to publish the final ruling to change 32 CFR Part 199 to ensure that every patient entering SUD treatment is evaluated for possible use of agonist and antagonist maintenance medications approved by the Food and Drug Administration for the treatment of opioid and alcohol use disorders, and that the TRICARE benefit covers such maintenance medications. Congress should review any such final rule to ensure that **Recommendation 7** in this report is appropriately represented in the changes to 32 CFR Part 199. Once the final rule has been accepted, DoD should move quickly to institute needed policy changes to revise the TRICARE benefit.

DoD should also move forward to propose a rule change to 32 CFR Part 199 to remove the restriction of care to SUDRFs and expand the TRICARE benefit coverage to include care provided in intensive outpatient treatment settings. Continued restriction of SUD treatment to SUDRFs is outdated. The range of SUD treatment services available in community settings has evolved substantially since the development of the regulation restricting care to SUDRFs. Inpatient and residential care is no longer the expected standard, and its use is restricted to the most severe, complex cases. Randomized controlled trials and retrospective cohort analyses comparing inpatient rehabilitation services with intensive outpatient services consistently have found little difference in outcomes. Patient placement criteria (Mee-Lee, 2007) encourage the use of appropriate levels of care and support a full continuum of services, including intensive outpatient services. The limited capacity for intensive outpatient services and office-based outpatient services forces TRICARE and the Military Health System to rely on the most intensive and restrictive levels of care. Employed and housed patients can usually be treated effectively in their community and need not be sent to geographically distant residential facilities.

Accessing TRICARE services can be difficult for military dependents because of the requirement to use SUDRFs. In **Finding 6-8,** the committee explained that DoD and branch policies are largely silent on SUD programs and services for dependents; expanded capacity for community-based outpatient services is a key to improving access to care for family members. The committee agrees with and supports efforts to better coordinate services in the VA and the Military Health System and strongly supports the recent extension of VA mental health personnel to serve veterans returning from Iraq and Afghanistan more promptly. Further, the committee agrees that TRICARE benefits for mental health disorders and SUDs should conform to the Mental Health Parity and Substance Abuse Equity Act, and quantitative and nonquantitative limits on behavioral health services should be eliminated. Evaluations of mental health parity have found little impact on the utilization and cost of health care, with the potential to reduce stigma and enhance access to care (Goldman et al., 2006; McConnell et al., 2012). In the update to the *Comprehensive Plan*, DoD notes that policy language is being drafted to revise the lifetime limits on SUD treatment episodes.[4] Currently, there is a lifetime limit of only three SUD treatment benefit periods per beneficiary (with additional benefit periods requiring a waiver). DoD should move forward expeditiously to enact this policy change and propose any needed rule change to 32 CFR Part 199.

The TRICARE SUD benefit is out of date with current standards for evidence-based care and needs to be revised without delay. If DoD fails to make the needed changes to the TRICARE SUD benefit in a timely manner, the committee recommends that Congress consider taking action to mandate that DoD make these changes.

Recommendation 8: DoD should encourage each service branch to provide options for confidential treatment of alcohol use disorders.

Finding 7-3 notes that low rates of self-referral to treatment corroborate reports of the perceived stigma of receiving treatment for SUDs, while **Finding 7-4** identifies various structural, social, and cultural barriers that inhibit access to SUD care, paramount among them being a lack of confidential services. The committee was impressed with the Army's implementation of the Confidential Alcohol Treatment and Education Pilot (CATEP)

[4] Personal communication, Alfred J. Ozanian, Ph.D., Addiction Medicine Program Manager, TRICARE Management Activity, June 6, 2012.

(discussed in Appendix D). CATEP attracts a broad range of patients, including officers who are not often seen in ASAP programs, and provides confidential treatment for alcohol use disorders (Gibbs and Rae Olmsted, 2011). The committee is not concerned that CATEP has a low treatment completion rate because the ASAP definition of treatment completion is an arbitrary number of sessions or weeks; many individuals benefit from brief treatment and need not complete a specified treatment regimen. The results of preliminary surveys of CATEP participants and commanders who were aware of their soldiers' participation in the program showed that there was broad support for expansion of the program and that career protections were seen as an important component. Referral rates to ASAP from postdeployment health assessments also increased at the pilot sites, presumably because of providers' increased willingness to refer to ASAP.[5] The committee recommends that programs such as CATEP be expanded to all ASAP sites within the Army, as well as to the other branches. Policies should be updated to facilitate Command support for recovery through these confidential programs.

Currently, CATEP functions by offering treatment services outside duty hours so soldiers can participate without informing their commander. CATEP encourages but does not require soldiers to disclose their participation in treatment to their commanders. A recent qualitative study found that participants in CATEP highly valued the provision of treatment services outside duty hours and the option to engage in confidential treatment (Gibbs and Rae Olmsted, 2011). The committee understands the need to balance health and discipline, and agrees with the approach CATEP has taken to providing confidential treatment outside of duty hours. Access to confidential brief counseling, brief treatment, and more intensive treatment promotes good care and builds resilience. Delivering these services without sanctions would promote an effective response to alcohol and other drug use problems as they emerge and foster a system in which individuals seek help instead of hiding problems. Service members should feel confident in disclosing problems to their commanders, who should then fully support service members' participation in treatment. In the absence of such support, it is essential that service members also have access to confidential systems of care.

Recommendation 9: DoD should establish a joint planning process with the VHA, with highly visible leadership (perhaps recently retired military personnel), to address the SUD needs and issues of access to care of reserve component personnel before and after mobilization.

[5]Personal communication, COL Charles S. Milliken, M.D., Walter Reed Army Institute of Research, May 3, 2011.

Over the last 10 years, the military has relied heavily on its reserve component forces in the ongoing military operations in Iraq and Afghanistan. In its review, the committee found a lack of access to SUD care for National Guard and Reserve members (**Finding 7-5**). These individuals are at high risk for developing SUDs and in many cases lack continuity of care for ongoing mental health problems once demobilized. Therefore, DoD should mount new programs to reach demobilized and discharged reserve component personnel and fund research to determine which strategies for doing so are most effective. A planning process should be used to establish new avenues for reaching or increase active outreach to all demobilized and discharged reserve component personnel if they have not enrolled in Veterans Health Administration (VHA) care within 6 months and if their VHA or alternative medical records do not contain a recent result from an alcohol or other drug use screening.

DoD also should make provisions for veterans with other than honorable discharges to receive referrals for outreach and continued SUD assessment and services by designated community-based providers. In addition, DoD should provide the option of receiving confidential screening and assessment in alternative venues to the VHA. Such venues include a telemedicine visit with a former DoD clinician with whom the service member had an established relationship or a community-based civilian program specifically designed to engage and serve demobilized and discharged reserve component veterans, innovative telehealth programs, smartphone and Web-based technology that can provide confidential self-assessment and motivational interviewing to address a reluctant veteran's concerns about visiting the VHA or seeking help, and active engagement in primary care settings at VHA programs when a reserve component member appears for medical services.

DoD should develop alternative procedures for demobilized and discharged reserve component veterans with elevated postdeployment health reassessment scores (indicating alcohol use and/or other high-risk behavior) to receive a "warm hand-off" to or facilitated appointment with a VHA or community-based provider with specialty training in serving veterans at risk of SUDs and/or suicide. DoD and the VHA should collaborate to contract with community providers or existing programs (e.g., Military OneSource) to perform some of the active outreach telephone contacts and facilitated linkage needed for particularly high-risk or difficult-to-contact reserve component members who have been demobilized or discharged. Additionally DoD should fund research and evaluation on the most effective technologies and strategies for active engagement of high-risk reserve component members in order to refine its future programming.

Recommendation 10: DoD and the individual service branches should evaluate the use of technology in the prevention, screening, diagnosis,

treatment, and management of SUDs to improve quality, efficiency, and access.

Finding 6-9 indicates that DoD and the service branches are infrequently using new technologies that could help standardize the delivery of evidence-based care and could also potentially reduce counselor workloads and increase access to care. Research is beginning to show support for various technological approaches to delivering health care screenings and interventions (Humphreys et al., 2011; Jackson et al., 2011; Tsoh et al., 2010) and SUD care in particular (Cunningham et al., 2009; Godley et al., 2010). DoD has an admirable track record in the implementation and adoption of technology, and while the effectiveness of these technological approaches is still somewhat unknown, DoD has a unique opportunity to participate in research designed to evaluate some of these approaches for use with service members and their families.

The committee found several promising examples of the use of technology in DoD's SUD programs, and sees value in further evaluation of the effectiveness of these efforts. The Air Force's use of the Substance Use Assessment Tool (SUAT) computerized assessment in all of its Alcohol and Drug Abuse Prevention and Treatment (ADAPT) programs is one example. The SUAT incorporates validated screening instruments in its assessment, and the committee found the content of the SUAT questions to be comprehensive. This tool may be useful for the other service branches, and DoD should explore this possibility further. Additionally, the use of Internet technology has the potential to provide patients with access to SUD care when deployed in settings where mental health providers are scarce. The Navy's use of Hazelden's My Ongoing Recovery Experience (MORE) (described in Appendix D) is a promising example of continuing aftercare being delivered in this manner, and its effectiveness for military populations should be evaluated systematically. DoD should evaluate whether the MORE program helps decrease counselor workloads in providing aftercare and therefore allows other screening and treatment services to receive greater priority.

STRENGTHENING THE SUD WORKFORCE

Nationally, the workforce that provides treatment for SUDs appears to be in transition. Alcohol and drug treatment emerged as freestanding residential services in the 1950s, 1960s, and 1970s. Many counselors used their personal experience in recovery to help patients initiate and maintain a stable recovery. State standards for counselors supported the nascent profession and did not require graduate degrees or professional licensure (IOM, 1990). Certification of alcohol and drug counselors emerged as an alternative to licensure and as documentation of specialty training and skill.

Since the 1970s, the SUD patient population has become considerably more complex; poly-substance use has become common, the rates and severity of psychiatric and medical comorbidities have increased, and services have increasingly been integrated with behavioral health and primary care services. Individuals in recovery no longer dominate the workforce; counselors with graduate degrees are prevalent, and health care reform is likely to demand counselors who are licensed independent practitioners. Although individuals certified as alcohol and drug counselors remain a key component of the civilian workforce treating SUDs, their role is increasingly limited and in the near future may disappear. Rather than continuing to use a 20th-century workforce to treat SUDs, DoD is challenged to structure and staff treatment services for alcohol and drug use disorders for the 21st century. The emerging model of care uses multidisciplinary treatment teams to create a varied workforce with carefully articulated roles and training. Individuals in recovery provide peer support instead of serving as primary counselors. Certified counselors work under the supervision of licensed independent practitioners. Treatment plans include evidence-based pharmacological and behavioral therapies and long-term continuing care with peer support. To increase caseloads and enhance productivity, services emphasize outpatient and intensive outpatient modalities, rely on group therapy, and use computer-assisted cognitive-behavioral techniques. The VA and leading fully integrated health plans provide models for the organization of services for optimal patient outcomes.

In reviewing DoD's SUD workforce requirements and comparing them with emerging models of care, the committee found shortages of SUD counselors across the branches (**Finding 8-5**), a conspicuous lack of physicians trained in addiction medicine or psychiatry (**Finding 8-3**), wide variation in training and credentialing requirements for SUD counselors across the branches (**Finding 8-1**), outdated training manuals for Air Force and Navy SUD counselors in particular (**Finding 8-2**), and a noticeable shortage of a workforce trained in SUD prevention (**Finding 8-6**). The committee makes the following recommendations for DoD to enhance its workforce providing SUD care.

Recommendation 11: The individual service branches should restructure their SUD counseling workforces, using physicians and other licensed independent practitioners to lead and supervise multidisciplinary treatment teams providing a full continuum of behavioral and pharmacological therapies to treat SUDs and comorbid mental health disorders.

The committee found high levels of comorbid mental health disorders among active duty service members and their dependents who seek care for alcohol and other drug use disorders. As noted above, moreover, emerging systems of care rely on multidisciplinary teams led by licensed independent practitioners (e.g., licensed clinical psychologists, licensed clinical social workers, licensed professional counselors). Licensed independent practitioners complete multidimensional assessments that include assessments of mental health and physical health disorders, develop comprehensive treatment plans, and provide active treatment using evidence-based pharmacological and behavioral therapies. Certified counselors and individuals in recovery may provide support and continuing care services under the direction of licensed practitioners. Additionally, the evolution from residential services to ambulatory treatment systems with continuing care requires a varied workforce.

Licensed independent practitioners with appropriate training and credentialing can provide active integrated treatment for both mental health disorders and SUDs. They can also be integrated into primary care settings as members of medical treatment teams. Care is likely to be more effective and efficient when integrated and coordinated. The workforce for SUD care also must have the capacity to provide ongoing monitoring and continuing care. Many individuals struggle to maintain a stable recovery. Chronic care models of treatment for SUDs are replacing time-limited acute care models. Physician support programs provide one model that DoD may choose to emulate.

The Air Force, Navy, and Marine Corps rely heavily on certified alcohol and drug counselors to staff their treatment programs. A transition to licensed independent practitioners could be phased so that credentialed counselors could complete graduate education and obtain professional licensure. The committee recognizes that hiring licensed practitioners may be particularly challenging for military bases located in rural areas and encourages increased use of Internet technology to promote access to appropriately trained and licensed counselors. The committee recommends that DoD begin planning to restructure the counselor workforce and strategize ways of responding to treatment needs among active duty service members and their dependents.

Recommendation 12: DoD should incorporate complete data on SUD encounters into the MDR database and recalculate the PHRAMS estimates for SUD counselors.

The committee's charge included proving guidance on how to calculate appropriate ratios of physicians and licensed practitioners for the population of DoD beneficiaries to provide sufficient services for alcohol and other drug use disorders. Calculating these ratios is an imprecise process. There is wide variation in the ratios in civilian health plans, reflecting the organization of care, productivity expectations, and the balance of group versus individual therapy. Systems that rely on residential and inpatient care require more intensive staffing ratios than those that emphasize ambulatory care. Integration of SUD care with primary care and behavioral health services requires different ratios than freestanding care. Treatment systems that build automated tools and information technology infrastructure require fewer staff. Population needs and the prevalence of SUDs affect staffing needs as well. Finally, continuing care and peer support services require different staffing patterns than acute care services.

DoD built the Psychological Health Risk-Adjusted Model for Staffing (PHRAMS) to help in making decisions about needed staffing ratios for behavioral health care. PHRAMS estimates staffing needs using service utilization data by encounter type from the Military Health System Data Repository (MDR) files. The encounter-based staffing requirement divides the anticipated number of clinical encounters by the productivity expectation. The encounter estimate reflects the population covered in the Defense Health Plan, multiplied by the prevalence rate of the specific psychological health needs, multiplied by the encounter rate. Separate estimates are generated for each risk group and 12 diagnostic groups. Non-encounter-based staffing requirements are the sum of enrollee-based requirements, plus structural unit requirements, plus support staff requirements, and reflect work requirements in addition to clinical productivity (encounters).

In **Finding 8-4,** the committee suggests that PHRAMS provides a reasonable starting point for determining the quantitative relationship between the need for SUD care and staffing levels. Yet while the PHRAMS estimates are careful and logical, they are far below the number of existing counselors. The individual branches, moreover, report needing more counselors. The underestimate appears to reflect incomplete data on SUD services in the MDR database, which excludes encounters in specialty SUD treatment programs. Consequently, the estimates are based on incomplete data and are inaccurate estimates of the number of needed counselors and physicians. Therefore, while the approach is strong, the wrong data are being used. Services provided by substance use counselors, moreover, may fall outside the definition of "psychological health provider" used for PHRAMS estimates. To apply PHRAMS to estimating the workforce required to address SUDs, DoD needs to modify the PHRAMS model and estimating procedures. An update to the *Comprehensive Plan on Prevention, Diagnosis, and Treatment of Substance Use Disorders and Disposition of Substance Use Offenders in the Armed Forces* notes that DoD is aware of this limitation in the PHRAMS model and is currently reviewing options for increasing the accuracy of PHRAMS estimates for SUD staffing requirements.[6]

---

[6]Personal communication, Alfred J. Ozanian, Ph.D., Addiction Medicine Program Manager, TRICARE Management Activity, June 6, 2012.

CONCLUSION

SUDs are a serious threat to force fitness and resilience. Greater integration with primary care, routine screening for unhealthy alcohol use, full implementation of the *VA/DoD Clinical Practice Guideline for Management of Substance Use Disorders* (VA and DoD, 2009), enhanced data systems and performance measurement, and a well-trained workforce that specializes in preventing and treating SUDs and comorbid physical health and mental health problems would strengthen the Military Health System and improve the lives and careers of active duty and reserve component and retired service members and their dependents.

REFERENCES

Bray, R. M., M. R. Pemberton, L. L. Hourani, M. Witt, K. L. Olmsted, J. M. Brown, B. Weimer, M. E. Lance, M. E. Marsden, and S. Scheffler. 2009. *Department of Defense survey of health related behaviors among active duty military personnel.* Research Triangle Park, NC: RTI International.

Cunningham, J. A., T. C. Wild, J. Cordingley, T. Van Mierlo, and K. Humphreys. 2009. A randomized controlled trial of an Internet-based intervention for alcohol abusers. *Addiction* 104(12):2023-2032.

Defense Health Board. 2011. *Psychotropic medication prescription practices and use and complementary and alternative medicine use.* Falls Church, VA: Defense Health Board.

DoD (Department of Defense). 2007. *An achievable vision: Report of the Department of Defense Task Force on Mental Health.* Washington, DC: DoD Task Force on Mental Health.

DoD. 2011a. *Instruction 6490.08: Command notification requirements to dispel stigma in providing mental health care to service members.* Washington, DC: DoD.

DoD. 2011b. *Comprehensive plan on prevention, diagnosis, and treatment of substance use disorders and disposition of substance use offenders in the armed forces.* Washington, DC: Office of the Under Secretary of Defense.

DoD. 2011c. TRICARE: Removal of the prohibition to use addictive drugs in the maintenance treatment of substance dependence in TRICARE beneficiaries. *Federal Register.* https://www.federalregister.gov/articles/2011/12/29/2011-33106/tricare-removal-of-the-prohibition-to-use-addictive-drugs-in-the-maintenance-treatment-of-substance#p-3 (accessed August 6, 2012).

DuPont, R. L., A. T. McLellan, W. L. White, L. J. Merlo, and M. S. Gold. 2009. Setting the standard for recovery: Physicians' health programs. *Journal of Substance Abuse Treatment* 36(2):159-171.

Gibbs, D. A., and K. L. Rae Olmsted. 2011. Preliminary examination of the confidential alcohol treatment and education program. *Military Psychology* 23(1):97-111.

Godley, M. D., V. H. Coleman-Cowger, J. C. Titus, R. R. Funk, and M. G. Orndorff. 2010. A randomized controlled trial of telephone continuing care. *Journal of Substance Abuse Treatment* 38(1):74-82.

Goldman, H. H., R. G. Frank, M. A. Burnam, H. A. Huskamp, M. S. Ridgely, S. L. T. Normand, A. S. Young, C. L. Barry, V. Azzone, A. B. Busch, S. T. Azrin, G. Moran, C. Lichtenstein, and M. Blasinsky. 2006. Behavioral health insurance parity for federal employees. *New England Journal of Medicine* 354(13):1378-1386.

Humphreys, J., J. Y. Tsoh, M. A. Kohn, and B. Gerbert. 2011. Increasing discussions of intimate partner violence in prenatal care using Video Doctor plus provider cueing: A randomized, controlled trial. *Women's Health Issues* 21(2):136-144.

IOM (Institute of Medicine). 1990. *Broadening the base of treatment for alcohol problems.* Washington, DC: National Academy Press.

IOM. 1994. *Under the influence? Drugs and the American work force.* Washington, DC: National Academy Press.

Jackson, R. A., N. E. Stotland, A. B. Caughey, and B. Gerbert. 2011. Improving diet and exercise in pregnancy with Video Doctor counseling: A randomized trial. *Patient Education and Counseling* 83(2):203-209.

Kaner, E. F. S., H. O. Dickinson, F. R. Beyer, F. Campbell, C. Schlesinger, N. Heather, J. B. Saunders, B. Burnand, and E. D. Pienaar. 2009. Effectiveness of brief alcohol interventions in primary care populations. *Cochrane Database of Systematic Reviews* 1.

Martell, B. A., P. G. O'Connor, R. D. Kerns, W. C. Becker, K. H. Morales, T. R. Kosten, and D. A. Fiellin. 2007. Systematic review: Opioid treatment for chronic back pain: Prevalence, efficacy, and association with addiction. *Annals of Internal Medicine* 146(2):116-127.

McConnell, K. J., S. H. Gast, M. S. Ridgely, N. Wallace, N. Jacuzzi, T. Rieckmann, B. H. McFarland, and D. McCarty. 2012. Behavioral health insurance parity: Does Oregon's experience presage the national experience with the Mental Health Parity and Addiction Equity Act? *American Journal of Psychiatry* 169(1):31-38.

McLellan, A. T., G. S. Skipper, M. Campbell, and R. L. DuPont. 2008. Five year outcomes in a cohort study of physicians treated for substance use disorders in the United States. *British Medical Journal* 337(7679):1154-1156.

Mee-Lee, D., ed. 2007. *ASAM patient placement criteria for the treatment of substance-related disorders* (2nd ed. rev.). Chevy Chase, MD: American Society of Addiction Medicine.

NQF (National Quality Forum). 2007. *National voluntary consensus standards for the treatment of substance use conditions: Evidence-based treatment practices.* Washington, DC: NQF.

NRC (National Research Council) and IOM. 2009. *Preventing mental, emotional, and behavioral disorders among young people: Progress and possibilities.* Washington, DC: The National Academies Press.

Polen, M. R., E. P. Whitlock, J. P. Wisdom, P. Nygren, and C. Bougatsos. 2008. *Screening in primary care settings for illicit drug use: Staged systematic review for the United States Preventive Services Task Force.* Rockville, MD: Agency for Healthcare Research and Quality.

Tsoh, J. Y., M. A. Kohn, and B. Gerbert. 2010. Promoting smoking cessation in pregnancy with Video Doctor plus provider cueing: A randomized trial. *Acta obstetricia et gynecologica Scandinavica* 89(4):515-523.

U.S. Army. 2010. *Pain Management Task Force: Final report.* Falls Church, VA: Office of the Army Surgeon General.

U.S. Army Surgeon General. 2011. *ALARACT 062/2011: Changes to length of authorized duration of controlled substance prescriptions in MEDCOM regulation 40-51.* Washington, DC: Department of the Army.

VA and DoD. 2009. *VA/DoD clinical practice guideline for management of substance use disorders.* Washington, DC: VA and DoD.

VA and DoD. 2010. *VA/DoD clinical practice guideline for management of opioid therapy for chronic pain.* Washington, DC: VA and DoD.

Weinick, R. M., E. B. Beckjord, C. M. Farmer, L. T. Martin, E. M. Gillen, J. D. Acosta, M. P. Fisher, J. Garnett, G. C. Gonzalez, T. C. Helmus, L. H. Jaycox, K. A. Reynolds, N. Salcedo, and D. M. Scharf. 2011. *Programs addressing psychological health and traumatic brain injury among U.S. military service members and their families.* Santa Monica, CA: RAND Corporation.

Whitlock, E. P., C. A. Green, M. R. Polen, A. Berg, J. Klein, A. Siu, and C. T. Orleans. 2004. *Behavioral counseling interventions in primary care to reduce risky/harmful alcohol use.* Rockville, MD: Agency for Healthcare Research and Quality.

Appendix A

Study Activities

The committee held data-gathering sessions that were open to the public at four of its five meetings. Committee members also visited several military installations, including Camp Pendleton, California; Fort Belvoir, Virginia; Keesler Air Force Base, Mississippi; San Diego Naval Base, California; and Fort Hood, Texas. The agendas for the open sessions of the committee's meetings and for the site visits are presented below.

MEETING ONE

Committee on Prevention, Diagnosis, Treatment and Management of Substance Use Disorders in the U.S. Armed Forces
March 30-31, 2011
Hotel Monaco
700 F Street, NW
Washington, DC

10:00 a.m. **Welcome and Introductory Remarks**
Charles O'Brien, M.D., Ph.D., Committee Chair, University of Pennsylvania

10:10 a.m. **The Charge to the Committee: A Discussion with the Sponsor**
Capt. Robert DeMartino, TRICARE Management Activity
Alfred Ozanian, Ph.D., TRICARE Management Activity

12:00 p.m. **Lunch**

1:00 p.m. **Introduction to SUD Prevention, Diagnosis, Treatment, and Management in the Armed Forces: What Is the Status Quo?**
Alfred Ozanian, Ph.D., TRICARE Management Activity
Les McFarling, Ph.D., Army Center for Substance Abuse Programs
Charles Gould, U.S. Navy Bureau of Medicine and Surgery
Lt. Col. Mark S. Oordt, Ph.D., Air Force Medical Operations Agency

3:30 p.m. **Break**

3:45 p.m. **Responding to Substance Use Disorders in Military Personnel and Their Dependents**
Keith Humphreys, Ph.D., Stanford University

5:00 p.m. **Public Comment Period**

5:30 p.m. **Meeting Close**

MEETING TWO

Committee on Prevention, Diagnosis, Treatment and
Management of Substance Use Disorders in the U.S. Armed Forces
May 3, 2011
DoubleTree Hotel
1515 Rhode Island Avenue, NW
Washington, DC

8:50 a.m.-9:00 a.m. **Welcome and Introduction**
Charles O'Brien, M.D., Committee Chair, University of Pennsylvania

9:00 a.m.-9:30 a.m. **Q&A on MHS and TRICARE**
Don Jansen, Congressional Research Service

9:30 a.m.-10:00 a.m. **The Reserve Components and Access to Care**
Brig. Gen. Margaret Wilmoth, Ph.D., Office of the Assistant Secretary of Defense for Health Affairs

	SUD Prevention, Diagnosis, Treatment, and Management in the Armed Forces: The Medical Perspective
10:00 a.m.-10:50 a.m.	*Barbara Marin, Ph.D., Walter Reed Army Medical Center* *Col. John J. Stasinos, M.D., Dept. of the Army, Office of the Surgeon General*
10:50 a.m.-11:20 a.m.	*Capt. Mary Rusher, M.D., Naval Medical Center San Diego*
11:20 a.m.-11:40 a.m.	*Lt. Col. Mark S. Oordt, Air Force Medical Operations Agency*
11:40 a.m.-12:00 p.m.	**Q&A**
12:00 p.m.-1:00 p.m.	**Lunch**
1:00 p.m.-1:45 p.m.	**SUDs in the Military: Medical vs. Personnel** *Vladimir Nacev, Ph.D., Defense Centers of Excellence*
1:45 p.m.-2:30 p.m.	**Prescription Drug Misuse Among Active Duty Service Members** *Diana D. Jeffery, Ph.D., TRICARE Management Activity*
2:30 p.m.-2:45 p.m.	**Break**
2:45 p.m.-3:45 p.m.	**Access to SUD Care: Confidentiality and Stigma** *Col. Charles Milliken, M.D., Walter Reed Army Institute of Research*
3:45 p.m.-4:30 p.m.	**Substance Use Disorders in the Military: The NIDA Perspective** *Wilson Compton, M.D., National Institute on Drug Abuse* *Eve Reider, Ph.D., National Institute on Drug Abuse*
4:30 p.m.-5:00 p.m.	**Public Comment Period**
5:00 p.m.	**Meeting Close**

SITE VISIT: MARINE CORPS BASE CAMP PENDLETON, CALIFORNIA

Committee on Prevention, Diagnosis, Treatment and Management of Substance Use Disorders in the U.S. Armed Forces
July 18, 2011
Marine Corps Consolidated Substance Abuse Counseling Center (CSACC) & The Navy Substance Abuse and Rehabilitation Program

7:45 a.m.-8:00 a.m.	**Check-In at Camp Pendleton Main Gate**
8:00 a.m.-8:30 a.m.	**Meet with CSACC Director John Veneziano**
8:30 a.m.-9:30 a.m.	**Meet with CSACC Staff**
9:30 a.m.-10:00 a.m.	**Break**
10:00 a.m.-12:00 p.m.	**Meet with Drug Demand Reduction Coordinators**
12:00 p.m.-1:00 p.m.	**Lunch**
1:00 p.m.-2:00 p.m.	**Meet with Staff from Navy Drug and Alcohol Counselor School**
2:00 p.m.-3:00 p.m.	**Meet with Marines Assigned for Temporary Duty at CSACC**
3:00 p.m.-4:00 p.m.	**Debrief with John Veneziano**

MEETING THREE

Committee on Prevention, Diagnosis, Treatment and Management of Substance Use Disorders in the U.S. Armed Forces
July 19, 2011
Beckman Center of the National Academies
100 Academy Way
Irvine, California

9:10 a.m.-9:30 a.m.	**Welcome and Introduction** *Charles O'Brien, M.D., Committee Chair, University of Pennsylvania*

9:30 a.m.-10:15 a.m.	**Purchased Care for Service Members and Their Families: The TRICARE SUD Benefit** *John Sparks, TRICARE Regional Office-West* *Frank Maguire, M.D., TriWest* *Andrea Brooks Tucker, TRICARE Regional Office-South* *Debbie Del Rosario and Gary Proctor, M.D., ValueOptions* *Marie Mentor, TRICARE Regional Office-North* *Ian Schaffer, M.D., and John Wagoner, M.D., Healthnet Federal Services*
10:15 a.m.-10:30 a.m.	**Break**
10:30 a.m.-11:15 a.m.	**Panel: Prevention for Members of the Armed Forces and Their Families** *John M. Morrow, Ph.D., Substance Abuse and Mental Health Services Administration* *Abigail Gewirtz, Ph.D., University of Minnesota* *Ron Astor, Ph.D., University of Southern California*
11:15 a.m.-11:45 a.m.	**Substance Abuse and Military Families** *Barbara Cohoon, Ph.D., National Military Family Association*
11:45 a.m.-12:15 p.m.	**Seeking Safety: Therapy for Comorbid PTSD and SUD** *Lisa Najavits, Ph.D., Harvard University*
12:15 p.m.-1:15 p.m.	**Lunch**
1:15 p.m.-1:45 p.m.	**Workforce Training** *Anthony Hassan, Ph.D., University of Southern California*
1:45 p.m.-2:15 p.m.	**Prescription Drug Monitoring in the Military** *Eugene Moore, PharmD, TRICARE Pharmacy Operations* *Cdr. Joseph B. Lawrence, PharmD, M.B.A., TRICARE Pharmacy Operations*

	Josh Devine, PharmD, TRICARE Pharmacy Operations *Libby Hearin, PharmD, TRICARE Pharmacy Operations*
2:15 p.m.-2:45 p.m.	**Alcohol Abuse in the Military: Findings from the Millennium Cohort Study** *Isabel Jacobson, M.P.H., Naval Health Research Center*
2:45 p.m.-3:00 p.m.	**Break**
3:00 p.m.-3:45 p.m.	**A General's Story** *Lt. Gen. David Fridovich, Dept. of the Army*
3:45 p.m.-4:45 p.m.	**Advancements in the Treatment of Pain: Efforts to Prevent Opioid Dependence** *Lt. Col. Kevin Galloway, Army Pain Management Task Force* *Col. Chester Buckenmaier, M.D., Walter Reed Army Medical Center* *Col. John J. Stasinos, M.D., Dept. of the Army, Office of the Surgeon General*
4:45 p.m.-5:00 p.m.	**Public Comment Period**
5:00 p.m.	**Meeting Close**

SITE VISIT: FORT BELVOIR, VIRGINIA, ADDICTION PROGRAMS

Committee on Prevention, Diagnosis, Treatment and Management of Substance Use Disorders in the U.S. Armed Forces
November 15, 2011

8:00 a.m.	**Arrive at Fort Belvoir Tulley Gate**
8:30 a.m.-9:00 a.m.	**Tour of the Fort Belvoir Community Hospital** *Anthony H. Dekker, D.O., Chief, Addiction Medicine at Fort Belvoir Community Hospital*

9:00 a.m.-9:30 a.m.	**Tour of the Residential Treatment Center, Fort Belvoir Community Hospital** (4 South) *Anthony H. Dekker, D.O., Chief, Addiction Medicine at Fort Belvoir Community Hospital*
9:30 a.m.-10:00 a.m.	**Tour of the Inpatient Residential Treatment Program, Fort Belvoir Community Hospital** (4 North) *Maj. Brunt, M.D., Staff Psychiatrist*
10:00 a.m.-11:00 a.m.	**The Pain Clinic at Fort Belvoir** *Ben Krepps, M.D., Director of the Pain Clinic at Fort Belvoir Community Hospital*
11:00 a.m.-11:30 a.m.	**Inpatient Residential Treatment Program, Fort Belvoir Community Hospital** (4 North) *Jennifer Weaver, M.D., Program Director*
11:30 a.m.-12:15 p.m.	**Lunch**
12:30 p.m.-12:45 p.m.	**Shuttle to the Dewitt Army Hospital Warrior Zone**
12:45 p.m.-1:30 p.m.	**Co-Occurring Program, Dewitt Army Hospital, Warrior Transition Brigade** *Chideha Ohuoha, M.D., M.P.H., Program Director*
1:30 p.m.-2:00 p.m.	**Army Substance Abuse Program, Dewitt Army Hospital** *Doryan Dixon, Program Manager for ASAP* *Dr. Jorge Grandella, ASAP Clinical Supervisor*
2:00 p.m.-3:45 p.m.	**Army Substance Abuse Program, Dewitt Army Hospital** *Ms. Susan Jessup, LCSW, LCAS, Clinical Program Manager*
3:45 p.m.	**Return to the Fort Belvoir Community Hospital River Garage**

MEETING FOUR

Committee on Prevention, Diagnosis, Treatment and Management of Substance Use Disorders in the U.S. Armed Forces
November 16, 2011
Keck Center of the National Academies
500 Fifth Street, NW
Washington, DC

9:00 a.m.-9:15 a.m.	**Welcome and Introduction** *Charles O'Brien, M.D., Committee Chair, University of Pennsylvania*
9:15 a.m.-9:45 a.m.	**NIAAA Update on Treatment for Alcohol Problems Among Active Duty Military Personnel and Veterans** *Bob Huebner, Ph.D., National Institute on Alcohol Abuse and Alcoholism*
9:45 a.m.-10:30 a.m.	**Improving Population Care of Substance Use Disorders in the Military: The Primary Care Imperative** *Col. Charles Engel, M.P.H., M.D., Department of Defense Deployment Health Clinical Center*
10:30 a.m.-10:45 a.m.	**Break**
10:45 a.m.-11:30 a.m.	**A Systems Perspective of Substance Use and Abuse in the Military** *Harold Holder, Ph.D., Prevention Research Center of the Pacific Institute for Research & Evaluation*
11:30 a.m.-12:15 p.m.	**Implementing Evidence-Based Practices for Identification and Management of Substance Use Conditions in the Veterans Health Administration** *Daniel Kivlahan, Ph.D., Office of Mental Health Services, Veterans Health Administration*
12:15 p.m.-12:30 p.m.	**Public Comment Period**
12:30 p.m.	**Meeting Close**

SITE VISIT: KEESLER AIR FORCE BASE, MISSISSIPPI

Committee on Prevention, Diagnosis, Treatment and Management of Substance Use Disorders in the U.S. Armed Forces
January 27, 2012

7:30 a.m.	**Arrive at White Avenue Gate** *Meet 1Lt. Julianna Petrone at Visitors Center*
7:45 a.m.-8:15 a.m.	**Tour of Mental Health Flight Clinics**
8:30 a.m.-9:15 a.m.	**ADAPT Drunk Busters Presentation at the Triangle** *1Lt. Julianna Petrone, LISW, ADAPT Program Manager* *SSgt. Cecilia Cardenas, ADC in Training, ADAPT NCOIC Prevention Activity at Keesler AFB*
9:30 a.m.-10:15 a.m.	**Alcohol and Drug Abuse Prevention and Treatment (ADAPT)** *1Lt. Petrone, LISW, ADAPT Program Manager* *Paul Ahlberg, ADC, ADAPT Counselor* *SrA. Stephanie Tipton, ADC in training, ADAPT Counselor* *SSgt. Cecilia Cardenas, ADC in Training, ADAPT NCOIC*
10:15 a.m.-10:45 a.m.	**Families OverComing Under Stress (FOCUS)** *Kim Perez, LPC, Family Resiliency Trainer* *Eva Shinka, LSCW-C, Assistant Site Director*
10:45 a.m.-11:00 a.m.	**Behavioral Health Optimization Program (BHOP)** *Maj. David Cordry, Clinical Neuropsychologist, Mental Health Flight Commander* *Dr. Myron Horn, Clinical Psychologist, BHOP Consultant*
11:00 a.m.-11:45 a.m.	**Question and Answer Session**

SITE VISIT: SAN DIEGO NAVAL AIR STATION, CALIFORNIA

Committee on Prevention, Diagnosis, Treatment and Management of Substance Use Disorders in the U.S. Armed Forces
March 1, 2012

8:00 a.m.-8:30 a.m.	**Welcome/In-Brief** *Warren Peter Klam, M.D., M.S.(MM), CAPT MC USN (r), Director, Mental Health Services, and Chairman, Psychiatry, General, Child, Adolescent and Addiction Psychiatry, Naval Medical Center, San Diego*
8:30 a.m.-9:30 a.m.	**Substance Abuse Rehabilitation Program (SARP)** *Mary K. Rusher, M.D., CAPT MC USN, Department Head, Substance Abuse Rehabilitation Program, Naval Medical Center, San Diego* *Joanne Rigoloso, Social Worker, Clinic Head at SARP* *Charlie Gould, Director of SARP at Navy Bureau of Medicine (BUMED)*
9:30 a.m.-10:15 a.m.	**Center for Personal and Professional Development** *Tara Leverett, Chief Yeoman (YNC), Prevention and Outreach, Center for Personal and Professional Development West*
10:15 a.m.-10:30 a.m.	**Break**
10:30 a.m.-11:15 a.m.	**DAPA/Command Master Chief NMCSD—CMDCM Duberek** *Valerie Sudduth, Hospital Corpsman (HM1), Assistant Command Drug and Alcohol Program Administrator, Naval Medical Center, San Diego* *Nelson Ferrer, Hospital Corpsman Chief (HMC), Command Drug and Alcohol Program Administrator, Naval Medical Center, San Diego*
11:15 a.m.-12:00 p.m.	**Fleet and Family Services** *Mr. Richard Arriaga, Director, Fleet and Family Support Center, San Diego*

12:00 p.m.-1:00 p.m.	**Lunch**
1:00 p.m.-1:45 p.m.	**Primary Care** *Steven Sovich, M.D., Primary Care Physician, Naval Medical Center, San Diego*
1:45 p.m.-2:30 p.m.	**Pain Management Specialist** *Steven Hanling, M.D., CDR MC USN, Pain Management Provider, Naval Medical Center, San Diego*
2:30 p.m.-2:45 p.m.	**Break**
2:45 p.m.-3:30 p.m.	**Substance Abuse Rehabilitation Program (SARP)** *Mary K. Rusher, M.D., CAPT MC USN, Department Head, Substance Abuse Rehabilitation Program San Diego, Naval Medical Center, San Diego*
3:30 p.m.-4:00 p.m.	**Out-Brief** *Warren Peter Klam, M.D., M.S.(MM), CAPT MC USN (r), Director, Mental Health Services, and Chairman, Psychiatry, General, Child, Adolescent and Addiction Psychiatry, Naval Medical Center, San Diego*

SITE VISIT: CARL R. DARNALL ARMY MEDICAL CENTER, FORT HOOD, TEXAS

Committee on Prevention, Diagnosis, Treatment and Management of Substance Use Disorders in the U.S. Armed Forces
March 15, 2012

7:00 a.m.	**Arrive at Fort Hood Main Gate** *Check into Visitor's Center*
8:00 a.m.-8:30 a.m.	**Introduction to Department of Behavioral Health** *LTC Gray, M.D., Chief, Department of Behavioral Health* *Ms. Nicolette Dennis, LCSW, Acting Chief of Intensive Outpatient Program* *MAJ Agius, M.D., Chief, Hospital & Administrative Psychiatry*

8:30 a.m.-10:30 a.m.	**Intensive Outpatient Program (IOP)** *Ms. Dennis, LCSW, Acting Chief of IOP program* *Dr. Shehan, Staff Psychiatrist for IOP program and ASAP* *Ms. Barnard, Administrator, IOP*
10:30 a.m.-11:30 a.m.	**Primary Care/Respect-Mil** *Dr. Ingram, Chief of Family Medicine* *Dr. Borah, Staff Psychiatrist (Respect-Mil representative, dept BH)* *Ms. April Arrington, Administrator, DFCM*
1:00 p.m.-5:00 p.m.	**Army Substance Abuse Program (ASAP)** *Ms. Pickering, LMFT, LCDC, Clinical Program Director* *Ms. Thompson, Administrator, ASAP*

Appendix B

S. 459 (111th): SUPPORT for Substance Use Disorders Act

S 459 IS

111th CONGRESS

1st Session

S. 459

To improve and enhance substance use disorder programs for members of the Armed Forces, and for other purposes.

IN THE SENATE OF THE UNITED STATES

February 24, 2009

Mrs. MCCASKILL (for herself and Mr. CORKER) introduced the following bill; which was read twice and referred to the Committee on Armed Services

---

A BILL

To improve and enhance substance use disorder programs for members of the Armed Forces, and for other purposes.

Be it enacted by the Senate and House of Representatives of the United States of America in Congress assembled,

SECTION 1. SHORT TITLE.

This Act may be cited as the 'Supporting Uniformed Personnel by Providing Oversight and Relevant Treatment for Substance Use Disorders Act' or the 'SUPPORT for Substance Use Disorders Act'.

SEC. 2. FINDINGS.

Congress makes the following findings:

(1) The Armed Forces is comprised of more than 1,400,000 members in the regular components and more than 1,080,000 members in the Reserves. More than 1,800,000 members of the Armed Forces have been deployed in Operation Iraqi Freedom,

Operation Enduring Freedom, and the Global War on Terrorism since 2001.

(2) Substance use disorders are chronic diseases that can be prevented, treated, and managed effectively. Failure to prevent or treat these conditions results in severe and widespread consequences, including increased risk of suicide, exacerbation of mental and physical health disorders, increased risk of domestic violence and family discord, and increased risk of unemployment and homelessness.

(3) According to the 2005 Department of Defense Survey of Health Related Behaviors Among Active Duty Personnel, 24 percent of the members of the Armed Forces surveyed reported symptoms of alcohol dependence and nearly 11 percent of the members surveyed reported use of an illicit drug. Misuse of controlled prescription drugs, particularly narcotic painkillers, is a significant and growing problem among members of the Armed Forces as well.

(4) Substance abuse disorders often co-occur with other health problems. According to the 2007 Report of the Department of Defense Task Force on Mental Health, 17 percent of soldiers from brigade combat teams are at risk of developing clinically significant symptoms of post-traumatic stress disorder (PTSD), major depression, or anxiety after deployment, and an even higher percentage of such soldiers, 28 percent, would experience symptoms based upon broader screening criteria. The prevalence of post-traumatic stress disorder within a year of combat deployment was estimated to range from 10 to 25 percent.

(5) According to the 2007 Report of the Department of Defense Task Force on Mental Health, symptoms of disorders such as post-traumatic stress disorder often include complex disinhibitory behaviors such as self-medicating with alcohol, other medications, or illicit drugs in an attempt to return to 'normalcy'.

(6) According to the 2007 Report of the Department of Defense Task Force on Mental Health, of the 686,306 veterans separated from active duty between 2002 and December 2006 who were eligible for care from the Department of Veterans Affairs, 229,015 (or 33 percent) accessed care at a Department facility. Of those veterans who accessed such care since 2002, 83,889 (or 37 percent) were diagnosed with or were evaluated for a mental disorder, including post-traumatic stress disorder (39,243 or 17 percent), nondependent abuse of drugs (33,099 or 14 percent), and depressive disorder (27,023 or 12 percent).

(7) According to the 2007 Report of the Department of Defense Task Force on Mental Health, 20 percent of married soldiers planned to separate or divorce.

(8) According to the 2007 Report of the Department of Defense Task Force on Mental Health, relationship problems are the top risk factor for suicide. Mental disorders, alcohol and substance use disorders, and significant stress are other significant risk factors for suicide. The National Violent Death Reporting System of the Centers for Disease Control and Prevention determined that, of a group of former or current military personnel who died by suicide in 2005, 17.2 percent had an alcohol problem and 7.7 percent had a problem with other substances. The suicide prevention action network (SPAN) reports a 20 percent increase in suicide among members of the Armed Forces on active duty, 89 suicides in 2007 with 32 deaths under investigation, and a rise of attempted suicides by soldiers by 6 times higher than it was at the start of Operation Iraqi Freedom.

(9) While some commands and facilities in the Armed Forces provide outstanding services for members of the Armed Forces for substance use disorders, the prevention, diagnosis, mitigation, treatment, and management of, and research on, substance use disorders in members of the Armed Forces is inconsistent in availability, structure, and success among the various Armed Forces.

SEC. 3. COMPREHENSIVE PLAN ON PREVENTION, DIAGNOSIS, MITIGATION, TREATMENT, AND MANAGEMENT OF SUBSTANCE USE DISORDERS IN MEMBERS OF THE ARMED FORCES.

(a) Review and Assessment of Current Capabilities-

(1) IN GENERAL- Not later than 180 days after the date of the enactment of this Act, the Secretary of Defense shall, in consultation with the Secretaries of the military departments and the Secretary of Veterans Affairs, conduct a comprehensive review of the programs and activities of the Department of Defense for the prevention, diagnosis, mitigation, treatment, and management of, and research on, substance use disorders in members of the Armed Forces.

(2) ELEMENTS- The review conducted under paragraph (1) shall include, but not be limited to, an assessment of each of the following:

(A) The current state and effectiveness of the programs of the Department of Defense and the military departments relating to the prevention, diagnosis, mitigation, treatment, and management of, and research on, substance use disorders in members of the Armed Forces.

(B) The adequacy of the availability of and access to care for substance use disorders in military medical treatment facilities and under the TRICARE program.

(C) The adequacy of oversight by the Department of programs relating to the prevention, diagnosis, mitigation, treatment, and management of substance use disorders in members of the Armed Forces.

(D) The adequacy and appropriateness of current credentials and other requirements for healthcare professionals treating members of the Armed Forces with substance use disorders, including an assessment of the advisability of adopting uniform credentials and requirements for such treatment for healthcare professionals who are members of organizations such as the Association for Addiction Professionals (NAADAC), the American Society of Addiction Medicine (ASAM), the American Psychiatric Association (APA), and the National Board for Certified Counselors (NBCC).

(E) The advisable ratio of physician and non-physician care providers for substance use disorders to members of the Armed Forces with such disorders.

(F) The adequacy and appropriateness of protocols for the diagnosis, treatment, and management of substance use disorders in members of the Armed Forces.

(G) The adequacy of the availability of and access to care for substance use disorders for members of the reserve components of the Armed Forces when compared with the availability of and access to care for substance use disorders for members of the regular components of the Armed Forces, including an identification of any obstacles that are unique to the prevention, diagnosis, mitigation, treatment, and management of substance use disorders in members of the reserve components of the Armed Forces.

(H) The adequacy of the prevention, diagnosis, mitigation, treatment, and management of substance use disorders and related distress in dependent family members of members of the Armed Forces, whether such family members suffer from their own substance use disorder or because of the substance use disorder of a member of the Armed Forces.

(I) Any gaps in the current capabilities of the Department of Defense for the prevention, diagnosis, mitigation, treatment, and management of, and research on, substance use disorders in members of the Armed Forces.

(3) REPORT- Not later than 180 days after the date of the enactment of this Act, the Secretary of Defense shall submit to the congressional defense committees a report setting forth the findings and recommendations of the Secretary as a result of the review conducted under paragraph (1). The report shall--

(A) set forth the findings and recommendations of the Secretary regarding each element of the review set forth in paragraph (2);

(B) set forth relevant statistics on the frequency of substance use disorders in members of the regular components of the Armed Forces, members of the reserve component of the Armed Forces, and dependents of such members (including spouses and children); and

(C) include such other findings and recommendations on improvements to the current capabilities of the Department of Defense for the prevention, diagnosis, mitigation, treatment, and management of, and research on, substance use disorders in members of the Armed Forces as the Secretary considers appropriate.

(b) Plan for Improvement and Enhancement of Programs-

(1) PLAN REQUIRED- Not later than 180 days after the date of the enactment of this Act, the Secretary of Defense shall, in consultation with the Secretaries of the military departments and the Secretary of the Department of Veterans Affairs, submit to the congressional defense committees a comprehensive plan for the improvement and enhancement of the programs and activities of the Department of Defense for the prevention, diagnosis, mitigation, treatment, and management of, and research on, substance use disorders in members of the Armed Forces and their dependent family members.

(2) BASIS- The comprehensive plan required by paragraph (1) shall take into account the following:

(A) The results of the review and assessment conducted under subsection (a).

(B) Any preliminary results of the study required by section 4.

(C) Similar initiatives of the Secretary of Veterans Affairs to expand and improve care for substance use disorders among veterans, including the programs and activities conducted under title I of the Veterans' Mental Health and Other Care Improvements Act of 2008 (Public Law 110-387; 112 Stat. 4112).

(3) COMPREHENSIVE STATEMENT OF POLICY- The comprehensive plan required by paragraph (1) shall include a comprehensive statement of the policy of the Department of Defense regarding the prevention, diagnosis, mitigation, treatment, and management of, and research on, substance use disorders in members of the Armed Forces and their dependent family members.

(4) AVAILABILITY OF SERVICES AND TREATMENT- The comprehensive plan required by paragraph (1) shall include mechanisms to ensure the availability to members of the Armed Forces and their dependent family members of services and treatment for substance use disorders, including, but not limited to, services and treatment as follows:

(A) Screening for substance use disorder in all settings, including primary care settings.

(B) Short-term motivational counseling services.

(C) Marital and family counseling.

(D) Inpatient, intensive outpatient, or other residential care services.

(E) Private medical, psychiatric, and professional counseling services.

(F) Relapse prevention services.

(G) Ongoing aftercare and outpatient counseling services.

(H) Pharmacological treatments aimed at treating substance use disorders, including treating cravings for drugs and alcohol.

(I) Detoxification and stabilization services.

(J) Coordination with groups providing peer-to-peer counseling.

(K) Such other services as the Secretary considers appropriate.

(5) PREVENTION AND REDUCTION OF DISORDERS- The comprehensive plan required by paragraph (1) shall include mechanisms to facilitate the prevention and reduction of substance use disorders in members of the Armed Forces through science-based initiatives, including education programs, for members of the Armed Forces and their families.

(6) SPECIFIC INSTRUCTIONS- The comprehensive plan required by paragraph (1) shall include each of the following

(A) SUBSTANCES OF ABUSE- Instructions on the prevention, diagnosis, mitigation, treatment, and management of substance use disorders in members of the Armed Forces, including the abuse of alcohol, illicit drugs, and nonmedical use and abuse of prescription drugs (including addiction to prescription drugs that is an unintended consequence of otherwise required and medically appropriate pain treatment).

(B) HEALTHCARE PROFESSIONALS- Instructions on--

(i) appropriate training of healthcare professionals in the prevention, screening, diagnosis, mitigation, treatment, and management of substance use disorders in members of the Armed Forces;

(ii) appropriate staffing levels for healthcare professionals at military medical treatment facilities for the prevention, screening, diagnosis, mitigation, treatment, and management of substance use disorders in members of the Armed Forces; and

(iii) such uniform training and credentialing requirements for physician and non-physician healthcare professionals in the prevention, screening, diagnosis, mitigation, treatment, and management of substance use disorders in members of the Armed Forces as the Secretary considers appropriate.

(C) SERVICES FOR DEPENDENTS- Instructions on the availability of services for substance use disorders to military dependents (including services for dependents suffering from their own substance use disorder and dependents suffering because of the substance use disorder of a member of the Armed Forces), including instructions on making such services available to such dependents to the maximum extent practicable.

(D) PREVENTION MATERIALS- Instructions on the dissemination of materials regarding substance abuse prevention, including, at a minimum, materials on the following:

(i) The dangers of alcohol abuse.

(ii) The risks of self-medication, and the potential co-occurrence of drug use or abuse with illnesses such as Post Traumatic Stress Disorder (PTSD).

(iii) The risks associated with abuse of prescription medications and the signs of inadvertent addiction to prescription medications that may occur as a consequence of otherwise prescribed treatment plans, as well as the need to properly secure and dispose of such substances to safeguard such substances from third parties such as children.

(iv) The risks of substance abuse faced by military dependents due to the stresses of having a spouse or parent deployed, as well as other factors relating to substance abuse that are unique to military families.

(v) Strategies for prevention of drug and alcohol abuse among children of military families, and suggestions for military parents on how to intervene and find help for a child with a substance use disorder.

(E) DIFFERENTIATION OF DISCIPLINARY ACTION AND TREATMENT- Instructions on the separation of disciplinary actions from prevention and treatment of substance use disorders in members of the Armed Forces.

(F) CONFIDENTIALITY- Instructions on confidentiality for members of the Armed Forces in seeking or receiving services or treatment for substance use disorders.

(G) PARTICIPATION OF CHAIN OF COMMAND- Instructions on appropriate consultation, reference to, and involvement of the chain of command of members of the Armed Forces in matters relating to the diagnosis, treatment, and management substance use disorders in such members.

(H) CONSIDERATION OF GENDER- Instructions on gender specific requirements in the prevention, diagnosis, mitigation, treatment, and management of substance use disorders in members of the Armed Forces, including gender specific care and treatment requirements.

(I) COORDINATION WITH OTHER HEALTHCARE INITIATIVES- Instructions on the integration of efforts on the prevention, diagnosis, mitigation, treatment, and management of substance use disorders in members of the Armed Forces with efforts to address co-occurring health care disorders (such as post-traumatic stress disorder (PTSD) and depression) and suicide prevention.

(7) OTHER ELEMENTS- In addition to the matters specified in paragraph (3), the comprehensive plan required by paragraph (1) shall include the following:

(A) LEAD AGENT- The designation by the Assistant Secretary of Defense for Health Affairs of a lead agent to coordinate implementation of the plan.

(B) MILESTONES AND SCHEDULES- Milestones and schedules for the achievement of the goals of the plan, including goals relating to the following:

(i) Enhanced education of members of the Armed Forces regarding substance use disorders.

(ii) Enhanced and improved identification and diagnosis of substance use disorders in members of the Armed Forces.

(iii) Enhanced and improved access of members of the Armed Forces to services and treatment for and management of substance use disorders.

(iv) Appropriate staffing of military medical treatment facilities and other facilities for the treatment of substance use disorders in members of the Armed Forces.

(C) BEST PRACTICES- The incorporation of evidence-based best practices utilized in current military and civilian approaches to the prevention, diagnosis, mitigation, treatment, and management of substance use disorders.

(D) AVAILABLE RESEARCH- The incorporation of applicable results of available studies, research, and academic reviews on the prevention, diagnosis, mitigation, treatment, and management of substance use disorders.

(8) UPDATE IN LIGHT OF INDEPENDENT STUDY- Upon the completion of the study required by section 4, the Secretary of Defense shall--

(A) in consultation with the Secretaries of the military departments and the Secretary of the Department of Veterans Affairs, make such modifications and improvements to the comprehensive plan required by paragraph (1) as the Secretary of Defense considers appropriate in light of the findings and recommendations of the study; and

(B) submit to the congressional defense committees a report setting forth the comprehensive plan as modified and improved under subparagraph (A).

SEC. 4. INDEPENDENT REPORT ON SUBSTANCE USE DISORDERS IN MEMBERS OF THE ARMED FORCES.

(a) Study Required- The Secretary of Defense shall provide for a study on substance use disorders in members of the Armed Forces to be conducted by the Institute of Medicine of the National Academies of Sciences or such other independent entity as the Secretary shall select for purposes of the study.

(b) Elements- The study required by subsection (a) shall include a review and assessment of the following:

(1) The current state and effectiveness of the programs of the Department of Defense and the military departments relating to the prevention, diagnosis, mitigation, treatment, and management of, and research on, substance use disorders in members of the Armed Forces.

(2) The adequacy of the availability of and access to care for substance use disorders in military medical treatment facilities and under the TRICARE program.

(3) The adequacy of the oversight by the Department of Defense of programs related to the prevention, diagnosis, mitigation, treatment, and management of substance use disorders in members of the Armed Forces.

(4) The adequacy and appropriateness of current credentials and other requirements for physician and non-physician healthcare professionals treating members of the Armed Forces with substance use disorders.

(5) The advisable ratio of physician and non-physician care providers for substance use disorders to members of the Armed Forces with such disorders.

(6) The adequacy and appropriateness of protocols for the diagnosis, treatment, and management of substance use disorders in members of the Armed Forces.

(7) The adequacy of the availability of and access to care for substance use disorders for members of the reserve components of the Armed Forces when compared with the availability of and access to care for substance use disorders for members of the regular components of the Armed Forces.

(8) The adequacy of the prevention, diagnosis, mitigation, treatment, and management of substance use disorders in dependent family members of members of the Armed Forces, whether such family members suffer from their own substance use disorder or because of the substance use disorder of a member of the Armed Forces.

(9) The need for and appropriate provision of confidentiality for members of the Armed Forces who seek services or treatment for a substance use disorder.

(10) Such other matters as the Secretary considers appropriate for purposes of the study.

(c) Report- Not later than one year after the date of the enactment of this Act, the entity conducting the study required by subsection (a) shall submit to the Secretary of Defense and the congressional defense committees a report on the results of the study. The report shall set forth the findings and recommendations of the entity as a result of the study.

SEC. 5. CENTER OF EXCELLENCE IN THE PREVENTION, DIAGNOSIS, MITIGATION, TREATMENT, AND MANAGEMENT OF SUBSTANCE USE DISORDERS.

(a) In General- The Secretary of Defense shall establish within the Department of Defense a Center of Excellence in the Prevention, Diagnosis, Mitigation, Treatment, and Management of Substance Use Disorders.

(b) Partnerships- The Secretary of Defense shall ensure that the Center collaborates to the maximum extent practicable with the Department of Veterans Affairs, institutions of higher education, and other appropriate public and private entities (including international entities) to carry out the responsibilities specified in subsection (c).

(c) Responsibilities- The Center shall have responsibilities as follows:

(1) To implement the comprehensive plan of the Department of Defense for the prevention, diagnosis, mitigation, treatment, and management of substance use disorders under section 3, including the performance of research on gender and ethnic group-specific health needs related to substance use disorders.

(2) To provide for the development, testing, and dissemination within the Department of evidence-based best practices for the prevention, diagnosis, mitigation, treatment, and management of substance use disorders.

(3) To provide guidance for healthcare professionals and support service staff of the health system of the Department in providing quality health care for members of the Armed Forces with substance use disorders, and their dependents, when possible, who are suffering from the effects of substance use disorders.

(4) To provide guidance for healthcare professionals and support service staff to make members of the Armed Forces receiving prescription pain medications aware of the potential for abuse of or addiction to such substances, and to provide such members education on ways of properly securing such substances and disposing of such substances when no longer needed.

(5) To recommend uniform credentials and other requirements for healthcare professionals and support service staff who provide care and support for members of the Armed Forces and their dependents who suffer from substance use disorders.

(6) To establish, implement, and oversee a uniform and comprehensive program to train physician and non-physician healthcare professionals and support staff in the Department in the screening, intervention, treatment, and management of substance use disorders.

(7) To coordinate research, data collection, and data dissemination on the prevention, diagnosis, mitigation, treatment, and management of substance use disorders, and to maintain a database of information for that purpose.

(8) To facilitate advancements in the study of the short-term and long-term physical and psychological effects of substance use disorders.

(9) To disseminate evidence-based best practices within the military medical treatment facilities for training healthcare professionals and support staff with respect to substance use disorders.

(10) To conduct basic science and translational research on substance use disorders in members of the Armed Forces for the purposes of understanding the etiology of substance use disorders and developing preventive interventions and new treatments.

(11) To develop programs and outreach strategies for families of members of the Armed Forces with substance use disorders to address and to mitigate the impact of substance use disorders on such family members and to support the recovery of such members from substance use disorders.

(12) To conduct research on the health needs of families of members of the Armed Forces with substance use disorders and develop protocols to address any needs identified through such research.

(13) To disseminate information to families of members of the Armed Forces regarding ways to help prevent alcohol and drug abuse among their children, as well as educational materials to address how situations unique to military families, such as having a parent deployed, can increase stress levels and put a child at increased risk of abusing drugs or alcohol.

(14) To develop and oversee a long-term plan to increase the number of healthcare professionals and support personnel within the Department in order to facilitate the meeting by the Department

of the needs of members of the Armed Forces with substance use disorders while they remain on active duty and until their transition to care and treatment from the Department of Veterans Affairs.

(15) To develop and deploy an education and awareness training initiative designed to reduce the negative stigma associated with substance use disorders and treatment.

(16) Such other responsibilities as the Secretary shall specify.

SEC. 6. CONGRESSIONAL DEFENSE COMMITTEES DEFINED.

In this Act, the term 'congressional defense committees' means--

(1) the Committee on Armed Services and the Committee on Appropriations of the Senate; and

(2) the Committee on Armed Services and the Committee on Appropriations of the House of Representatives.

Appendix C

Sec. 596 of Public Law 111-84, October 28, 2009

SEC. 596. <<NOTE: 10 USC 1071 note.>> COMPREHENSIVE PLAN ON PREVENTION, DIAGNOSIS, AND TREATMENT OF SUBSTANCE USE DISORDERS AND DISPOSITION OF SUBSTANCE ABUSE OFFENDERS IN THE ARMED FORCES.

(a) Review and Assessment of Current Capabilities.--

(1) In general.-- <<NOTE: Deadline.>> Not later than 180 days after the date of the enactment of this Act, the Secretary of Defense, in consultation with the Secretaries of the military departments, shall conduct a comprehensive review of the following:

(A) The programs and activities of the Department of Defense for the prevention, diagnosis, and treatment of substance use disorders in members of the Armed Forces.

(B) The policies of the Department of Defense relating to the disposition of substance abuse offenders in the Armed Forces, including disciplinary action and administrative separation.

(2) Elements.--The review conducted under paragraph (1) shall include an assessment of each of the following:

(A) The current state and effectiveness of the programs of the Department of Defense and the military departments

[[Page 123 STAT. 2340]]

relating to the prevention, diagnosis, and treatment of substance use disorders.

(B) The adequacy of the availability of care, and access to care, for substance abuse in military medical treatment facilities and under the TRICARE program.

(C) The adequacy of oversight by the Department of Defense of programs relating to the prevention, diagnosis, and treatment of substance abuse in members of the Armed Forces.

(D) The adequacy and appropriateness of current credentials and other requirements for healthcare professionals treating members of the Armed Forces with substance use disorders.

(E) The advisable ratio of physician and nonphysician care providers for substance use disorders to members of the Armed Forces with such disorders.

(F) The adequacy and appropriateness of protocols and directives for the diagnosis and treatment of substance use disorders in members of the Armed Forces and for the disposition, including disciplinary action and administrative separation, of members of the Armed Forces for substance abuse.

(G) The adequacy of the availability of and access to care for substance use disorders for members of the reserve components of the Armed Forces, including an identification of any obstacles that are unique to the prevention, diagnosis, and treatment of substance use disorders among members of the reserve components, and the appropriate disposition, including disciplinary action and administrative separation, of members of the reserve components for substance abuse.

(H) The adequacy of the prevention, diagnosis, and treatment of substance use disorders in dependents of members of the Armed Forces.

(I) Any gaps in the current capabilities of the Department of Defense for the prevention, diagnosis, and treatment of substance use disorders in members of the Armed Forces.

(3) Report.--Not later than 180 days after the date of the enactment of this Act, the Secretary of Defense shall submit to the Committees on Armed Services of the Senate and the House of Representatives a report setting forth the findings and recommendations of the Secretary as a result of the review conducted under paragraph (1). The report shall--

(A) set forth the findings and recommendations of the Secretary regarding each element of the review specified in paragraph (2);

(B) set forth relevant statistics on the frequency of substance use disorders, disciplinary actions, and administrative separations for substance abuse in members of the regular components of the Armed Forces, members of the reserve component of the Armed Forces, and to the extent applicable, dependents of such members (including spouses and children); and

[[Page 123 STAT. 2341]]

(C) include such other findings and recommendations on improvements to the current capabilities of the Department of Defense for the prevention, diagnosis, and treatment of substance use disorders in members of the Armed Forces and the policies relating to the disposition, including disciplinary action and administrative separation, of members of the Armed Forces for substance abuse, as the Secretary considers appropriate.

(b) Plan for Improvement and Enhancement of Programs and Policies.--

(1) Plan required.-- <<NOTE: Deadline.>> Not later than 270 days after the date of the enactment of this Act, the Secretary of Defense shall submit to the congressional defense committees a comprehensive plan for the improvement and enhancement of the following:

(A) The programs and activities of the Department of Defense for the prevention, diagnosis, and treatment of substance use disorders in members of the Armed Forces and their dependents.

(B) The policies of the Department of Defense relating to the disposition of substance abuse offenders in the Armed Forces, including disciplinary action and administrative separation.

(2) Basis.--The comprehensive plan required by paragraph (1) shall take into account the following:

(A) The results of the review and assessment conducted under subsection (a).

(B) Similar initiatives of the Secretary of Veterans Affairs to expand and improve care for substance use disorders among veterans, including the programs and activities conducted under title I of the Veterans' Mental Health and Other Care Improvements Act of 2008

(Public Law 110-387; 112 Stat. 4112).

(3) Comprehensive statement of policy.--The comprehensive plan required by paragraph (1) shall include a comprehensive statement of the following:

(A) The policy of the Department of Defense regarding the prevention, diagnosis, and treatment of substance use disorders in members of the Armed Forces and their dependents.

(B) The policies of the Department of Defense relating to the disposition of substance abuse offenders in the Armed Forces, including disciplinary action and administrative separation.

(4) Availability of services and treatment.--The comprehensive plan required by paragraph (1) shall include mechanisms to ensure the availability to members of the Armed Forces and their dependents of a core of evidence-based practices across the spectrum of medical and non-medial services and treatments for substance use disorders, including the reestablishment of regional long-term inpatient substance abuse treatment programs. The Secretary may use contracted services for not longer than three years after the date of the enactment of this Act to perform such inpatient substance abuse treatment until the Department of Defense reestablishes this capability within the military health care system.

[[Page 123 STAT. 2342]]

(5) Prevention and reduction of disorders.--The comprehensive plan required by paragraph (1) shall include mechanisms to facilitate the prevention and reduction of substance use disorders in members of the Armed Forces through science-based initiatives, including education programs, for members of the Armed Forces and their dependents.

(6) Specific instructions.--The comprehensive plan required by paragraph (1) shall include each of the following:

(A) Substances of abuse.--Instructions on the prevention, diagnosis, and treatment of substance abuse in members of the Armed Forces, including the abuse of alcohol, illicit drugs, and nonmedical use and abuse of prescription drugs.

(B) Healthcare professionals.--Instructions on--

(i) appropriate training of healthcare professionals in the prevention, screening, diagnosis, and treatment of substance use disorders in members of the Armed Forces;

(ii) appropriate staffing levels for healthcare professionals at military medical treatment facilities for the prevention, screening, diagnosis, and treatment of substance use disorders in members of the Armed Forces; and

(iii) such uniform training and credentialing requirements for physician and nonphysician healthcare professionals in the prevention, screening, diagnosis, and treatment of substance use disorders in members of the Armed Forces as the Secretary considers appropriate.

(C) Services for dependents.--Instructions on the availability of services for substance use disorders for dependents of members of the Armed Forces, including instructions on making such services available to dependents to the maximum extent practicable.

(D) Relationship between disciplinary action and treatment.--Policy on the relationship between disciplinary actions and administrative separation processing and prevention and treatment of substance use disorders in members of the Armed Forces.

(E) Confidentiality.--Recommendations regarding policies pertaining to confidentiality for members of the Armed Forces in seeking or receiving services or treatment for substance use disorders.

(F) Participation of chain of command.--Policy on appropriate consultation, reference to, and involvement of the chain of command of members of the Armed Forces in matters relating to the diagnosis and treatment of substance abuse and disposition of members of the Armed Forces for substance abuse.

(G) Consideration of gender.--Instructions on gender specific requirements, if appropriate, in the prevention, diagnosis, treatment, and management of substance use disorders in members of the Armed Forces, including gender specific care and treatment requirements.

(H) Coordination with other healthcare initiatives.--Instructions on the integration of efforts on the

[[Page 123 STAT. 2343]]

prevention, diagnosis, treatment, and management of substance use disorders in members of the Armed Forces with efforts to address co-occurring health care disorders (such as post-traumatic stress disorder and depression) and suicide prevention.

(7) Other elements.--In addition to the matters specified in paragraph (3), the comprehensive plan required by paragraph (1) shall include the following:

(A) Implementation plan.--An implementation plan for the achievement of the goals of the comprehensive plan, including goals relating to the following:

(i) Enhanced education of members of the Armed Forces and their dependents regarding substance use disorders.

(ii) Enhanced and improved identification and diagnosis of substance use disorders in members of the Armed Forces and their dependents.

(iii) Enhanced and improved access of members of the Armed Forces to services and treatment for and management of substance use disorders.

(iv) Appropriate staffing of military medical treatment facilities and other facilities for the treatment of substance use disorders in members of the Armed Forces.

(B) Best practices.--The incorporation of evidence-based best practices utilized in current military and civilian approaches to the prevention, diagnosis, treatment, and management of substance use disorders.

(C) Available research.--The incorporation of applicable results of available studies, research, and academic reviews on the prevention, diagnosis, treatment, and management of substance use disorders.

(8) Update in light of independent study.--Upon the completion of the study required by subsection (c), the Secretary of Defense shall--

(A) in consultation with the Secretaries of the military departments, make such modifications and improvements to the comprehensive plan required by paragraph (1) as the Secretary of Defense considers appropriate in light of the findings and recommendations of the study; and

(B) <<NOTE: Reports.>> submit to the congressional defense committees a report setting forth the comprehensive plan as modified and improved under subparagraph (A).

(c) Independent Report on Substance Use Disorders Programs for Members of the Armed Forces.--

(1) Study required.--Upon completion of the policy review required by subsection (a), the Secretary of Defense shall provide for a study on substance use disorders programs for members of the Armed Forces to be conducted by the Institute of Medicine of the National Academies of Sciences or such other independent entity as the Secretary shall select for purposes of the study.

(2) Elements.--The study required by paragraph (1) shall include a review and assessment of the following:

(A) The adequacy and appropriateness of protocols for the diagnosis, treatment, and management of substance use disorders in members of the Armed Forces.

[[Page 123 STAT. 2344]]

(B) The adequacy of the availability of and access to care for substance use disorders in military medical treatment facilities and under the TRICARE program.

(C) The adequacy and appropriateness of current credentials and other requirements for physician and non-physician healthcare professionals treating members of the Armed Forces with substance use disorders.

(D) The advisable ratio of physician and non-physician care providers for substance use disorders to members of the Armed Forces with such disorders.

(E) The adequacy of the availability of and access to care for substance use disorders for members of the reserve components of the Armed Forces when compared with the availability of and access to care for substance use disorders for members of the regular components of the Armed Forces.

(F) The adequacy of the prevention, diagnosis, treatment, and management of substance use disorders programs for dependents of members of the Armed Forces, whether such dependents suffer from their own substance use disorder or because of the substance use disorder of a member of the Armed Forces.

(G) Such other matters as the Secretary considers appropriate for purposes of the study.

(3) Report.--Not later than two years after the date of the enactment of this Act, the entity conducting the study required by paragraph (1) shall submit to the Secretary of Defense and the congressional defense committees a report on the results of the study. The report shall set forth the findings and recommendations of the entity as a result of the study.

Appendix D

Program Reviews

This appendix summarizes programs identified in the *Comprehensive Plan on Prevention, Diagnosis, and Treatment of Substance Use Disorders and Disposition of Substance Use Offenders in the Armed Forces* (*Comprehensive Plan*) (DoD, 2011) as pertaining to the prevention, diagnosis, treatment, and management of substance use disorders (SUDs). Summary tables on each program[1] are followed by descriptive analyses based on the committee's review of relevant information gathered from policies, responses to information requests, the published literature, public meetings, and site visits. In addition to the programs discussed in the Department of Defense (DoD) report, the committee learned during the course of its research about additional pertinent programs worthy of inclusion here. These programs are reviewed at the end of the section on each branch. Several DoD programs are cited by the individual branches in the *Comprehensive Plan* as programs they implement; additionally, the branches occasionally make use of each other's programs. To avoid redundancy, these programs are reviewed in the sections on the branches responsible for their development and/or initial implementation and referenced in the sections on the other branches that utilize them.

[1]The summary tables are excerpted from the *Comprehensive Plan* (Appendix C). The elements in the tables and the subsequent findings on each program contained within were generated by DoD for the *Comprehensive Plan*. Based on the information presented in the *Comprehensive Plan*, the committee noted that when evidence-based practices (EBPs) are identified for a program, it is in many cases unclear to what extent they are being used or how specifically they are implemented.

DEPARTMENT OF DEFENSE

Red Ribbon Campaign

Purpose and Goals	*Clinical Focus*	*Program Evaluation/ Outcomes*	*Target Population*	*EBPs*
• The national Red Ribbon campaign raises public awareness and mobilizes communities to combat tobacco, alcohol and drug use among military personnel, civilians and their families.	• Prevention	• N/A	• Active Duty • Dependents	• N/A*

NOTE: EBP = evidence-based practice; N/A = not applicable.
*Note that the entry on the Red Ribbon campaign in the DoD section of Appendix C of the *Comprehensive Plan* lists "N/A" in the "EBP" column, while the entry in the Air Force section suggests that the campaign does, in fact, employ EBPs, including "community-based processes, environmental strategies, information dissemination, alternative activities, education and problem recognition and referral."

Red Ribbon Week is an annual campaign that is conducted nationwide in the United States every October both at the community level and on military bases. Consequently, it has the capacity to reach service members and their families at all stages of military involvement except deployment outside of the United States. Within DoD, the targets are active duty service members (ADSMs) and their families, as well as the community at large. The focus is on raising awareness about SUD prevention and risk factors (DEA, 2012). The program's website indicates that "Red Ribbon Week educates individuals, families, and communities on the destructive effects of alcohol and drugs and encourages the adoption of healthy lifestyle choices." The program is a universal prevention campaign aimed at addressing peer pressure and prosocial bonding in youth, as well as parent monitoring. Thus, it is most developmentally appropriate for young military members with families. The primary setting for delivery is the community, although as noted, the campaign can be implemented on base. The committee finds there is no evidence on this program's effectiveness, and both military bases and communities vary widely in the activities they sponsor under the auspices of the campaign. There is presently no published information on Red Ribbon's theoretical basis or on its outcomes.

That Guy Alcohol Abuse Prevention Education Campaign

Purpose and Goals	*Clinical Focus*	*Program Evaluation/ Outcomes*[a]	*Target Population*[b]	*EBPs*[c]
• That Guy is a multi-media campaign designed to reduce binge drinking among military enlisted personnel ages 18-24. • The campaign includes online and offline advertising and promotions, viral marketing, a website, www.thatguy.com, public service announcements, and branded collateral materials.	• Prevention	• Number of personnel joining social network sites • Change in drinking behavior where implemented • Overall awareness of campaign • Change in drinking attitudes	• Active Duty	• N/A

NOTE: EBP = evidence-based practice; N/A = not applicable.
[a] The table on this program in the Navy section of Appendix C of the *Comprehensive Plan* lists the following under "Program Evaluation/Outcomes": "Total number of visits per month to website per Service, Average number of minutes per visit spent on website per Service, Total number of public service announcements per Service, and Number of promotional items distributed."
[b] The table on this program in the Navy section identifies Reserves as an additional target population.
[c] The table on this program in the Navy section lists "CSAP [Center for Substance Abuse Prevention] prevention strategies" under EBPs.

The That Guy campaign uses on- and offline public service announcements, a website with animated risk scenarios and modeling of prevention techniques, and prevention marketing. Because of its accessibility by Internet, the campaign can reach National Guard and Reserve members, although its primary focus is on ADSMs. In a typical animated scenario, a service member is shown exhibiting socially inappropriate behavior after drinking. The scenario is designed to show negative consequences of binge drinking, including negative reactions from military peers. Alternative scenarios with positive decision making and outcomes also are depicted. This campaign is most developmentally appropriate for younger ADSMs. The overall aims are to increase awareness about the hazards of excessive drinking and shift attitudes toward this behavior. This represents a change from the precontemplation to the contemplation stage of substance use behavior according to Prochastka and Velicer's (1997) transtheoretical stage of change model.

In reviewing this program, the committee found that it uses evidence-based practices of modeling, rehearsal, discussion, and practice and focuses primarily on negative perceived consequences, negative social consequences, and peer pressure. Because it is an Internet-based campaign, its setting can be anywhere. Repeat use is dependent on the user. The March 2012 That Guy newsletter (That Guy Campaign, 2012) reports several statistics on reach and usage for 2011, including

- There were more than 1.3 million ThatGuy.com sessions.
- Users spent an average of 9 minutes on the site.
- The That Guy Facebook page had more than 26,000 fans.
- More than 2.7 million branded materials were being used by all of the branches.
- More than 4,200 points of contact were engaged across the globe.
- More than 800 installations, ships, fleets, submarines, and units had engaged in the campaign.
- Forty-seven states and 22 countries had a That Guy presence.

According to a recent RAND report, an annual DoD survey of forces indicated that awareness of the campaign had increased over time, and attitudes toward excessive drinking had changed (Weinick et al., 2011). DoD, TRICARE Management Activity, and Fleishmann-Hillard released a paper on That Guy in 2009 that mentions a "statistically significant increase in awareness of That Guy and a positive shift in attitudes toward excessive drinking," but does not describe an evaluation methodology or provide outcome data (DoD et al., 2009, p. 2). There has as yet been no formal outcome evaluation of the That Guy campaign in a peer-reviewed journal, and based on its findings, the committee cannot determine whether the program is effective at preventing risky drinking and alcohol misuse.

Health Assessments

Periodic Health Assessment (PHA) Screening				
Purpose and Goals	*Clinical Focus*	*Program Evaluation/ Outcomes*	*Target Population*	*EBPs*
• Personnel are screened annually for substance use related issues during the annual preventive health assessment. Services vary as to their use of screening instruments.	• Screening	• Percent of ADSM who complete annual PHA	• Active Duty • Reserve • National Guard	• Screening typically by AUDIT-C, but screening tools choice can vary*

Force Health Protection and Readiness Post-Deployment Health Assessment (PDHA) and Post-Deployment Health Reassessment (PDHRA) Program				
Purpose and Goals	*Clinical Focus*	*Program Evaluation/ Outcomes*	*Target Population*	*EBPs*
• To review each service's member's current health, mental health/ substance abuse or psychosocial issues commonly associated with deployments, special medications taken during deployment, possible deployment-related occupational/ environmental exposures, and to discuss deployment related health concerns. Positive responses require use of supplemental assessment tools and/or referrals for medical consultation. The provider documents concerns available to help resolve any post-deployment issues. • The new DoD policy mandates person-to-person mental health assessments prior to deployment and then three times after return from deployment. These assessments include use of the Alcohol Use Disorders Identification Test-Consumption (AUDIT-C), as well as intervention by a primary care provider, based on the number of positive responses made by the Service member on the AUDIT-C.	• Prevention • Screening	• Comprehensive quality assurance program	• Active Duty • Reserve • National Guard	• AUDIT-C

NOTE: ADSM = active duty service member; AUDICT-C = Alcohol Use Disorders Identification Test-Consumption; DoD = Department of Defense; EBP = evidence-based practice; N/A = not applicable; PHA = periodic health assessment.
*In the Air Force, all service members are assessed for hazardous drinking and alcohol abuse and dependence based on the AUDIT-C.

Health assessments of military members are conducted during active military duty service on a yearly basis, as well as pre- and postdeployment. Health assessment could be considered a prevention strategy to the extent that the provider discusses SUD risk factors or the service member raises questions about risk factors or strategies for preventing SUDs, but its primary focus is on screening.

DoD's pre- and postdeployment health assessments have three stages. Stage 1 is based on self-report and has the objective of defining high-risk groups. The first three questions of the Alcohol Use Disorders Identification Test-Consumption (AUDIT-C) are used to detect risky drinking as part of Stage 1. Stage 2 collects additional information if Stage 1 screening is positive for posttraumatic stress disorder (PTSD) or depression. If Stage 1 screening with AUDIT-C is positive, Stage 3 consists of a provider interview in which brief intervention for risky drinking is administered or a referral is made. The provider training for the deployment health assessments instructs the provider to do the following in the brief intervention: bring attention to the elevated level of drinking; recommend limiting use or abstaining; inform about the effects of alcohol on health; explore and help/support in choosing a drinking goal; and follow up and refer for specialty treatment, if indicated (Vythilingam et al., 2010). Referral is recommended when the service member requires further evaluation of use, has tried and has been unable to change on his/her own, has had prior treatment, has had a recent problem with alcohol that resulted in counseling or referral to treatment, or has an AUDIT-C score equal to or greater than 8. Referral options vary with the service member's status, and include emergency behavioral health referral and referral to a provider in a military treatment facility, a TRICARE purchased care provider, a Department of Veterans Affairs (VA) medical center, a Veterans (VET) center, or Military OneSource (DoD, 2010; Vythilingam et al., 2010).

The committee finds that the use of AUDIT-C for pre- and postdeployment health assessments is an appropriate means of screening for excessive and hazardous alcohol use; AUDIT-C is well known and has been well validated for use in a variety of settings. Unfortunately, the only service branch to require the use of AUDIT-C in periodic health assessments is the Air Force. The other branches recommend screening by a clinician but do not identify specific screening tools to be used. The committee would prefer to see AUDIT-C used uniformly across all the branches and in all health assessments, independently of whether they are related to deployment.

A second important consideration in evaluating screening in both periodic and deployment-related health assessments is that positive screening should lead to further intervention depending on the severity of the condition being screened for. In the case of alcohol, identification of excessive use should lead to a more detailed assessment and brief intervention, with referral to treatment as indicated. Indeed, as described above, Stage 3 of the pre- and postdeployment assessments follows this procedure. However, studies have found that while positive screening rates for alcohol misuse can be as high as 27 percent among Army soldiers in postdeployment health assessments (Santiago et al., 2010), only a small proportion of those who screen positive ever receive treatment. For instance, Milliken and colleagues (2007) report that 12 percent of soldiers screened positive for alcohol misuse in postdeployment assessments, but only 0.2 percent were referred to the Army Alcohol Safety Action Program (ASAP), and only 0.05 percent were actually seen at ASAP within 90 days of referral. This situation is critical because members who screen positive for alcohol misuse are likely also to be engaged in risky behaviors such as drinking and driving and illicit drug use (Santiago et al., 2010).

The committee finds this low rate of referral and treatment for those who screen positive to be related to the stigma associated with substance abuse treatment in the military. Such stigma also exists in the larger society, but it is stronger in the military in part because of the requirement to inform Command when service members are admitted for SUD treatment. Many service members fear that Command knowledge of their need for treatment will negatively impact their career (Gibbs et al., 2011). The committee finds that the low rates of referral resulting from a positive screen for alcohol misuse in pre- and postdeployment health assessments represent a threat to public health and force readiness.

Military Pathways

Purpose and Goals	*Clinical Focus*	*Program Evaluation/ Outcomes*	*Target Population*	*EBPs*
• Program offers service personnel and their families the opportunity to take anonymous, mental health and alcohol use self-assessments online, via the phone, and through special events held at installations. Program is designed to help individuals identify their own symptoms and access assistance before a problem becomes serious.	• Prevention • Screening	• Numbers of screenings • Quantities of promotional materials distributed • Customer satisfaction	• Active Duty • Reserve • National Guard • Dependents	• EBPs are utilized

Purpose and Goals	*Clinical Focus*	*Program Evaluation/ Outcomes*	*Target Population*	*EBPs*
• The self-assessments address posttraumatic stress disorder (PTSD), depression, generalized anxiety disorder, alcohol use, and bipolar disorder. After completing a self-assessment, individuals receive referral information including services provided by TRICARE, Military OneSource, and Vet Centers.				

NOTE: EBP = evidence-based practice.

Military Pathways encompasses a multifaceted set of program components aimed primarily at universal prevention. The program also includes a self-assessment/self-screening component that can serve as secondary prevention for military members who identify themselves as being at personal risk for SUD and subsequently seek help. Designed by the nonprofit organization Screening for Mental Health, the program has as its primary goals to "reduce stigma, raise awareness about mental health, and connect those in need to available resources" (Military Pathways, 2012, p. 1). The multiple components of the program (described in the table above) enable repetition of prevention education. A theoretical basis is implied by program content that includes empowerment building and social and family support seeking. The empowerment content is consistent with military life and institutional goals of fitness. A RAND report estimates that this intervention reaches more than 305,000 ADSMs and their families each year (Weinick et al., 2011). The program targets ADSMS and their families primarily at entry into the military and predeployment. However, it is assumed that the online, telephone, and video components of the program can be accessed at any stage of military life. The family resiliency kit and a special program for youth (Signs of Suicide, or SOS) are special components aimed directly at military family members (although they do not apply specifically to the prevention of substance abuse); trained paraprofessionals deliver the family kit, and school professionals (not specified) deliver the SOS program to youth in schools. The RAND report (Weinick et al., 2011) cites ongoing trials to evaluate the effectiveness of the self-screening and youth program components, but no outcome data have yet been published on the alcohol, PTSD, or mental health screening components. Without such data, the committee cannot comment on the extent to which the program is evidence based or effective at preventing and screening for SUDs.

Real Warriors Campaign

Purpose and Goals	*Clinical Focus*	*Program Evaluation/ Outcomes*	*Target Population*	*EBPs*
• A multimedia public education initiative designed to address the stigma associated with seeking psychological health care and encourage service members and their families to reach out to resources. • The Real Warriors Campaign website, public service announcements and broadcasts on Armed Services Radio encourage service members and their families to seek help for psychological health issues including SUD. • The website includes original articles focused specifically on substance misuse and providing individuals multiple avenues to care.	• Prevention	• Numbers of calls or hits • Customer satisfaction	• Active Duty • Dependents	• N/A

NOTE: EBP = evidence-based practice; N/A = not applicable; SUD = substance use disorder.

The Real Warriors Campaign is an initiative launched by the Defense Centers of Excellence for Psychological Health and Traumatic Brain Injury (DCoE). While its goal is to "promote the processes of building resilience, facilitating recovery and supporting reintegration of returning service members, veterans and their families" (DCoE, 2012, p. 1), the program is not specifically aimed at the prevention of substance abuse. The campaign was developed in response to recommendations of the 2007 DoD Task Force on Mental Health designed to remove the barriers that often prevent service members from obtaining treatment for psychological health issues and traumatic brain injury (Weinick et al., 2011). Utilizing print materials, media outreach, an interactive website, and social media, the campaign features stories of actual service members who have sought treatment and continue to maintain successful military or civilian careers. In developing the program, DCoE did a thorough job of analyzing the characteristics of the service members who would be seeking treatment, and conducted literature searches and focus groups to determine the most effective content to include in the campaign (Acosta et al., 2012; DCoE, 2012). While RAND did conduct a recent study to assess the content, design, and dissemination of the campaign (Acosta et al., 2012), to date, no outcome evaluation has been conducted. DCoE does require the collection of various process indicators, such as the number of visitors to the website, but without further evaluation the committee cannot determine if this program is effective at preventing SUDs.

Military and Civilian Drug Testing Program

Purpose and Goals	*Clinical Focus*	*Program Evaluation/ Outcomes*	*Target Population*	*EBPs*
• The military and civilian drug testing programs are a primary component of the installation Drug Demand Reduction Programs. The program works to ensure a drug-free workplace.	• Prevention	• Percentage of mandated population testing per year • Rate of untestable samples • Rate of verified positive samples	• Active Duty • Reserve	• EBPs are utilized

NOTES: This table is included in the section on Air Force programs in Appendix C of the *Comprehensive Plan*, but is, in fact, a DoD-wide initiative. In addition, the Navy makes use of a software tool called the Navy Drug Screening Program that randomizes testing. EBP = evidence-based practice.

The Military and Civilian Drug Testing Program is identified in the *Comprehensive Plan* as both a prevention and screening program. The program is guided by policy (DoD, 1994), and the stated prevention aim is deterrence. The implied prevention mediator is increasing the perceived negative consequences of positive drug testing rather than drug use per se. As described in Chapter 5, however, there is no clear evidence from controlled studies that drug testing is an effective prevention strategy. While the decline in rates of substance use in the military correlates temporally with the inception of drug testing for specific substances (see Chapter 2), there have been no studies assessing the causal relationship between the two; therefore, the committee cannot report on the effectiveness of the drug testing program in preventing SUDs.

Adolescent Substance Abuse Counseling (ASAC) Program

Purpose and Goals	*Clinical Focus*	*Program Evaluation/ Outcomes*	*Target Population*	*EBPs*
• The ASAC program provides substance abuse counseling services including outreach, prevention, education, and referral services to adolescents in selected OCONUS middle and high schools.	• Prevention • Screening • Diagnosis • Treatment	• Total number of prevention classes • Total number of students referred • Total number of students enrolled • Total number of students screened but not enrolled	• Dependents	• ASAC counselors are trained in EBPs such as outcome-informed counseling, solution-focused counseling, brief interventions, and ASAM Patient Placement Criteria

NOTES: The ASAC program is listed as an Air Force program in Appendix C of the *Comprehensive Plan*, but the committee learned during the course of its research that it is used by other branches as well, and therefore listed it here in the section on DoD programs. ASAC = Adolescent Substance Abuse Counseling; ASAM = American Society of Addiction Medicine; EBP = evidence-based practice; OCONUS = outside of contiguous United States.

ASAC was initially listed as a Science Applications International Corporation contract with the Army, but now also includes Air Force (where ASAC is listed under "DoD/Service Branch" programs), Navy, and Marine Corps dependents. The focus is on children of military families in 6th through 12th grades who are considered at risk for substance use and who are authorized to use military treatment facilities. Contracted providers who include licensed and certified counselors deliver early intervention counseling with adolescents and their parents and, if necessary, make referrals to additional services (U.S. Army, 2011). The counselors may include social workers, substance use counselors, family therapists, and psychologists. The program is delivered in DoD-dependent schools, in civilian schools, and within other existing substance abuse programs for the military. Services specified in the contract include treatment, identification and referral, and prevention education (U.S. Army, 2011).

The ASAC prevention education program includes information and skill-building activities designed to increase protective factors such as life skills, decision-making skills, and prosocial support for dealing with parental deployment, reintegration, and transition, as well as to minimize risk factors related to transition. Prevention is delivered both in the classroom for whole groups of students and in a counseling format for subgroups and individuals within a school. Students identified as at further risk based on a request for help, a reported behavioral or substance use event, or a substance use assessment are referred for additional intervention. The prevention education component of ASAC is relevant to all stages of military involvement, with the possible exception of the postmilitary stage. While the program does not specify a theoretical basis in its standard operating procedures, it draws from Substance Abuse and Mental Health Services Administration (SAMHSA) guidelines for addressing risk and protective factors in school-based skills training programs.

Beyond prevention activities, the ASAC program provides extensive assessments to determine whether individuals need more intensive services. Counselors use the American Society of Addiction Medicine (ASAM) criteria to determine the appropriate level of care for referral if further intervention is needed. The standard operating procedures also detail many quality-assurance activities that are built into the program, including completing utilization reviews of all activities and maintaining a clinical quality-assurance plan (U.S. Army, 2011).

The committee finds that this contracted program provides a comprehensive set of services that meet standards of care for SUD prevention and early interventions for youth. The committee is unaware of the availability of the ASAC program across different branches and military sites. Also unknown is the effectiveness of the program as no formal outcome evaluations have been conducted with the target population.

Additional Programs and Initiatives

Military OneSource is an online source of information on many topics, including 800 telephone numbers of "consultants," the National Suicide Prevention Lifeline, and the Safe Helpline for Sexual Assault Support. DoD describes Military OneSource as

> a free service provided by the Department of Defense to service members and their families to help with a broad range of concerns including money management, spouse employment and education, parenting and child care, relocation, deployment, reunion, and the particular concerns of families with special-needs members. They can also include more complex issues like relationships, stress, and grief. Services are available 24 hours a day—by telephone and online. Many Military OneSource staff members have military experience (veterans, spouses, Guardsmen, Reservists), and

> all receive ongoing training on military matters and military lifestyle. The program can be especially helpful to service members and their families who live at a distance from installations. (DoD, 2012, p. 1)

Military OneSource also provides basic information on alcohol abuse and Web links for the Army's Substance Abuse Program, Cocaine Anonymous, TRICARE Alcohol Awareness, and other related sources (DoD, 2012). In response to the committee's request for information, the program manager of Military OneSource explained the scope of services available. The counseling provided by Military OneSource's contracted providers is nonmedical in nature (e.g., connecting people to resources; counseling on relationship issues, readjustment, and stress). Individuals presenting with an issue that warrants a mental health diagnosis or pharmacotherapy are referred to services through the Military Health System or their health insurance. In July 2011, in response to concern that providers were counseling people beyond their scope,[2] an internal policy clarification was sent to Military OneSource providers specifying the nonmedical nature of the counseling that should be provided. The committee finds that while Military OneSource provides a confidential means for service members and their families to be screened for SUDs and referred to resources, the lack of any clinical counseling indicates that the service is not designed to provide actual treatment for mental health issues.

AIR FORCE

Alcohol and Drug Abuse Prevention and Treatment (ADAPT) Program

Purpose and Goals	*Clinical Focus*	*Program Evaluation/ Outcomes*	*Target Population*	*EBPs*
• The ADAPT Program provides substance related assessment, preventative education, clinical treatment and referral services for Airmen, civilian employees, and family members.	• Prevention • Diagnosis • Treatment	• Access time to substance assessment and clinical treatment • Proportion of participants completing treatment program (tracked locally only)	• Active Duty • Reserve • National Guard • Dependents	• Substance Abuse Counselors are trained in motivational interviewing and cognitive-behavioral interventions

[2]Personal communication, Dave Kennedy, Program Manager of Military OneSource, August 11, 2011 (Office of the Secretary of Defense, Personnel and Readiness, Military Community and Family Policy).

Purpose and Goals	*Clinical Focus*	*Program Evaluation/ Outcomes*	*Target Population*	*EBPs*
• The objectives of the ADAPT program are to promote readiness, health, and wellness through the prevention and treatment of substance abuse; minimize the negative consequences of substance abuse to the individual, family, and organization; provide comprehensive education and treatment to individuals who experience problems attributed to substance abuse; and to return identified substance abusers to unrestricted duty status or assist them in their transition to civilian life.		• Assessment of drinking behavior and duty performance at 3, 6, and 12 months post discharge from intensive outpatient, partial hospitalization, variable length of stay, or inpatient treatment programs (tracked locally only)		

NOTE: ADAPT = Alcohol and Drug Abuse Prevention and Treatment; EBP = evidence-based practice.

ADAPT is described in Air Force Instruction (AFI) 44-121 (U.S. Air Force, 2011), which is discussed in Chapter 6. The purpose of the program is to restore function and return personnel to duty or assist them in returning to civilian life. ADAPT has four tiers of activities according to AFI 44-121: Tier I—primary prevention and education, Tier II—secondary/targeted prevention, Tier III—tertiary care/treatment, and Tier IV—training.

According to AFI 44-121, Tier I activities center around primary prevention and education, which have a different focus depending on the individual being targeted (e.g., service member, health care professional, Air University student, commander). Program activities related to primary prevention appear to focus exclusively on the individual level, without including prevention at the environmental level (e.g., alcohol control policies).

Tiers II and III focus on secondary/targeted prevention and tertiary care/treatment, respectively. The targeted prevention program, Alcohol Brief Counseling (described below), is correctly directed at individuals who are at high risk because of heavy alcohol use but who do not qualify for a full diagnosis of abuse or dependence. All individuals seen in the ADAPT program also receive an Alcohol Education Module, which reinforces Air Force policies on use of substances and also focuses on clarification of values and anxiety and anger management.

For screening, all ADAPT sites make use of the Substance Use Assessment Tool (SUAT). The SUAT, developed for use in the Air Force in 2007, is a comprehensive mental health and substance use assessment and case management tool that is designed to be self-administered by the service member and is used across all ADAPT sites. It provides a preliminary diagnosis (to then be confirmed or revised by a licensed mental health provider), a level-of-care recommendation, and motivational interviewing feedback.

ADAPT treatment programs are designed to ensure that the individual acquires and applies an understanding of the disease of alcoholism, communication and coping skills, and mechanisms for establishing goals that reinforce an alcohol-free lifestyle. Abstinence from alcohol is required in the initial treatment phase of ADAPT. ADAPT staff evaluate any service members who have problems with abstaining from alcohol to determine appropriate interventions and, if necessary, change the treatment plan to help clients meet their goals and return to full duty status. Treatment is planned according to ASAM placement criteria. In ADAPT Level I treatment, which usually last 8 weeks, service members participate in both individual and group counseling sessions weekly. Counselors offer interventions based on motivational interviewing, as well as cognitive-behavioral treatment. The treatment team includes not only mental health professionals involved in the clinical care being provided but also the service member's immediate supervisor and the commander and/or first sergeant. The ADAPT staff at each base coordinate with local TRICARE providers to arrange treatment for those service members requiring inpatient residential treatment, a level of care not provided within ADAPT. Upon completion of residential or nonresidential treatment off base, service members normally return to their duty stations and enter the aftercare phase. Failure to complete treatment successfully may lead to administrative separation.

ADAPT staff design individualized aftercare plans providing continued support with at least monthly monitoring. During this phase of treatment, service members demonstrate their ability to meet Air Force standards and develop the skills and resources needed to maintain a substance-free lifestyle. Normally, individuals remain in aftercare for 6 months to a year after entering the ADAPT program. Procedures also include assessment of drinking behavior and duty performance at 3, 6, and 12 months after discharge from treatment at higher levels of care. The treatment team evaluates the individual's progress quarterly and keeps the commander informed (U.S. Air Force, 2011). The committee did not have access to information about treatment success rates.

Finally, ADAPT works closely with the Behavioral Health Optimization Program (BHOP) (described further below), which provides brief intervention in a primary care setting to respond to behavioral health needs. Clients are referred by primary care physicians and are seen for three to four sessions. These sessions focus, for example, on planned behavior change, screening for depression, and planning for relapse prevention. The committee found that BHOP does not see a large number of clients with substance abuse problems because primary care providers often refer these patients directly to ADAPT for further assessment. Nevertheless, the existence of BHOP and its relationship with ADAPT are a strength of the Air Force's approach to addressing behavioral health concerns, including substance abuse.

Overall, the committee finds that ADAPT offers a comprehensive array of services, providing interventions at different levels of intensity and complexity depending on the initial assessment of individuals referred to the program. Thus, brief intervention is available for high-risk individuals as is more intensive treatment, with the latter ranging from outpatient to day treatment to inpatient care. Aftercare plans, which include relapse prevention, also are offered.

Alcohol Brief Counseling (ABC)

Purpose and Goals	*Clinical Focus*	*Program Evaluation/ Outcomes*	*Target Population*	*EBPs*
• ABC is an individualized, targeted preventive intervention for members seen in ADAPT who are not diagnosed with a substance use disorder.	• Prevention	• Outcome survey to track self-reported impact of intervention on substance use and program quality monitoring (tracked locally only)	• Active Duty • Reserve • National Guard	• ABC utilizes standardized assessment tools (AUDIT, CEOA, SIP, RTCQ) and motivational interviewing

Purpose and Goals	*Clinical Focus*	*Program Evaluation/ Outcomes*	*Target Population*	*EBPs*
• ABC's process is conducted within 10 days of the initial assessment. ABC components include a brief consultation and feedback, an alcohol education module and one or more follow-up session(s) to track progress on a personalized change plan.				

NOTE: ABC = Alcohol Brief Counseling; ADAPT = Alcohol and Drug Abuse Prevention and Treatment; AUDIT = Alcohol Use Disorders Identification Test; CEOA = Comprehensive Effects of Alcohol; EBP = evidence-based practice; RTCQ = Readiness to Change Questionnaire; SIP = Short Index of Problems.

If individuals assessed by ADAPT do not meet diagnostic criteria for an SUD, they receive ABC as an indicated prevention measure. Counseling sessions last about 45 minutes, and service members participate in one to four sessions, depending on an assessment of risk level. If a diagnosis is assigned during the course of ABC, an individual can then enter a treatment program, with the level of treatment being determined according to ASAM criteria. The Air Force reported to the committee that it tracks recidivism rates for those who undergo the ABC intervention, but no formal evaluations are conducted to assess the program's effectiveness.[3] The Air Force Medical Operations Agency reported to the committee outcome measures related to recidivism for fiscal year (FY) 2008-2010. Of the 5,960 service members referred to ABC in FY 2010, 1,137 (19 percent) were defined as recidivists; recidivism rates were similar for FY 2008 and 2009. The implementation of ABC is assessed during the Air Force Inspection Agency's Health Services Inspection.[4]

The committee finds that the use of ABC conforms to the evidence-based practice of providing brief intervention and education to those at risk for developing SUDs. The Air Force appropriately uses ABC as an initial intervention aimed at preventing more serious alcohol use in the future, and applies it to individuals who are drinking in a hazardous way but have not been diagnosed with an alcohol use disorder. The committee cannot comment on the program's effectiveness based on the limited outcome data reported on recidivism.

[3] Personal communication, Air Force Medical Operations Agency, October 25, 2011.
[4] Personal communication, Air Force Medical Operations Agency, October 25, 2011.

Behavioral Health Optimization Program (BHOP)

Purpose and Goals	*Clinical Focus*	*Program Evaluation/ Outcomes*	*Target Population*	*EBPs*
• BHOP providers are integrated into primary care clinics to provide consultation to medical providers and focused assessment and interventions for patients with substance abuse concerns. • BHOP providers provide patient advice, education, and facilitate referrals to ADAPT for substance abuse assessment when appropriate.	• Prevention • Screening • Diagnosis	• None identified	• Active Duty • Reserve • National Guard • Dependents	• Training in EBPs is included in the basic and advanced BHOP training • AUDIT and AUDIT-C for screening • VA/DoD clinical practice guidelines • Motivational interviewing • 5-A's model

NOTE: ADAPT = Alcohol and Drug Abuse Prevention and Treatment; AUDIT = Alcohol Use Disorders Identification Test; AUDIT-C = AUDIT-Consumption; BHOP = Behavioral Health Optimization Program; DoD = Department of Defense; EBP = evidence-based practice; VA = Department of Veterans Affairs.

BHOP providers are psychologists who work in integrated in primary care clinics, consulting on cases that involve either behavioral health (e.g., PTSD) exclusively or dual diagnoses of a physical health problem with a behavioral health component (e.g., hazardous drinking). BHOP providers also offer brief advice and refer service members to the ADAPT program if they need more intensive substance abuse assessment. The structure of the BHOP program allows for a degree of confidential screening for SUDs, as well as brief advice, in a way that counters the stigma associated with service members disclosing and discussing personal issues related to their alcohol and other drug use. This brief intervention within primary care practices is an important model for identifying and resolving SUD issues early. With this new model, the Air Force is building the capacity to provide confidential screening, brief intervention, and referral to treatment (SBIRT) for those at risk of developing SUDs.

Consistent with national trends toward the integration of behavioral health care into primary care services, the Air Force has moved aggressively toward integrated care. The committee finds that BHOP is an important step toward fully integrated care, particularly as it evolves from identification of

SUDs and referral to specialty care toward care that includes the provision of early and brief intervention for SUDs by primary care providers. BHOP is a model for expanding integrated care in all military treatment facilities.

Culture of Responsible Choices (CoRC)

Purpose and Goals	*Clinical Focus*	*Program Evaluation/ Outcomes*	*Target Population*	*EBPs*
• CoRC is a commander's program consisting of a four-tiered approach with emphasis on leadership, individual, base, and community-level involvement—underscoring responsible behaviors including alcohol and drug abuse, the prevention of accidents, tobacco cessation, obesity and fitness, health and wellness, prevention of STDs, etc. CoRC initiatives include Assessment/ Screening of risk in all personnel, education/ awareness programs, brief interventions and treatment when needed, top down emphasis on responsibility and commitment. Components also include base and local community opportunities for change such as developing a range of alternate activities, media campaign promoting responsibility, coalition with community agencies, and monitoring of locally identified metrics.	• Prevention • Screening • Diagnosis • Treatment	• Alcohol-Related Misconduct (ARM) incidences per 1,000 SMs • Drug positives per 1,000 SMs	• Active Duty • Dependents	• Use EBPs (e.g., screening instruments) recommended by the National Institute of Alcohol Abuse and Alcoholism (NIAAA)

NOTE: CoRC = Culture of Responsible Choices; EBP = evidence-based practice; SM = service members; STD = sexually transmitted disease.

The CoRC program trains commanders to promote wellness at four levels: (1) leadership, (2) individual, (3) base, and (4) community. Several of the program components are designed as "toolkits." At the leadership level, commanders and health care providers who deliver prevention (i.e., ADAPT providers, BHOP consultants, and Life Skills Support Center [LSSC] personnel) are trained annually on the purpose, use, and measurement of prevention program components. Toolkits are used to supplement Command training.

Toolkits 1-4 address the individual level. Toolkit 1 is a universal prevention program targeting population-wide screening for alcohol use using the AUDIT instrument, with the option of an additional social norms survey. It targets primarily ADSMs but can also include civilians and contract employees at Command's discretion. Anonymous surveys are administered annually at major Command-involved activities such as Commander's Calls. The prevention focus includes deterrence and surveillance, as well as educational feedback about consequences of alcohol misuse and perceived social norms for use. To the extent that screening and social norms surveys are used for educational feedback, this toolkit could be considered evidence based. Toolkit 2 is a selected prevention program component that trains Command on the purpose of preventive health assessment and routine care, as well as on procedures for referring ADSMs who have been or are at risk for being involved in alcohol-related incidents to appropriate selective prevention and intervention. Annual screening using AUDIT-C is recommended. Referral channels are specified; for example, individuals with comorbid behavioral health conditions should be referred to an LSSC for further intervention after screening. To the extent that referral channels and procedures are clear, this toolkit could be considered to accord with evidence-based practices (EBPs) for screening and referral. Whether Command or providers are responsible for initial identification of high-risk individuals for screening is not specified. Toolkits 1 and 2 are used at the base as well as the individual level. The six components of the Enforcing Underage Drinking Laws (EUDL) program (discussed further below) apply to both levels.

Toolkit 3 is a procedural guide for service providers in behavioral health clinics and LSSCs in use of the AUDIT screening tool. This toolkit is used as indicated prevention for service members with alcohol problems. Toolkit 4 is a training and resource guide aimed at Command, ADAPT staff, and Drug Demand Reduction staff, with the purpose of building community collaborations for prevention. This toolkit includes training in prevention concepts, screening, social norms, consulting to the community, and prevention program management. It follows EBPs for community implementation processes and prevention operating systems (Hawkins and Catalano, 1992).

The committee does not agree with the designation of CoRC in the above table as having a clinical focus in treatment.

Drug Education for Youth (DEFY)

Purpose and Goals	*Clinical Focus*	*Program Evaluation/ Outcomes*	*Target Population*	*EBPs*
• DEFY's goals are to produce 9- to 12-year-olds with character, leadership, and confidence so that they are equipped to engage in positive, healthy lifestyles as drug-free citizens, and have the necessary skills to be successful in their lives through coordinated community participation, commitment, and leadership thereby empowering military youth to make positive life choices. • DEFY is operated world-wide and consists of a summer leadership camp (Phase 1) and a school-year mentoring program (Phase 2). The program curriculum provides youth with a variety of topics including substance abuse prevention and other vital life skills including conflict resolution, self-management skills, study skills, leadership, and community service.	• Prevention	• Knowledge • Skills • Attitudes	• Dependents	• EBPs from the National Institute of Drug Abuse are incorporated within the DEFY curriculum

NOTE: DEFY = Drug Education for Youth; EBP = evidence-based practice.

The DEFY program was started by the Navy in 1993, and although it is also used by the Air Force, the discussion is on this program is in the section on Navy programs below.

Enforcing Underage Drinking Laws (EUDL) Program

Purpose and Goals	*Clinical Focus*	*Program Evaluation/ Outcomes*	*Target Population*	*EBPs*
• EUDL is a pilot prevention program being conducted in conjunction with the Department of Justice (DOJ) and the National Institute of Alcohol Abuse and Alcoholism (NIAAA). • EUDL is designed to reduce the availability of alcoholic beverages to and the consumption of alcoholic beverages by underage service members using environmental approaches and community coalitions.	• Prevention	• DWIs/DUIs • Traffic accidents • Compliance checks • Crimes	• Active Duty • Dependents	• Development of EUDL was predicated on the use of EBPs such as increased enforcement of underage drinking laws, increased DWI/DUI checks, increased compliance checks, covert underage buys, party patrols, etc.

NOTE: DUI = driving under the influence; DWI = driving while intoxicated; EBP = evidence-based practice; EUDL = Enforcing Underage Drinking Laws.

The EUDL program was a pilot that showed significant reductions in underage drinking (Spera and Franklin, 2010). A grant initiative funded by the Office of Juvenile Justice and Delinquency Prevention resulted in the development and testing of the EUDL program at five Air Force sites. The program used evidence-based strategies advocated by the Office of Juvenile Justice and Delinquency Prevention and the National Institute on Alcohol Abuse and Alcoholism (NIAAA). Its six components were (1) enforcement aimed at reducing the social availability of alcohol, (2) compliance checks at alcohol establishments, (3) driving under the influence (DUI) checks, (4) education of state legislatures and development of local policies, (5) a media awareness campaign, and (6) provision of alternative activities to alcohol use. Results from the five sites showed significant reductions in rates of problem drinking both within sites and compared with control communities (Spera and Franklin, 2010; Spera et al., 2012). The committee learned during an information gathering session that EUDL was a demonstration project and that there are currently no plans to expand it to all Air Force bases; however, some of its components will be implemented within other Air Force–wide initiatives.[5] The committee finds the EUDL program to be a promising example of an effective approach to SUD prevention in military settings.

Air Force Reserve Component Substance Abuse Prevention Specialist Training (SAPST)

Purpose and Goals	*Clinical Focus*	*Program Evaluation/ Outcomes*	*Target Population*	*EBPs*
• The SAPST program aims to increase knowledge and improve skills of Drug Demand Reduction Program technicians and program managers in substance abuse prevention, facilitate full-scale adaptation and implementation of the SAPST model, and provide preliminary direction to the identification of related training and technical assistance needs.	• Prevention	• None identified	• Reserve	• EBPs are utilized

NOTE: EBP = evidence-based practice; SAPST = Substance Abuse Prevention Specialist Training.

A September 2011 evaluation of a SAPST session sponsored by SAMHSA in cooperation with the U.S. Air Force Reserve Command, held June 27 to July 1, 2011, measured trainees' reactions to the training. The trainees gave high marks to the training's design and materials and its usefulness, and expressed confidence that they could carry out the prevention programs covered. However, no follow-up outcome evaluations were conducted to determine whether the trainees actually carried out the prevention programs as they were trained to do, or to evaluate whether the programs

[5]Personal communication, Lt. Col. Mark S. Oordt, Ph.D., USAF ADAPT Program, October 25, 2011.

reduced the prevalence of SUDs in the populations to whom they were delivered. Therefore, the committee cannot determine whether the program is effective at preventing SUDs.

ARMY

Army Substance Abuse Program (ASAP)

The Army Center for Substance Abuse Programs (ACSAP) manages ASAP, which provides nonclinical prevention services (e.g., universal education, deterrence, identification/detection, referral) and clinical rehabilitation services (assessment and treatment). These services and related activities are reviewed below.

Prevention, Education, and Training Program

Purpose and Goals	*Clinical Focus*	*Program Evaluation/ Outcomes*	*Target Population*	*EBPs*
• The program provides soldiers with substance abuse prevention and awareness training to include at a minimum: Army Substance Abuse Program (ASAP) policies and services, consequences of alcohol and other drug abuse, incompatibility of alcohol and other drug abuse with physical and mental fitness, combat readiness, Army Values, and the Warrior Ethos.	• Prevention	• Screening Enrollment Report by Installation and Command • Education/ Training Report by Unit • UPL Certification Database by Individual Command • Resource and Performance Report by Installation and Command	• Active Duty • Reserve • Dependents	• ADAPT curriculum utilizes EBPs

NOTE: ADAPT = Alcohol and Drug Abuse Prevention and Treatment; EBP = evidence-based practice; UPL = unit prevention leader.

The Army employs designated personnel called unit prevention leaders (UPLs) who oversee each unit's prevention plan. They monitor substance abuse training, ensuring that all active soldiers meet the mandatory minimum requirement to complete 4 hours of substance abuse awareness training per year (2 hours per year for Reserve and National Guard members) (U.S. Army, 2009). UPLs also monitor how commanders identify high-risk populations. UPLs are certified after a 2-week training program (U.S. Army, undated). The most noteworthy Army prevention programs are Prime for Life (PFL) and myPRIME.

PFL is based on the Lifestyle Risk Reduction Model, the Transtheoretical Model, and persuasion theory and has demonstrated efficacy in young adults and adults up to age 55 (SAMHSA, 2010). It is listed as a universal, selective, and indicated prevention program. The program's classroom-based training, offered by certified PFL instructors (ACSAP, 2012b), focuses on the adverse effects and consequences of alcohol and other drug abuse. Designed as a motivational group intervention to prevent alcohol and other drug problems or provide early intervention, PFL emphasizes changing participants' perceptions of the risks of alcohol and other drug use and related attitudes and beliefs. It also has been used with military personnel, college students, middle and high school students, and parents. Different versions of the program, ranging from 4.5 to 20 hours in duration, and optional activities are available for use with various populations. While PFL is listed as an evidence-based approach in the National Registry of Evidence-Based Programs and Practices (SAMHSA, 2010) and widely used throughout the United States, very few studies have been conducted that demonstrate the efficacy of PFL. It should also be noted that no studies have been conducted to evaluate the efficacy of PFL with the U.S. military population. Therefore, the committee cannot determine whether the use of this program with Army service members is effective at preventing SUDs.

The myPrime prevention program, designed specifically for use in the military, is based on the PFL curriculum. It is an indicated intervention intended for soldiers who present with issues with alcohol and/or other drugs while deployed. This online intervention-training tool enables deployed soldiers to self-assess their high-risk behaviors and is intended to influence changes in attitudes, beliefs, and behaviors (ACSAP, 2012b).

The ACSAP website (ACSAP, 2012a) identifies training appropriate at the squad to unit level. When a soldier who completed myPRIME while deployed returns to his/her home station, the commander must send the soldier to the garrison ASAP office for completion of care. The myPRIME adaptation for military personnel is generic in nature; it includes no military-specific information, nor has it been adapted for the contexts of substance use among military personnel. As with PFL, there is no evidence that this program is effective at preventing SUDs in the Army.

Risk Reduction Program

Purpose and Goals	*Clinical Focus*	*Program Evaluation/ Outcomes*	*Target Population*	*EBPs*
• The Army Risk Reduction Program (RRP) is a commander's tool designed to identify and reduce soldiers' high-risk behaviors in the areas of substance abuse, spouse and child abuse, sexually transmitted diseases, suicide, crimes against people, crimes against property, absence without leave (AWOL), traffic violations, accidents and injuries, and financial problems. RRP focuses on effective use of installation resources and a coordinated effort between commanders and installation agencies to implement intervention and prevention programs.	• Prevention	• Regression Analysis by Risk Factors by Unit, Installation, Region, and Command • Unit Risk Inventory (URI) Survey Administrated at Unit Level with Upper Level Comparisons, Installation, Region, and Command • Reintegration-URI Survey Administrated at Unit Level with Upper Level Comparisons, Installation, Region, and Command	• Active Duty • Reserve	• N/A

NOTE: EBP = evidence-based practice; N/A = not applicable.

The Army Risk Reduction Program is a Command prevention tool aimed at reducing high-risk behaviors such as substance abuse among soldiers. It began in 1994 at Fort Campbell and has since been implemented at Army sites around the world. The program is designed to collect data on high-risk behaviors at the installation level and then bring together an Installation Prevention Team to create interventions targeting the high-risk behaviors thus identified. The program's data systems allow commanders to track trends in the incidence of high-risk behaviors and to compare those rates between specific units or with Army-wide rates (ACSAP, 2012c).

During its site visit to Fort Hood, the committee learned that the Risk Reduction Program had helped lead to the decision to close on-base liquor stores at 9:00 PM instead of 12:00 AM in an effort to reduce risky drinking behaviors on base. The committee finds that this program could assist commanders in allocating prevention resources to the highest-risk behaviors, in making decisions about implementing environmental prevention strategies (such as the earlier closing of liquor stores at Fort Hood), and in tracking outcome trends after specified interventions have been delivered. The extent to which commanders are held accountable for the results of the program's risk analyses and the extent to which the program's tools are utilized across Army sites is unknown.

Employee Assistance Program (EAP)

Purpose and Goals	*Clinical Focus*	*Program Evaluation/ Outcomes*	*Target Population*	*EBPs*
• The Army's Employee Assistance Program (EAP) provides a wide variety of services for various adult living problems. These services include but are not limited to screening, short-term counseling, and referral for all adult living problems.	• Prevention • Screening	• EAP reports by Installation and User • Screening and Enrollment Report by Installation and Command	• Dependents	• N/A

NOTE: EBP = evidence-based practice; N/A = not applicable.

Civilian employers frequently offer EAPs as a human resources benefit to provide assessment and brief intervention services for employees seeking behavioral health assistance. The EAPs offered in the Army are located within ASAP and provide a multitude of services, including short-term counseling and referral to care providers for more intensive needs. The Army supports EAP services for ADSMs, members of the National Guard and Reserves, and civilian employees. Unlike ADSMs, Guard and Reserve members can access treatment programs through the EAP without having to notify their Command. While the Army's EAP services may provide some early intervention and referral services for SUDs (particularly for Guard and Reserve members who may need assistance with finding care options outside of the TRICARE network), the committee finds the location of these services within ASAP to be problematic because of the stigma associated with accessing care for SUDs. The committee did not receive enough information on the Army's EAP to comment on the quality or effectiveness of these services in preventing and screening for SUDs.

Rehabilitation Program

Purpose and Goals	*Clinical Focus*	*Program Evaluation/ Outcomes*	*Target Population*	*EBPs*
• The objective of the Rehabilitation Program is to return soldiers to full duty as soon as possible; identify and refer soldiers who cannot be rehabilitated in the Army Substance Abuse Program (ASAP) to a rehabilitation facility in the vicinity where they reside after discharge from the Army; help resolve alcohol and other drug abuse problems in the family, with the ultimate goal of enabling the soldier to perform more effectively; and for civilian employees to restore them to effective duty performance.	• Screening • Diagnosis • Treatment	• Screening and Enrollment Report by Installation and Command • Rehabilitation Summary • Rehabilitation Caseload • DAMIS dynamic ad hoc query capability	• Active Duty • Reserve • Dependents	• N/A

NOTE: DAMIS = Drug and Alcohol Management Information System; EBP = evidence-based practice; N/A = not applicable.

The ASAP Rehabilitation Program focuses on returning soldiers to full duty quickly by providing outpatient, intensive outpatient, and residential rehabilitation services for SUDs. Enrollment in rehabilitation services requires Command notification, and the commander is included on the treatment team. Most ASAP clinics provide outpatient treatment (with a few exceptions noted in the next section); more intensive services often are referred to TRICARE network providers. During a site visit to Fort Belvoir, the committee found that while ASAP treats many individuals with comorbid disorders, ASAP treatment counselors are credentialed through the military treatment facility only to provide treatment for SUDs. The result is that soldiers cannot receive care in ASAP that addresses comorbid disorders. Since the Army requires master's level counselors with independent licensure (see Chapter 8), the committee finds this limitation to be impractical. The committee is unaware of any formal evaluations of the ASAP rehabilitation program to determine its effectiveness.

Additional Programs and Initiatives

The committee reviewed two ongoing pilot programs within the Army—the Confidential Alcohol Treatment and Education Pilot (CATEP) and an Intensive Outpatient Program (IOP) pilot at Fort Hood. CATEP is a program for soldiers who self-refer to ASAP with alcohol problems *before* they are involved in an incident. Because participation in CATEP does not compromise one's military career, soldiers have improved access to treatment for alcoholism earlier in the course of their illness. The IOP program at Fort Hood, which began in February 2010, was designed to provide more intensive care than was available at the ASAP clinic on base, as well as to treat those with comorbid disorders. Currently, the program is providing ASAM Level II.5 care as a 4-weekday treatment program; therefore, the name of the program will be changing to reflect that it provides care beyond the IOP level. For further discussion of these two pilot programs, see Chapter 6.

A third initiative the committee examined is the Comprehensive Solider Fitness (CSF) program, a resiliency training program with four elements: (1) a global assessment tool (GAT), an online self-report measure of the ability to adapt to stress and challenge that is used as a measure of self-assessment and goal setting and as a guide for the selection of program modules that are tailored to an individual's needs; (2) comprehensive resilience modules, a set of self-development training modules that are accessed online and address specific resilience skills in four dimensions (social, emotional, spiritual, family) for a total of 24 hours; (3) a master resiliency train-the-trainer program that trains primarily noncommissioned officers (NCOs) to implement CSF with groups of soldiers at the unit or installation level, and requires a total of 10 days and 80 hours of training for certification; and (4) resiliency training, which is delivered by master trainers in groups to military members and their families. ADSMs are required to be trained in CSF, with a recommended implementation schedule of 2 hours/month; families and Army civilians can participate on a voluntary basis. Resiliency training can conceivably be delivered throughout the stages of military life, from entry through postdeployment.

The program, adapted from the Penn Resiliency Program, is based on resiliency theory (Rutter, 2006) and theories of positive psychology as an alternative to depression (Seligman, 1998). A special issue of *American Psychologist* described the CSF program and initial research results on military populations, which are focused on changes in GAT scores (Peterson et al., 2011). In addition, an internal military evaluation examined approximately 10,000 soldiers assigned by installation to one of two groups: intervention or control. Analyzing data from three GAT survey assessments conducted over a 15-month period, the evaluators concluded that the intervention group showed sustained, beneficial changes in resiliency, depression, and fitness compared with the control group (Lester et al., 2011b). However, assignment was not random; installations that could not schedule the program were assigned to the control group. Furthermore, it is unclear whether changes in either nonmilitary or military populations have translated to changes in substance use behavior. Thus, while CSF might be considered a promising approach to preparing and maintaining military fitness under stressful conditions, it is unclear whether this program prevents or reduces substance use.

NAVY

Substance Abuse Rehabilitation Program (SARP)

Purpose and Goals	*Clinical Focus*	*Program Evaluation/ Outcomes*	*Target Population*	*EBPs*
• Using the American Society of Addiction Medicine patient placement criteria, SARP matches the appropriate intensity of treatment to the individual's level of need. SARP covers a spectrum referred to as the continuum of care that ranges from early intervention, through outpatient, intensive outpatient, residential and medically managed care.	• Prevention • Screening • Diagnosis • Treatment	• Number of patients retained on Active Duty after 1 year • Percentage of patients completing treatment • Length of time to wait for a screening • Length of time before treatment begins	• Active Duty • Reserve • Dependents	• Motivational interviewing • Twelve-step facilitation • Living in Balance • Contingency management • Cognitive behavioral intervention

NOTE: EBP = evidence-based practice; SARP = Substance Abuse Rehabilitation Program.

SARP is the Navy's substance use treatment program. It provides prevention, screening, diagnosis, and treatment services. The Navy recognizes that SUDs are preventable and treatable. Command is trained to identify Navy members in need of treatment. Orders are written, and those identified are required to follow through with treatment orders or be at risk for loss of clearance and discharge.

The effectiveness of the Navy's prevention and treatment programs is monitored in part by the Alcohol and Drugs Management Information and Tracking System (ADMITS). ADMITS collects, maintains, analyzes, and disseminates data on all incidents and activities related to the Navy's drug and alcohol abuse prevention and control programs. It also provides screening numbers and documentation of treatment outcomes to SARP. ADMITS is able to track numbers of Drug and Alcohol Abuse Report submissions, screening results submitted accurately, and treatment results submitted accurately (DoD, 2011).

Aftercare also is provided to each individual seen in treatment. Typical aftercare includes ongoing participation in approved self-help groups and clinically monitored outpatient counseling groups, and enrollment in the Navy My Ongoing Recovery Experience (MORE) program (described in the following section). Recommendations are tailored to the individual, and Command is responsible for monitoring aftercare participation.

SARP has 40 sites plus 14 additional sites on ships to provide substance use treatment. More than 300 certified substance use counselors are available. The counselors follow the ASAM Patient Placement Criteria. Outpatient treatment consists of an 8-day program for those identified as alcohol abusers. Intensive outpatient treatment, consisting of a 3-week, full-day program, is available for individuals identified as dependent. Residential programs also are available for those who are dependent. Treatment includes programs for family members interested in learning how dependence impacts families. Evidence-based treatments provided include cognitive-behavioral therapy, motivational interviewing, and psychopharmacology.

The Navy also offers an indicated prevention program called Impact. This program was described to the committee during its visit to the naval base in San Diego. It is a 20-hour program designed for patients who have not been diagnosed with a significant substance-related disorder but whose use of substances has created concern for the patient or the patient's Command. The program includes participation in an interactive educational curriculum and exposure to 12-step recovery programs.

The San Diego SARP, the largest and most intensive, provides both residential care (34 days of around-the-clock care, including assessment, group counseling, workshops, fitness activity, and self-help meetings) and outpatient care. Instruction 5353.4A requires SARPs to provide a continuum of care that includes

- early intervention/education (20 hours of instruction) (ASAM Level 0.5)—Alcohol-AWARE and Alcohol-Impact (these programs are not classified as treatment, and initial completion of the programs does not require Command notification);
- outpatient treatment and continuing care (9 hours or less contact per week unless mission requirements necessitate more compressed

and intense clinical contact during the first 2 weeks of care) (ASAM Level I);

- intensive outpatient treatment and partial hospitalization (80 to 100 hours of clinical contact over a 4- to 6-week period) (ASAM Level II)—4 or more hours of care 3 to 5 days per week;
- clinically monitored residential treatment (variable lengths of stay, generally up to 4 weeks in duration) (ASAM Level III)—for patients who require a safe and stable living environment in which to develop recovery skills; and
- medically managed inpatient treatment (ASAM Level IV)—medical services for detoxification and comorbidities coordinated through military treatment facilities.

SARP is therefore a comprehensive treatment program that offers several therapeutic interventions with varying levels of intensity depending on ASAM placement criteria (Levels 0.5 to IV). Besides treatment, SARP's activities appropriately encompass prevention, early indicated intervention, screening and diagnosis, and aftercare. EBPs are applied throughout. The effectiveness of treatment is monitored, although no assessment of effectiveness with state-of-the-art randomized techniques has been conducted. The committee was particularly impressed with the focus, breadth, supervision, and operation of SARP's prevention, screening, diagnostic, and treatment services.

My Ongoing Recovery Experience (MORE)

Clinical Focus	*Clinical Focus*	*Program Evaluation/ Outcomes*	*Target Population*	*EBPs*
• MORE is a continuing care program that supports patients as they leave their primary treatment. Through the use of Web technology, MORE provides tailored support to patients during the first 18 months after treatment as a means to improve treatment outcomes and eliminate, reduce, or shorten episodes of relapse.	• Treatment	• Abstinence and retention rates of those actively involved/ completing the MORE program versus those who do not participate • Number of relapses during 18-month enrollment in MORE	• Active Duty • Reserve • Dependents	• Motivational interviewing • Twelve-step facilitation • Living in Balance • Contingency management • Cognitive behavioral intervention

Purpose and Goals	*Clinical Focus*	*Program Evaluation/ Outcomes*	*Target Population*	*EBPs*
• MORE allows for ongoing support wherever a patient is located to support continued engagement in a therapeutic effort that will enhance long-term abstinence and recovery from substance dependence.		• Length of relapses before returning to the path of recovery • Number of days patients are abstinent		

NOTE: EBP = evidence-based practice; MORE = My Ongoing Recovery Experience.

MORE is an 18-month online support program for individuals who complete SARP. The program connects these individuals to additional tools and resources to aid in their recovery. MORE was developed and is administered by the widely recognized Hazelden treatment program and is oriented toward 12-step recovery. Since August 2010, MORE has supported those in the early stages of aftercare by giving them a recovery coach who is a licensed addiction counselor and is available to provide electronic and telephone support. The program encourages individuals to designate goals for the week and promotes insight through journaling, the development of healthy coping strategies, reading of fact sheets, and participation in a serenity area of the MORE website to help manage stress. Hazelden has also created a new recovery support tool called Mobile MORE Field Guide to Life. This iPhone application, which builds on the MORE program, is being pilot tested by the Navy.

MORE is a positive example of the innovative use of the Internet and the provision of a confidential source of support for recovery. The evaluation and outcomes of the MORE program cited in the above table are likely based on research by Hazelden's Butler Center for Research (Klein et al., 2012). That study was conducted on a limited sample of residential patients discharged in 2006-2007 who met the diagnostic criteria only for dependence, so the study population does not appear to be comparable to the greater range of diagnostic severity encountered in discharged SARP patients. An evaluation of the outcomes of MORE with the Navy population is therefore needed.

Drug Detection and Deterrence Program

Purpose and Goals	*Clinical Focus*	*Program Evaluation/ Outcomes*	*Target Population*	*EBPs*
• The Drug Detection and Deterrence Program develop policies and provide guidance for all Navy urinalysis drug-screening programs. Provides policy guidance and ensures compliance with existing policies and directives of DoD, Department of the Navy, and other agencies in development, implementation, quality assurance, and evaluation of substance abuse prevention programs.	• Prevention	• Number of urine samples submitted to Navy Drug Screening Laboratories at San Diego, Great Lakes, and Jacksonville • Number of drug positives due to illicit drug use • Number of drug positives cleared due to prescribed medication • Number of drug positives retained due to innocent ingestion • Number of drug positives retained due to break in the chain of custody • Number of drug positives cleared due to ADMIN board/Court-Martial acquittal and Board of Inquiry retention	• Active Duty • Reserve	• N/A

NOTE: DoD = Department of Defense; EBP = evidence-based practice; N/A = not applicable.

The policies promulgated in relation to this program are reviewed in Chapter 6. In general, policies emphasize detection and deterrence and do not specify the need for evidence-based public health interventions focused on prevention. The program is driven by concerns of commanders rather than medical providers and thus discourages early identification and education to prevent SUDs.

Drug Education for Youth (DEFY)

Purpose and Goals	*Clinical Focus*	*Program Evaluation/ Outcomes*	*Target Population*	*EBPs*
• DEFY's goals are to produce 9- to 12-year-olds with character, leadership, and confidence so that they are equipped to engage in positive, healthy lifestyles as drug-free citizens, and have the necessary skills to be successful in their lives through coordinated community participation, commitment, and leadership thereby empowering military youth to make positive life choices. • DEFY is operated worldwide and consists of a summer leadership camp (Phase 1) and a school-year mentoring program (Phase 2). The program curriculum provides youth with a variety of topics including substance abuse prevention and other vital life skills, including conflict resolution, self-management skills, study skills, leadership, and community service.	• Prevention	• Number of DEFY program sites • Number of youth participants • Number of adult staff participants • Longevity of individual program sites (longer running program is considered more successful)	• Dependents	• CSAP prevention strategies

NOTES: Appendix C of the *Comprehensive Plan* provides information on DEFY in both the Air Force and Navy sections. The content pertaining to program outcomes/evaluation and EBPs differs in the two tables. CSAP = Center for Substance Abuse Prevention; DEFY = Drug Education for Youth; EBP = evidence-based practice.

DEFY is a comprehensive prevention program now shared by the Navy, Air Force, and Marine Corps. The Navy launched the DEFY prevention program in 1993. In 1999, the Air Force became a partner in the DEFY effort and began operating program sites at numerous installations worldwide. In addition, in 1996 the Attorney General's Weed & Seed program adopted DEFY, expanding it to any location with a U.S. attorney's office. Navy policy specifies that DEFY is a voluntary program, and local commanders should not mandate participation in any way (U.S. Navy, 2007). While DoD identifies in the *Comprehensive Plan* that DEFY incorporates EBPs in its curriculum, the committee is not aware of any formal outcome evaluations that have been conducted with military dependent participants. Therefore, it is unknown whether the program is effective at preventing SUDs for military dependents. The Air Force reported that DEFY administers surveys to youth participants and parents for purposes of evaluating the program.[6]

Right Spirit Campaign

Purpose and Goals	*Clinical Focus*	*Program Evaluation/ Outcomes*	*Target Population*	*EBPs*
• The Right Spirit Campaign enhances fleet readiness by the reduction of alcohol abuse and related incidents, and provides a safe and productive working environment while deglamorizing alcohol use. The campaign uses videos, posters, etc.	• Prevention	• Number of command and self-referrals for alcohol screenings • Number of participants in local events held to deglamorize alcohol use • Reduction in number of alcohol incidents fleet-wide	• Active Duty • Reserve	• CSAP prevention strategies

NOTE: CSAP = Center for Substance Abuse Prevention; EBP = evidence-based practice.

The Right Spirit Campaign was designed to change the Navy's attitude and culture regarding alcohol. The committee was informed that the Right

[6]Personal communication, Lt. Col. Mark Oordt, Air Force Medical Operations Agency, October 25, 2011.

Spirit Campaign will be phased out during FY 2012 and therefore did not request additional information on this program to review.

Alcohol Abuse Prevention Program

Purpose and Goals	*Clinical Focus*	*Program Evaluation/ Outcomes*	*Target Population*	*EBPs*
• A comprehensive alcohol abuse prevention and control program for all Navy military personnel that focuses on the responsible use of alcoholic beverages through education, training, and awareness. Assigns responsibility to all personnel and recognizes that alcohol abuse and dependency are preventable and treatable.	• Prevention	• Number of personnel with ARIs • Number of personnel with DUI/ DWI • Number of treatment failures • Number of self-referrals	• Active Duty • Reserve	• Community-based processes, environmental strategies, information dissemination, alternative activities, education, and problem recognition and referral

NOTE: ARI = Alcohol Related Incident; DUI = driving under the influence; DWI = driving while intoxicated; EBP = evidence-based practice.

This program is similar to the Drug Detection and Deterrence Program, discussed above. It assigns responsibility for alcohol abuse and dependency to all personnel and recognizes that they are preventable and treatable. The program has not been formally evaluated for effectiveness. However, alcohol misuse and abuse appear to remain highly prevalent among Navy personnel, as is the case with the other branches. Thus, the committee finds that there appears to be either a breakdown in implementation or some limitations in the materials used for the Navy's alcohol prevention programs. Further, the program relies on information dissemination rather than motivational interviewing messages and skill-building exercises that are part of evidence-based prevention programs.

Navy Drug and Alcohol Advisory Council (NDAAC)

Purpose and Goals	*Clinical Focus*	*Program Evaluation/ Outcomes*	*Target Population*	*EBPs*
• The NDAAC provides local and regional commanders with written plans of action to combat identified local and regional drug and alcohol threats.	• Prevention	• Quarterly meetings in area of responsibility • Number of prevention programs/events monitored • Number of ARIs at AOR • Number of DUIs/ DWIs at AOR • Number of days without ARI or DUI/DWI	• Active Duty • Reserve • Dependents	• N/A

NOTE: AOR = Area of Responsibility; ARI = Alcohol Related Incident; DUI = driving under the influence; DWI = driving while intoxicated; EBP = evidence-based practice; N/A = not applicable; NDAAC = Navy Drug and Alcohol Advisory Council.

The NDAAC is a local and regional mechanism by which commanders can monitor and communicate achievements or lack of success in attaining prevention goals related to alcohol-related incidents. Thus it is not a prevention program. While local monitoring is appropriate, it would be more effective to establish specific short- and long-term branch-level goals for reducing harmful alcohol use that are focused not just on incidents (i.e., getting caught) but also on changes in alcohol use behavior (e.g., reduced number of military personnel who binge drank during the last month; reduced number of underage personnel consuming any alcohol). The Navy also offers Commands a training course for drug and alcohol program advisers on all matters relating to alcohol or other drugs. This collateral duty Command position advises the commanding officer on all substance abuse matters, including administrative screenings, reports, prevention education, and monitoring of aftercare for service members who complete treatment programs.

Overall the committee finds that the program could be enhanced if specific short- and long-term behavior change targets were established at the branch level. Commanders should compare their progress with that of other installations and be held accountable for reaching prevention-related behavioral goals.

Training and Courses

Prevention Specialist Course				
Purpose and Goals	*Clinical Focus*	*Program Evaluation/ Outcomes*	*Target Population*	*EBPs*
• The Prevention Specialist Course provides education and training on how to design and implement evidence-based prevention programs at the local command level.	• Prevention	• Decreased number of Alcohol and Drug Related Incidents (ARIs/DRIs) at commands • Number of people successfully passing the certification examination and becoming certified • Prevention specialists • Number of prevention programs implemented at the command level	• Active Duty • Dependents	• Students are trained in CSAP strategies and learn to utilize the National Registry of Evidence-Based Programs and Practices (NREPP) in selecting prevention programs for their local community

Navy Drug and Alcohol Counselor School (NDACS)				
Purpose and Goals	*Clinical Focus*	*Program Evaluation/ Outcomes*	*Target Population*	*EBPs*
• NDACS provides education and training to Active Duty personnel who in turn provide treatment at SARP programs. This training ensures Active Duty personnel are providing high-quality patient care competently utilizing EBPs.	• Prevention • Screening • Diagnosis • Treatment	• Number of counselors certified following internship • Number of personnel passing certification examinations at various levels • Number of personnel screened out, deselected and dis-enrolled from the course	• Active Duty	• Adult learning model • Motivational interviewing • Twelve-step facilitation • Living in Balance

Clinical Preceptorship Program				
Purpose and Goals	*Clinical Focus*	*Program Evaluation/ Outcomes*	*Target Population*	*EBPs*
• The program provides counselors assigned to SARPs with the unique skills and training required of counselors engaged in substance use disorder treatment and education.	• Screening • Diagnosis • Treatment	• Number of counselors passing certification examinations and becoming certified • Hours provided and utilized at each SARP • Treatment Director/ Counselor's satisfaction annual quality assessment survey • Number of ethical complaints per year submitted to U.S. Navy Certification board	• Active Duty	• Motivational interviewing • Interpersonal recall model • In vivo supervision

Personal Responsibility and Values Education and Training (PREVENT) Course				
Purpose and Goals	*Clinical Focus*	*Program Evaluation/ Outcomes*	*Target Population*	*EBPs*
• A prevention education and health promotion course (24-hr course) specifically developed to target the 18- to 25-year age group. PREVENT deals with life choices related to alcohol and drug use; interpersonal relationships (including sexual responsibility); and health, fitness, and financial responsibility.	• Prevention	• Number of personnel who attend annually • 15,798 (3-year annual average throughput)	• Active Duty • Reserve	• N/A

Alcohol and Drug Abuse Management Seminar (ADAMS) for Supervisors Course				
Purpose and Goals	*Clinical Focus*	*Program Evaluation/ Outcomes*	*Target Population*	*EBPs*
• A course designed to provide Navy supervisors with knowledge and skills in alcohol and drug abuse prevention, recognition and documentation, intervention and aftercare. Because policy and programs are subject to change, ADAMS for Supervisors should be repeated every 5 years.	• Prevention	• Number of personnel who attend annually • 9,801 (3-year annual average throughput)	• Active Duty • Reserve	• N/A

Alcohol and Drug Abuse Management Seminar (ADAMS) for Leaders Course				
Purpose and Goals	*Clinical Focus*	*Program Evaluation/ Outcomes*	*Target Population*	*EBPs*
• A brief seminar designed for Commanding Officers, Executive Officers, Command Master Chiefs, Chiefs of the Boat, and other senior command personnel to provide an overview of what is taught in the ADAMS for Supervisors course.	• Prevention	• Number of personnel who attend annually • 723 (3-year annual average throughput)	• Active Duty • Reserve	• N/A

Alcohol-AWARE Course				
Purpose and Goals	*Clinical Focus*	*Program Evaluation/ Outcomes*	*Target Population*	*EBPs*
• Alcohol-AWARE is an alcohol-awareness training that provides basic information about alcohol use and associated risks, Navy policies, responsible drinking, and alternatives. • Course is a requirement for all personnel.	• Prevention	• Number of personnel who attend annually • 7,382 (3-year annual average throughput)	• Active Duty • Reserve	• N/A
Drug and Alcohol Program Advisor (DAPA) Course				
Purpose and Goals	*Clinical Focus*	*Program Evaluation/ Outcomes*	*Target Population*	*EBPs*
• This course provides training to Drug and Alcohol Program Advisors for commands on all matters relating to alcohol or other drugs. This collateral duty command position advises the CO on all substance abuse matters to include administrative screenings, reports, prevention education, and monitor aftercare of service members.	• Prevention	• Number of personnel who attend annually • 1,421 (3-year annual average throughput)	• Active Duty • Reserve	• N/A

NOTE: CO = commanding officer; CSAP = Center for Substance Abuse Prevention; EBP = evidence-based practice; N/A = not applicable; SARP = Substance Abuse Rehabilitation Program.

The Navy has made an extensive and impressive investment in a series of training initiatives ranging from prevention to intervention for the entire Navy workforce and their families to sophisticated leadership training for commanders. Among these courses are the Prevention Specialist Course, the Navy Drug and Alcohol Counselor School (NDACS), the Clinical Preceptorship Program, the Personal Responsibility and Values Education and Training (PREVENT) Course, the Alcohol and Drug Abuse Management Seminar (ADAMS) for Supervisors and the ADAMS for Leaders Courses, the Alcohol-AWARE Course, and the Drug and Alcohol Program Advisor (DAPA) Course.

The purpose of the **Prevention Specialist Course** is to prepare installation personnel who are responsible for prevention programming. Participants take a certification examination upon completing the course. These specialists then design their own programs at local installations under the commander's direction. Thus, training is provided to designated personnel in prevention programming at each installation. The committee finds that while the content of this course appears to be appropriate, directing prevention specialists to Center for Substance Abuse Prevention (CSAP) strategies and to a registry of evidence-based programs, the implementation of unique prevention programs at each installation is challenging and likely to erode overall quality. The committee also finds that it would be more cost-effective to have branch-wide initiatives in which the prevention specialists would receive training that could be modified to reflect local conditions. Fidelity to the evidence-based program models could be monitored.

NDACS is a 10-week program that is divided into 7 weeks of didactic training and 3 weeks of clinical rotation. The school convenes a new class five times per year for military personnel who will be working in various drug- and alcohol-related jobs, including outreach, screening, assessment, and treatment for alcohol and other drug addictions. In reviewing the NDACS student guide (U.S. Navy, 2011), the committee noted that basic psychosocial theory and its application to clinical practice and basic biology (as regards SUDs) are covered extensively. However, there is little medical information regarding evidence-based treatment approaches, and as is the case with virtually all training materials the committee reviewed, there is a lack of attention to, or in this case no coverage of, the role of medication in the treatment of SUDs.

Following their training at NDACS, graduates enter the **Clinical Preceptorship Program** as intern counselors. The Clinical Preceptorship Program is a structured internship intended to develop knowledge and skills under the mentorship of a person with advanced skills in drug and alcohol counseling. After a minimum 12-month internship, interns may apply for certification as alcohol and drug counselor (ADC) I.

The **PREVENT** Course focuses on sailors aged 18-25 and assists them in achieving their highest levels of personal development. It is believed that this will reduce risk-related behaviors and enhance mission readiness. Like the ADAMS and DAPA Courses, PREVENT has training goals and lesson plans; its facilitator guide was prepared by the Pacific Institute for Research and Evaluation, a group with sophisticated knowledge of prevention programs.

ADAMS, developed for E-5s and above, is divided into two courses, one directed at supervisors and the other at leaders, such as commanding officers and executive officers. These seminars are basically a practical leadership course and are highly regarded by Commands, as the committee learned on its site visit to the naval base at Point Loma, California. The current evaluation metrics appear to be limited to the number of people trained annually.

Alcohol-AWARE is a prevention-oriented course that provides anti-alcohol education intended for all sailors E-1 through E-4 and O-1 through O-3. The emphasis is on leadership, deglamorization, intervention, and accountability.

The **DAPA Course** trains advisers who manage and administer the Command's alcohol and drug abuse programs. During its San Diego site visit, the committee heard of the critical importance of this position in linking Command to effective SUD program and policy implementation.

Both the ADAMS and DAPA Courses have training guides, lesson plans, and case scenarios. The committee reviewed these materials and found them to be sound learning tools. Particularly impressive are the ADAMS scenarios directed at supervisors and commanders. The committee is aware of the crucial role of the Command structure in the implementation of SUD prevention and treatment programs. Hands-on training for that Command structure through ADAMS and DAPA is essential to the success of these programs. The committee believes the ADAMS and DAPA Courses are models worthy of adoption by all branches.

Additional Programs and Initiatives

In addition to the programs cited by the Navy in the *Comprehensive Plan*, the committee reviewed Families OverComing Under Stress (FOCUS). FOCUS is a family-centered program aimed at building resiliency among ADSMs; their spouses, children, and other family members; providers; and other community members. As a resiliency program, its primary clinical focus is on prevention. It is implemented and repeated over several developmental stages, including pre-, during, and postdeployment. While this large-scale demonstration project was initiated by the Navy's Bureau of Medicine and Surgery (BUMED), it has been expanded to 18 installations serving the Army, Air Force, Navy, and Marine Corps. Based on resiliency theory (Rutter, 1999) and multiple family and individual resiliency programs, FOCUS is considered evidence based. The committee reviewed two published articles on the implementation and evaluation of FOCUS (Lester et al., 2011a, 2012). Based on this review, the committee finds FOCUS to be a promising program that should be widely disseminated at military sites. Efforts to evaluate the program and document its effectiveness should also be continued.

MARINE CORPS

Marine Corps Substance Abuse Program

Purpose and Goals	*Clinical Focus*	*Program Evaluation/ Outcomes*	*Target Population*	*EBPs*
• The Marine Corps Substance Abuse Program provides screening and assessment, and treatment services for Active Duty military members and other eligible beneficiaries with substance abuse disorders.	• Prevention • Screening • Diagnosis • Treatment	• Number of completion of treatments • Number of treatment failures • Number of re-screens after completion of treatment	• Active Duty	• ASAM Patient Placement Criteria for the treatment of substance related disorders are used for alcohol treatment

NOTE: ASAM = American Society of Addiction Medicine; EBP = evidence-based practice.

The Marine Corps Substance Abuse Program operates under the Marine Corps Community Services Command and within the Marine and Family Programs Division "to provide timely, consistent and effective care for active duty military members and other eligible beneficiaries with substance abuse and dependency disorders which interfere with mission readiness and inter-personal functioning" (USMC, 2011a, p. 1). The program is responsible for prevention, screening, diagnosis, and treatment for SUDs. Three program elements (prevention, drug demand reduction, and treatment) form the core of the program. Prevention support services include prevention activities, urine testing, and indicated prevention programs. The Drug Demand Reduction program includes Command-level education and training, compulsory random drug testing with punitive consequences, assessments of illegal drug use, and training and action plans at installations as needed.

Substance Abuse Counseling Centers (SACCs) provide screening and assessment for alcohol and other drug problems. Outpatient education and counseling may include early intervention, outpatient care, and intensive outpatient services. Marine Corps Order 5300.17 details the requirements for SACCs: "The Marine Corps is required to identify, counsel, or treat Marines identified as alcohol or drug abusers or alcohol or drug dependent" (USMC, 2011b, p. 3-1). Individuals involved in a substance abuse incident are referred to a SACC for assessment. At the SACC, qualified personnel (generally certified substance abuse counselors), under the supervision of the medical officer (either a physician or a psychologist), provide necessary intervention and treatment services. The substance abuse counselor conducts the initial biopsychosocial assessment using a standard form contained in NAVMC 2931. The items on this form do not appear to reflect standardized screening instruments for assessing alcohol and other drug use. If the counselor determines that a Marine does not need formal assessment for treatment placement by a licensed independent practitioner, the Marine returns to duty or is assigned to the early intervention program offered through the SACC (Impact, which is also used by the Navy and was reviewed previously under Navy programs).

At the start of treatment, an individualized treatment plan is developed and approved by the medical officer. This plan addresses seven dimensions to determine the required level of care: potential for withdrawal, biomedical complications, emotional/behavioral complications, readiness to change, relapse potential, recovery/living environment, and operational commitment. An interdisciplinary team reviews the assessment, treatment plan, and treatment progress weekly and makes recommendations to the medical officer. The SACC treatment modalities include a 12-step program, motivational interviewing, group therapy, and other models depending on the individual counselors providing treatment. The committee learned that the treatment modalities provided at each SACC site vary, and there are no standardized or required methods.[7] The committee finds this lack of standardization and endorsement of evidence-based treatment modalities to be a weakness of the Marine Corps programs.

Marine Corps Order 5300.17 requires 1 year of aftercare for those who have engaged in treatment. This aftercare is not provided through the SACC but is delivered in the unit. It involves monitoring and documentation of progress on the individual's aftercare plan.

---

[7]Personal communication, Erik Hollins, Marine and Family Programs Division, December 26, 2011.

Substance Abuse Prevention and Intervention Program

Purpose and Goals	*Clinical Focus*	*Program Evaluation/ Outcomes*	*Target Population*	*EBPs*
• The Marine Corps Substance Abuse Prevention program provides prevention tools such as antidrug videos and games, substance abuse prevention tool kits, Command Summits, and the Battalion Alcohol Skill Intervention Curriculum that help commanders prevent problems that detract from unit performance and mission readiness. • To assist in the commander's prevention efforts, a Drug Demand Reduction Coordinator, Substance Abuse Control Officers, and Alcohol Abuse Prevention Specialists are available to provide support in the following areas: ○ Illegal drug use prevention activities ○ Drug testing ○ Implementing prevention programs ○ Coordinating treatment services with the SACC ○ Conducting aftercare	• Prevention	• Number of positive samples • Number of multiple positives • Number of prescription drug confirmed positives	• Active Duty • Reserve	• Prevention tools created specifically for the Marine Corps based on research by the Naval Health Research Center

NOTE: EBP = evidence-based practice; SACC = Substance Abuse Counseling Center.

Activities with the goal of preventing substance use and abuse among Marines generally are carried out in individual units and Commands. The specific content of the education delivered through these activities varies from site to site. One component of the Marine Corps Substance Abuse Prevention and Intervention Program is the Battalion Alcohol Skills Intervention Curriculum (BASIC), which is used across Marine Corps sites. Following a train-the-trainer model, SACC staff train battalion unit trainers, who then train their senior leadership and unit commanders in how to deliver the BASIC program within their units. The training focuses on building skills and providing information on alcohol use, challenging assumptions about the effects of alcohol, and reducing risk associated with alcohol use based on a harm reduction rather than an abstention approach. The program grew out of work done by contracted researchers from the University of Washington, San Diego State University, and the University of California, San Diego, to study the problem and make recommendations for possible interventions among Marines. The program is based on the BASICS (Brief Alcohol Screening and Intervention for College Students) program, an evidence-based prevention program originally developed by researchers from the University of Washington Addictive Behaviors Research Center for college students with problem drinking (Dimeff et al., 1999).

The original BASICS program is listed as an evidence-based prevention program in the National Registry of Evidence-Based Programs and Practices (SAMHSA, 2012). The committee finds that the use of the BASIC program in the Marine Corps shows promise for the implementation of an evidence-based prevention program. However, the only evaluation of BASIC showed that it did not have a significant overall effect on drinking behavior among Marines (Hurtado, 2003). Additional research is needed to determine the effectiveness of BASIC in the Marine Corps and perhaps identify modifications that would increase positive results.

The Impact program (described previously in the section on Navy programs) also falls under the umbrella of the Marine Corps Substance Abuse Prevention and Intervention Program. This indicated prevention program is delivered at the majority of SACC sites to those Marines identified as being at risk for developing SUDs because of their risky use of alcohol or other drugs. At the Marine Corps Base at Camp Pendleton, Impact has been modified to include the Marine Alcohol Awareness Course (MAAC),[8] a 1-day (8-hour) group educational course designed to raise individuals' awareness level when choosing to consume alcohol. Much like Impact, the course highlights many of the negative consequences and peripheral

[8]Personal communication, Erik Hollins, Marine and Family Programs Division, December 26, 2011.

problems that can result from consuming alcohol. The course focuses primarily on alcohol-related policies and consequences and how individuals can establish proper measures and responsible behavior (i.e., safety, environmental and situational awareness, and a solid plan) before deciding to drink alcohol. The program is based on a risk reduction model of alcohol use and designed for delivery to those individuals who have been involved in alcohol-related incidents.

Additional Programs

The Marine Corps utilizes the FOCUS program, described previously in the section on Navy programs. As a resiliency program, FOCUS places primary clinical emphasis on prevention. It is implemented and repeated over several developmental stages, including pre-, during, and postdeployment. FOCUS is considered to be a large-scale demonstration project that has been expanded to 18 installations serving the Army, Air Force, Navy, and Marine Corps (FOCUS Project, 2012). Based on resiliency theory (Rutter, 1999) and multiple family and individual resiliency programs, it is considered evidence-based.

REFERENCES

Acosta, J., L. T. Martin, M. P. Fisher, R. Harris, and R. M. Weinick. 2012. *Assessment of the content, design, and dissemination of the Real Warriors Campaign.* Santa Monica, CA: RAND Corporation.

ACSAP (Army Center for Substance Abuse Programs). 2012a. *ASAP public home.* http://www.acsap.army.mil/sso/pages/index.jsp (accessed June 8, 2012).

ACSAP. 2012b. *Overview ADAPT/myPRIME.* http://acsap.army.mil/sso/pages/public/resources/myprime.jsp (accessed June 8, 2012).

ACSAP. 2012c. *Risk reduction.* http://acsap.army.mil/sso/pages/public/resources/risk-reduction.jsp (accessed June 8, 2012).

DCoE (Defense Centers of Excellence). 2012. *The Real Warriors Campaign.* http://www.realwarriors.net/aboutus (accessed May 29, 2012).

DEA (Drug Enforcement Administration). 2012. *Red Ribbon Week factsheet.* http://www.justice.gov/dea/ongoing/redribbon_factsheet.html (accessed May 29, 2012).

Dimeff, L. A., J. S. Baer, D. R. Kivlahan, and G. A. Marlatt. 1999. *Brief Alcohol Screening and Intervention for College Students (BASICS): A harm reduction approach.* New York: Guilford Press.

DoD (Department of Defense). 1994. *Directive 1010.1: Health promotion.* Washington, DC: DoD.

DoD. 2010. *Training to administer DoD deployment mental health assessments: Office of Force Health Protection & Readiness and the Deployment Health Clinical Center.* Washington, DC: DoD.

DoD. 2011. *Comprehensive plan on prevention, diagnosis, and treatment of substance use disorders and disposition of substance use offenders in the armed forces.* Washington, DC: Office of the Undersecretary of Defense.

DoD. 2012. *Military one source.* http://www.militaryonesource.mil/MOS/f?p=MOS:HOME:0 (accessed May 29, 2012).

DoD, TRICARE Management Activity, and Fleishman-Hillard. 2009. *Don't be That Guy.* http://www.instituteforpr.org/wp-content/uploads/That_Guy_JFGRA.pdf (accessed July 23, 2012).

FOCUS Project. 2012. *FOCUS: Family resiliency training for military families.* http://www.focusproject.org (accessed June 15, 2012).

Gibbs, D. A., K. L. Rae Olmsted, J. M. Brown, and A. M. Clinton-Sherrod. 2011. Dynamics of stigma for alcohol and mental health treatment among army soldiers. *Military Psychology* 23(1):36-51.

Hawkins, J. D., and R. F. J. Catalano. 1992. *Communities that care.* San Francisco, CA: Jossey-Bass.

Hurtado, S. 2003. *Evaluation of an alcohol misuse prevention program in a military population.* San Diego, CA: Naval Health Research Center.

Klein, A. A., V. J. Slaymaker, K. L. Dugosh, and J. R. McKay. 2012. Computerized continuing care support for alcohol and drug dependence: A preliminary analysis of usage and outcomes. *Journal of Substance Abuse Treatment* 42(1):25-34.

Lester, P., C. Mogil, W. Saltzman, K. Woodward, W. Nash, G. Leskin, B. Bursch, S. Green, R. Pynoos, and W. Beardslee. 2011a. Families overcoming under stress: Implementing family-centered prevention for military families facing wartime deployments and combat operational stress. *Military Medicine* 176(1):19-25.

Lester, P. B., P. D. Harms, M. N. Herian, D. V. Krasikova, and S. J. Beal. 2011b. *The comprehensive soldier fitness program evaluation.* Anchorage, AK: TKC Global Solutions, LLC.

Lester, P., W. R. Saltzman, K. Woodward, D. Glover, G. A. Leskin, B. Bursch, R. Pynoos, and W. Beardslee. 2012. Evaluation of a family-centered prevention intervention for military children and families facing wartime deployments. *American Journal of Public Health* 102(Suppl 1):S48-S54.

Military Pathways. 2012. *Military mental health screening program.* http://www.militarymentalhealth.org/about.aspx (accessed May 29, 2012).

Milliken, C. S., J. L. Auchterlonie, and C. W. Hoge. 2007. Longitudinal assessment of mental health problems among active and reserve component soldiers returning from the Iraq war. *Journal of the American Medical Association* 298(18):2141-2148.

Peterson, C., N. Park, and C. A. Castro. 2011. Assessment for the U.S. Army comprehensive soldier fitness program: The global assessment tool. *American Psychologist* 66(1):10-18.

Prochastka, J. O., and W. F. Velicer. 1997. The transtheoretical model of health behavior change. *American Journal of Health Promotion* 12(1):38-48.

Rutter, M. 1999. Resilience concepts and findings: Implications for family therapy. *Journal of Family Therapy* 21(2):119-144.

Rutter, M. 2006. Implications of resilience concepts for scientific understanding. *Annals of the New York Academy of Sciences* 1094:1-12.

SAMHSA (Substance Abuse and Mental Health Services Administration). 2010. *Prime for life.* http://www.nrepp.samhsa.gov/ViewIntervention.aspx?id=12 (accessed June 8, 2012).

SAMHSA. 2012. *SAMHSA's national registry of evidence-based programs and practices.* http://www.nrepp.samhsa.gov (accessed June 18, 2012).

Santiago, P. N., J. E. Wilk, C. S. Milliken, C. A. Castro, C. C. Engel, and C. W. Hoge. 2010. Screening for alcohol misuse and alcohol-related behaviors among combat veterans. *Psychiatric Services* 61(6):575-581.

Seligman, M. E. P. 1998. *Learned optimism.* New York: Pocket Books (Simon and Schuster).

Spera, C., and K. Franklin. 2010. Reducing drinking among junior enlisted Air Force members in five communities: Early findings of the EUDL program's influence on self-reported drinking behaviors. *Journal of Studies on Alcohol and Drugs* 71(3):373-383.

Spera, C., F. Barlas, R. Z. Szoc, J. Prabhakaran, and M. H. Cambridge. 2012. Examining the influence of the Enforcing Underage Drinking Laws (EUDL) program on alcohol-related outcomes in five communities surrounding Air Force bases. *Addictive Behaviors* 37(4):513-516.

That Guy Campaign. 2012, March. *The buzz on That Guy: A newsletter for supporters of the That Guy campaign.* http://thatguy.com/newsletter/march2012/index.php (accessed May 29, 2012).

U.S. Air Force. 2011. *Instruction 44-121: Alcohol and Drug Abuse Prevention and Treatment (ADAPT) program.* Washington, DC: Department of the Air Force.

U.S. Army. 2009. *Army regulation 600-85: The Army substance abuse program.* http://www.apd.army.mil/pdffiles/r600_85.pdf (accessed July 23, 2012).

U.S. Army. 2011. *ASAC standard operating procedures* (revised). Cedar Rapids, IA: Area Substance Abuse Council.

U.S. Army. Undated. *Unit prevention leader handbook.* Washington, DC: Department of the Army.

U.S. Navy. 2007. *Instruction 5355.3: Drug Education for Youth (DEFY) Program.* Washington, DC: Department of the Navy.

U.S. Navy. 2011. *Student guide for Navy Drug and Alcohol Counselor School.* San Diego, CA: Navy Drug and Alcohol Counselor School.

USMC (U.S. Marine Corps). 2011a. *Substance abuse program.* http://www.usmc-mccs.org/subabuse/index.cfm?sid=ml (accessed June 8, 2012).

USMC. 2011b. *Order 5300.17: Marine Corps substance abuse program.* Washington, DC: Department of the Navy.

Vythilingam, M., J. Davison, C. Engel, and H. Ritschard. 2010. *Training to administer DoD deployment mental health assessments.* http://fhpr.osd.mil/pdfs/NDAA%20FHP_DHCC.pdf (accessed July 23, 2012).

Weinick, R. M., E. B. Beckjord, C. M. Farmer, L. T. Martin, E. M. Gillen, J. D. Acosta, M. P. Fisher, J. Garnett, G. C. Gonzalez, T. C. Helmus, L. H. Jaycox, K. A. Reynolds, N. Salcedo, and D. M. Scharf. 2011. *Programs addressing psychological health and traumatic brain injury among U.S. military service members and their families.* Santa Monica, CA: RAND Corporation.

Appendix E

Features of TRICARE and Related Purchased Care Plans

TRICARE Prime	TRICARE Standard
• Health maintenance organization • Active duty service members automatically enrolled • Some other beneficiary groups can choose to enroll • Some groups have annual enrollment costs • Based on a managed care model with an assigned primary care manager and referrals for specialty care • Limited co-payments for some beneficiary groups	• Fee-for-service for non–active duty beneficiaries • Does not require pre-enrollment • No annual enrollment costs • Beneficiary has most options for provider selection • Provider can charge usual fees • Benefit is a percentage of billed charges after an annual deductible • No referrals, some preauthorization • Does not require use of network
TRICARE Prime Remote	**TRICARE Extra**
• Similar to TRICARE Prime • For beneficiaries 50 miles or an hour's drive from a military treatment facility • Primary care manager selected from TRICARE civilian provider network • Referrals for specialty care • Limited to active duty service members and their dependents	• Preferred provider organization • Fee-for-service plan for non–active duty beneficiaries • Does not require pre-enrollment • No annual enrollment costs • Beneficiary chooses authorized TRICARE provider • Benefit is a percentage of allowable charges after an annual deductible • No referrals, some preauthorization

TRICARE Prime Overseas	TRICARE for Life
• Similar to TRICARE Prime when near an overseas military treatment facility • Requires enrollment • Limited to active duty service members and their Command-sponsored dependents who are living together in a nonremote overseas location (near a military treatment facility) • Primary care managers are assigned and make referrals for specialty care	• Medicare "wraparound" • Authorized in 2001 for Medicare beneficiaries who also were eligible for TRICARE benefits (generally retirees and their dependents) • Requires Medicare Parts A and B • Generally no out-of-pocket expenses
TRICARE Prime Remote Overseas	**TRICARE Plus**
• Provides TRICARE-like benefits for active duty service members and their dependents living in remote overseas locations (distant from a military treatment facility) • Requires enrollment to participate • Divided into Eurasia-Africa, Latin America, and Pacific regions • Requires primary care managers who also makes referrals • Coordinated by International SOS, a civilian corporation that coordinates overseas health care for DoD	• New program that allows TRICARE Extra and TRICARE for Life beneficiaries to enroll at a military treatment facility and receive their primary care there • No enrollment fees • Not all military treatment facilities participate
U.S. Family Health Plan for Non–Active Duty Beneficiaries	**TRICARE Young Adult**
• TRICARE Prime managed care option that evolved from the old Marine Hospital System/Public Health Service Hospitals in the early 1980s • Managed by six health care organizations • Available to beneficiaries in selected areas of the northeast United States, Washington State, southeast Texas, and southwest Louisiana	• Program for eligible dependents aged 21 (or 23 if enrolled in college full time) to 26 originating in the 2010 Patient Protection and Affordable Care Act
TRICARE Reserve Select	**Civilian Health and Medical Program of the Uniformed Services**
• Premium-based health plan available to Selected Reserve members of the Ready Reserve (and their dependents) who are not eligible for or enrolled in the Federal Employee Health Benefits program • Requires cost sharing • No referrals, some preauthorization	• Predecessor of TRICARE; began in 1966 • DoD secretary was authorized to contract with civilian providers to provide health care, primarily to non–active duty beneficiaries

TRICARE Reserve Retired	Federal Employee Health Benefits Program
• For certain retired Reserve members under age 60 • Premium-based worldwide health plan that may be purchased by qualified Reserve members and survivors • Covers member and dependents • Provides choice of providers although out-of-pocket costs vary • No referrals, some preauthorization	• Overall health insurance program available to federal civilian employees • Includes various options with a number of insurance carriers • Premium-based

Appendix F

Workforce Standards for Substance Use Disorder (SUD) Care

Addiction treatment is changing (McCarty et al., 2010): medications are increasingly effective, payers require treatment providers to use evidence-based behavioral therapies, and the workforce is changing to include more individuals with graduate degrees. At the same time, however, linkages with medical practice remain weak. The 2010 and 2011 National Drug Control Strategies promote a new vision for the U.S. addiction treatment system (ONDCP, 2010, 2011). Because the Patient Protection and Affordable Care Act of 2010 will reduce the numbers of uninsured and increase access to primary care, the Office of National Drug Control Policy (ONDCP) calls for the nation's primary care clinics and clinicians to become more active in the treatment of addiction. Addiction treatment services will be integrated into primary care, and ONDCP has directed the Health Resources and Services Administration and the Indian Health Service to allocate resources to support the expansion of addiction treatment services in primary care settings. This represents a major change in federal strategy. For the first time, addiction treatment resources are being directed to primary care rather than to specialty care settings. Health plans and Accountable Care Organizations will become the dominant payers for addiction treatment. These payers are unlikely to support the continued use of credentialed counselors; they will require that licensed practitioners deliver addiction treatment services.

HISTORICAL OVERVIEW

Addiction treatment has a legacy of segregation in nonmedical facilities because hospitals and health care practitioners had little interest in treating men and women who were dependent on alcohol and addicted to illicit drugs, many of whom were uninsured with a limited ability to afford professional care. Women and men who found stable recovery through participation in self-help became the foundation for the addiction treatment workforce. Their personal experience with recovery guided others seeking sobriety. Working with alcoholics and drug addicts, moreover, helped newly sober counselors maintain and enhance their commitment to recovery. Chapter 1 of the "Big Book" (Alcoholics Anonymous World Services, 1939, p. 14) briefly reiterates Bill W's vision and recipe for sobriety.

> While I lay in the hospital the thought came that there were thousands of hopeless alcoholics who might be glad to have what had been so freely given me. Perhaps I could help some of them. They in turn might work with others.

Bill W continues, noting that during his first 18 months of his sobriety, working with other alcoholics helped him maintain his sobriety.

> I was not too well at the time, and was plagued by waves of self-pity and resentment. This sometimes nearly drove me back to drink, but I soon found that when all other measures failed, work with another alcoholic would save the day. Many times I have gone to my old hospital in despair. On talking to a man there, I would be amazingly lifted up and set on my feet. It is a design for living that works in rough going. (Alcoholics Anonymous World Services, 1939, p. 14)

Maintaining sobriety by helping others gain sobriety continues to be an essential facet of recovery for many women and men. They freely volunteer assistance and provide support both through personal commitment to 12-step programming and through training and employment as alcohol and drug counselors.

When Prohibition ended in 1933 in the United States, an addiction treatment system did not exist. There was little demand for alcohol treatment. Rates of problem drinking and cirrhosis declined dramatically in the United States during Prohibition (Blocker, 2006). The Federal Narcotic Treatment programs in Lexington, Kentucky, and Fort Worth, Texas, were in development. Alcoholics and addicts were sometimes treated in psychiatric hospitals, but in most cases, the drunk tank and the county work farm were the primary system of care. Beginning in 1935 in Akron, Ohio, Alcoholics Anonymous offered a self-help approach to recovery. Individuals in recovery reached out to help others seeking recovery. These early pioneers became the roots of the recovery movement. During the 1950s and 1960s, Councils on Alcoholism formed and evolved from public advocacy organizations to treatment services offering detoxification, residential care, and outpatient treatment. Men and women with personal experience in recovery were the primary workforce.

Independent grassroots initiatives became systems of care when the Comprehensive Alcohol Abuse and Alcoholism Prevention, Treatment and Rehabilitation Act of 1970 (Public Law 91-616) formed the National Institute on Alcohol Abuse and Alcoholism, mandated the development of Single State Agencies to plan and support alcohol prevention and treatment services, and authorized federal funding for alcohol prevention and treatment services. The Drug Abuse Office and Treatment Act of 1972 established the Special Action Office for Drug Abuse Prevention (SAODAP) and authorized federal funding for drug abuse treatment. SAODAP morphed into the National Institute on Drug Abuse in 1974.

States used federal funding to stimulate the development of alcohol and drug treatment systems and used their regulatory authority to set minimum standards for treatment services. In most states, programs must be licensed or approved to provide services, but in some states, compliance with the standards may have voluntary elements. The regulations establish minimum criteria for qualifying as a treatment facility. These criteria are intended to protect consumers from unqualified providers, and program licensure or approval usually is required to qualify for state contracts and third-party reimbursement.

Program rather than practitioner licensure has been the primary regulatory mechanism because of the reliance of the alcohol and drug treatment workforce on men and women in recovery. Counselors with experiential training (their personal recovery) strengthen services with a pragmatic orientation and the ability to provide role models for recovery. Individuals seeking services often express a preference for a counselor in recovery. Some consumers and many payers, however, are concerned that individuals who counsel without the benefit of formal training and advanced degrees may not be appropriately qualified to provide services for patients. Counselor certification emerged as a way to recognize individuals with work experience and training in the absence of professional licensure.

Counselor certification has been an important strategy to legitimize the field and document that individuals are qualified to provide treatment and counseling services. In the early 1980s, with support from the National Institute on Alcohol Abuse and Alcoholism, a coalition of trade and advocacy groups collaborated to develop credentialing guidelines and specify 12 core competency areas (Birch and Davis Associates, Inc., 1984). For the most part, credentialing is a trade group activity, and the federal and state roles tend to be more indirect. Certification requirements vary by state; the Addiction Technology Transfer Center website summarizes state requirements (Addiction Technology Transfer Center Network, 2012).

Nationally, two professional trade organizations seek to standardize certification standards for alcohol and drug counselors. The International Certification and Reciprocity Consortium (IC&RC) and the National Certification Commission provide nationally recognized certification. According to the IC&RC website, IC&RC certification is recognized in 44 states, the District of Columbia, and three branches of the U.S. armed forces; more than 40,000 individuals hold IC&RC certification (IC&RC, 2012). IC&RC grew out of a coalition of regional state certification boards in 1981, expanded nationally in 1989, and became international in 1992 with the participation of boards in Canada. The National Certification Commission began in 1990 as an independent entity affiliated with the National Association of Alcohol and Drug Abuse Counselors (National Certification Commission, 2012). Both certification bodies offer basic and advanced certification; certification requires completing verified hours of work experience with supervision and passing a written exam.

An analysis of state requirements found that, compared with requirements for mental health counselors, states require less formal education and more work experience for alcohol and drug counselors (Kerwin et al., 2006). Twenty-five states require alcohol and drug counselors to have a license or certification (44 states require licensure for mental health counselors), and licensure or credentialing is not available in 11 states. To become an alcohol and drug counselor, only 3 states require a master's degree (47 states require a master's degree for mental health counselors). The substantial disparity in state requirements for certification and licensure suggests that substance abuse counselors as a group are less trained and perhaps less qualified than mental health counselors to work effectively with the most complex patients.

THE SUD WORKFORCE

Assessments of the alcohol and drug abuse treatment workforce began in the 1970s. They described a workforce with few licensed professionals and estimated the proportion of counselors with a graduate degree as ranging between one in five (Camp and Kurtz, 1982) and one in three (Birch and Davis Associates, Inc., 1984). A comparison of the workforce in 1976 and 1991 found little change in the presence of psychiatrists (1 percent), other physicians (1 percent), psychologists (3 percent), social workers (6 percent), and nurses (9 percent) (Brown, 1997). Yet change is apparent. More recent analyses suggest that counselors with graduate degrees are more prominent in the workforce, representing about 50 percent of counselors (Gallon et al., 2003; McCarty et al., 2007; Mulvey et al., 2003).

The workforce survey completed within the National Drug Abuse Treatment Clinical Trials Network offers the most complete description of the contemporary addiction treatment workforce (McCarty et al., 2007). Counselors (n = 1,757), managers and supervisors (n = 511), medical staff (n = 522), and support staff (n = 908) completed a survey that captured demographics and assessed attitudes toward the use of evidence-based practices (EBPs). Two of three (66 percent) individuals were women, and women were overrepresented among support staff (74 percent). The diverse workforce included African Americans (22 percent), Hispanics (11 percent), and other minorities (6 percent); African Americans were overrepresented among support staff (33 percent). Individuals with a master's or doctoral degree were most common among counselors (42 percent) and managers/supervisors (58 percent); counselors working in outpatient settings (53 percent) were more likely than their counterparts in residential programs (30 percent) to hold a graduate degree. Professional licensure was most common among medical staff (93 percent). Managers/supervisors (57 percent) and counselors (42 percent) were less likely to have licenses but more likely to hold state certification: counselors = 44 percent, managers/supervisors = 47 percent. Analyses of attitudes found that increased education was associated with more positive attitudes toward the use of medication and other EBPs. Managers/supervisors were most supportive of motivational interviewing, the use of treatment manuals, and the use of contingency management. Medical staff tended to have positive attitudes toward the use of medication in the treatment of addiction. Support personnel, in contrast, were more likely to support discharges for noncompliance and the use of confrontation.

Because of the historical segregation of treatment for alcohol and drug use disorders from mainstream health care, relatively few physicians, psychiatrists, and other health care professionals specialize in addiction treatment. Targeted training, specialized credentialing, and continuing education for health care professionals would enhance the integration of SUD treatment into medical care settings.

Three organizations support physicians and provide certification in addiction medicine: the American Society of Addiction Medicine (ASAM), the American Academy of Addiction Psychiatry, and the American Osteopathic Academy of Addiction Medicine. Each organization is relatively small and reflects the paucity of physicians who specialize in treating alcohol and drug use disorders.

ASAM traces its roots to the founding of the New York City Medical Committee on Alcoholism in 1951 within the National Council on Alcoholism. Currently, ASAM has about 3,000 members (ASAM, 2012). ASAM has offered a certification examination in addiction medicine since 1983 that is widely recognized by state agencies and insurance carriers as a credible measure of knowledge; more than 4,500 physicians are ASAM-certified. The examination was transferred in 2009 to the newly formed

American Board of Addiction Medicine (ABAM). One reason for the formation of ABAM was the eventual goal of attaining recognition by the American Board of Medical Specialties (ABMS) (ABAM, 2012). ABAM, incorporated in 2007, accredited its first diplomates in 2009. As of 2011, 2,000 had been designated fellows of ABAM. Of these, 38 percent are psychiatrists, and about the same number are in primary care specialties. A rough estimate by the ABAM Foundation is that more than 6,000 physicians trained in addiction medicine will be needed by 2020, assuming 1 for every 1,000 patients in need. However, current levels of fellowship training are inadequate to meet this need (Tontchev et al., 2011). In an effort to foster fellowship training in addiction medicine, ABAM formally recognized 10 such fellowship programs in 2011.

The American Academy of Addiction Psychiatry began in 1985 to promote quality care, excellence in addiction psychiatry, public education, and research on addiction (AAAP, 2012). Its current membership is about 2,100. After finishing a psychiatric residency and a year of specialized training, psychiatrists may take an ABMS-approved subspecialty examination in addiction psychiatry. The American Board of Psychiatry and Neurology's Subspecialty Board Certification in Addiction Psychiatry is officially recognized by ABMS.

The American Osteopathic Academy of Addiction Medicine seeks to improve the health of individuals and families burdened with the disease of addiction (AOAAM, 2011). A small number of osteopaths have completed the American Osteopathic Association's certification in addiction medicine, and several hundred have completed the ASAM certification.

There is also limited expertise among other health professions. With support from the Health Resources and Services Administration and the Substance Abuse and Mental Health Services Administration, the Association for Medical Education and Research in Substance Abuse drafted a strategic plan for interdisciplinary faculty development (Haack and Adger, 2002). The plan heightened the visibility of the need for increased training in addiction across all of the professions working in health care. Recommendations addressed training for allied health professionals, dentists, physicians, midwives, nurse practitioners, nurses, pharmacists, physician assistants, psychologists, social workers, and public health workers. In the ensuing decade, however, the incorporation of required SUD curricula into health professions education has been minimal. Graduates in these professions have little experience with and training in treating alcohol and drug use disorders.

Certification for expertise in addiction treatment is available for psychologists and nurses. In 1996, the American Psychological Association began offering a Certificate of Proficiency in the Treatment of Alcohol and other Psychoactive Substance Use Disorders. More than 1,000 have been certified. The International Nurses Society on Addictions (IntNSA) is a specialty organization founded in 1975 for nurses committed to prevention, intervention, treatment, and management for addictive disorders. IntNSA's mission is to advance excellence in nursing care for the prevention and treatment of addictions for diverse populations across all practice settings. With the American Nurses Association, IntNSA has established the *Scope and Standards of Addictions Nursing Practice* (IntNSA et al., 2004), a foundation upon which the certification in addiction nursing (Certified Addictions Registered Nurse [CARN] and CARN-Advanced Practice) is based. IntNSA has about 700 members (IntNSA, 2012).

REFERENCES

AAAP (American Academy of Addiction Psychiatry). 2012. *Mission statement.* http://www2.aaap.org/about-aaap/mission-statement (accessed June 15, 2012).

ABAM (American Board of Addiction Medicine). 2012. *About ABAM.* http://www.abam.net/about (accessed June 15, 2012).

Addiction Technology Transfer Center Network. 2012. *Certification information.* http://www.attcnetwork.org/find/certinfo (accessed June 15, 2012).

Alcoholics Anonymous World Services. 1939. *Alcoholics Anonymous.* New York: Works Publishing, Inc.

AOAAM (American Osteopathic Academy of Addiction Medicine). 2011. *Mission statement.* http://www.aoaam.org/content.php?pg=11 (accessed June 15, 2012).

ASAM (American Society of Addiction Medicine). 2012. *Membership.* http://www.asam.org/membership (accessed June 15, 2012).

Birch and Davis Associates, Inc. 1984. *Development of model professional standards for counselor credentialing* (Vol. 1). Rockville, MD: U.S. Department of Health and Human Services, Public Health Service, Alcohol, Drug Abuse, and Mental Health Administration, National Institute on Alcohol Abuse and Alcoholism.

Blocker, J. S., Jr. 2006. Did prohibition really work? Alcohol prohibition as a public health innovation. *American Journal of Public Health* 96(2):233-243.

Brown, B. S. 1997. Staffing pattern and services for the war on drugs. In *Treating drug abusers effectively,* edited by J. A. Egertson, D. M. Fox, A. I. Leshner, and M. M. Fund. Malden, MA: Blackwell. Pp. 99-124.

Camp, J. M., and N. R. Kurtz. 1982. Redirecting manpower for alcoholism treatment. In *Prevention, intervention and treatment: Concerns and models.* Rockville, MD: U.S. Department of Health and Human Services, Public Health Service, Alcohol, Drug Abuse, and Mental Health Administration, National Institute on Alcohol Abuse and Alcoholism. Pp. 371-397.

Gallon, S. L., R. M. Gabriel, and J. R. W. Knudsen. 2003. The toughest job you'll ever love: A Pacific Northwest Treatment Workforce Survey. *Journal of Substance Abuse Treatment* 24(3):183-196.

Haack, M. R., and H. Adger, Jr., eds. 2002. *Strategic plan for interdisciplinary faculty development: Arming the nation's health professional workforce for a new approach to substance use disorders.* Providence, RI: Association for Medical Education and Research in Substance Abuse.

IC&RC (International Certification and Reciprocity Consortium). 2012. *Setting global standards for addiction professionals.* http://internationalcredentialing.org (accessed May 28, 2012).

IntNSA (International Nurses Society on Addictions). 2012. *Our mission*. http://www.intnsa.org/home/index.asp (accessed June 15, 2012).

IntNSA, ANA (American Nurses Association), and NNSA (National Nurses Society on Addictions). 2004. *Scope and standards of addictions nursing practice*. Washington, DC: Nursesbooks.org, NNSA, ANA.

Kerwin, M. E., K. Walker-Smith, and K. C. Kirby. 2006. Comparative analysis of state requirements for the training of substance abuse and mental health counselors. *Journal of Substance Abuse Treatment* 30(3):173-181.

McCarty, D., B. E. Fuller, C. Arfken, M. Miller, E. V. Nunes, E. Edmundson, M. Copersino, A. Floyd, R. Forman, R. Laws, K. M. Magruder, M. Oyama, K. Prather, J. Sindelar, and W. W. Wendt. 2007. Direct care workers in the National Drug Abuse Treatment Clinical Trials Network: Characteristics, opinions, and beliefs. *Psychiatric Services* 58(2):181-190.

McCarty, D., K. J. McConnell, and L. A. Schmidt. 2010. Priorities for policy research on treatments for alcohol and drug use disorders. *Journal of Substance Abuse Treatment* 39(2):87-95.

Mulvey, K. P., S. Hubbard, and S. Hayashi. 2003. A national study of the substance abuse treatment workforce. *Journal of Substance Abuse Treatment* 24(1):51-57.

National Certification Commission. 2012. *National certification program*. http://www.naadac.org/index.php?option=com_content&view=article&id=478&Itemid=129 (accessed June 15, 2012).

ONDCP (Office of National Drug Control Policy). 2010. *National drug control strategy, 2010*. Washington, DC: ONDCP.

ONDCP. 2011. *National drug control strategy, 2011*. Washington, DC: ONDCP.

Tontchev, G. V., T. R. Housel, J. F. Callahan, M. M. Miller, and R. D. Blondell. 2011. Specialized training on addictions for physicians in the United States. *Substance Abuse* 32:84-92.

Appendix G

Access Standards for TRICARE Prime Enrollees

In the military's purchased care system, access to substance use disorder (SUD) care by family members and retirees[1] differs somewhat by TRICARE program. This appendix describes policies of TRICARE Prime, the largest program used by Active and Reserve Component family members when their military sponsor is called to active duty, as well as by retirees. Access standards for TRICARE Prime that apply to all health care needs of beneficiaries also apply to their behavioral health needs with few exceptions.

INITIAL ASSESSMENT

TRICARE Prime policy states that the initial visit to evaluate a new or recurring behavioral health problem is considered primary care, and the beneficiary should be evaluated by a provider who is professionally capable or specifically privileged to perform behavioral health assessments. Family members and retirees may choose whether to receive the initial assessment from their primary care provider, an integrated mental health provider within their primary care clinic, or a behavioral health care provider.

ROUTINE APPOINTMENT: NEW CONDITION

Policy states that beneficiaries requesting an appointment for a new or recurring behavioral health condition must be seen by an appropriately

[1] If retirees obtain Medicare Parts A and B they are no longer eligible for TRICARE Prime, but would instead be eligible for TRICARE for Life secondary coverage to Medicare.

trained provider within 7 calendar days and within 30 minutes' travel time of the beneficiary's residence. All TRICARE Prime beneficiaries have access to a primary care provider representative by telephone around the clock.

SPECIALTY APPOINTMENTS

Following an initial behavioral health assessment, referrals for additional care are to be provided within the access standard for specialty care, which is 4 weeks (28 days), unless the referring provider determines that care is needed more urgently. Beneficiaries must be offered an appointment with an appropriately trained provider within 1 hour's travel time from the beneficiary's residence. Military treatment facilities have first priority for providing referred specialty care or inpatient care for behavioral health conditions for all TRICARE Prime beneficiaries.

PRIOR APPROVAL

Referral by a primary care provider is not required for family members and retirees for the first eight outpatient behavioral health visits.

Appendix H

Levels of Care

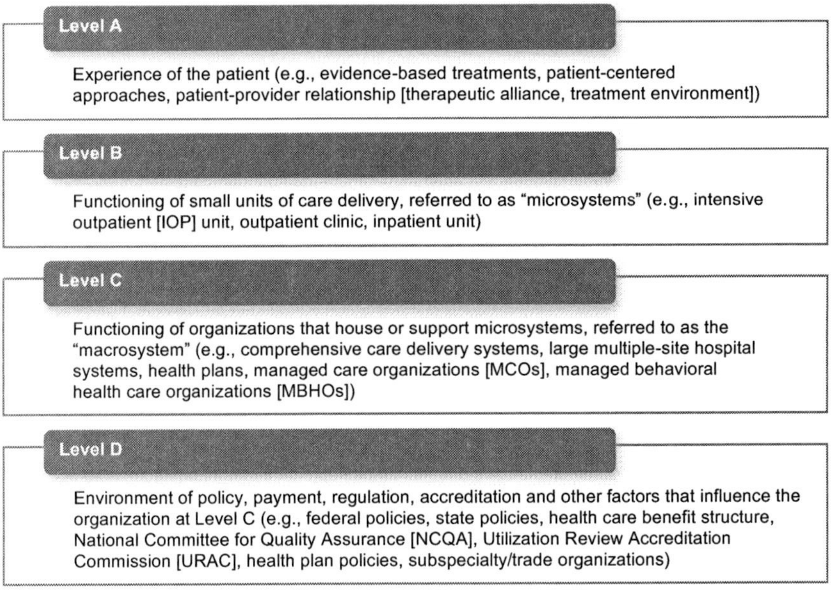

FIGURE H-1 Components of health care delivery systems.
SOURCE: Adapted from Berwick, 2002.

Figure H-1 depicts how the health care environment (i.e., policies, regulation, financing [Level D]), the organizational setting (i.e., health plans and health systems [Level C]), and the delivery of care (i.e., clinics [Level B]) combine to affect patient care (i.e., the patient experience [Level A]). The committee suggests that these four levels of care provide a blueprint applicable to the development of a 21st-century system of substance use disorder (SUD) prevention and treatment services within the U.S. military.

REFERENCE

Berwick, D. M. 2002. A user's manual for the IOM's "quality chasm" report. *Health Affairs* 21(3):80-90.

Appendix I

Summary of Policy-Relevant Strategies for the Prevention of Alcohol-Related Problems

TABLE I-1 Ratings of Policy-Relevant Strategies and Interventions

Strategy or Intervention	Effectiveness	Breadth of Research Support	Cross-National Testing	Cost to Implement or Sustain	Comments
Pricing and Taxation					**Generally evaluated in terms of how price changes affect population level alcohol consumption, alcohol-related problems and beverage preferences.**
Alcohol taxes	+++	+++	+++	Low	Increased taxes reduce alcohol consumption and harm. Effectiveness depends on government oversight and control of the total alcohol supply.
Minimum price	?	+	+	Low	Logic based on price theory, but there is very little evidence of effectiveness. Competition regulations and trade policies may restrict implementation.
Bans on price discounts and promotions	?	+	+	Low	Only weak studies in general populations of the effect of restrictions on consumption or harm; effectiveness depends on availability of alternative forms of cheap alcohol.
Differential price by beverage	+	+	++	Low	Higher prices for distilled spirits shifts consumption to lower alcohol content beverages resulting in less overall consumption. Evidence for the impact of tax breaks on low alcohol products is suggestive, but not comprehensive.
Special or additional taxation on alcopops and youth-oriented beverages	+	+	++	Low	Evidence that higher prices reduce consumption of alcopops by young drinkers without complete substitution; no studies of impact on harms.
Regulating Physical A vailability					Generally evaluated in terms of how changes in availability affect population level alcohol consumption and alcohol-related problems.
Ban on sales	+++	+++	++	High	Can reduce consumption and harm substantially, but often with adverse side-effects from black market, which is expensive to suppress. Ineffective without enforcement.

Bans on drinking in public places	?	+	++	Moderate	Generally focused on young or marginalized high-risk drinkers; may displace harm without necessarily reducing it.
Minimum legal purchase age	+++	+++	++	Low	Effective in reducing traffic fatalities and other harms with minimal enforcement but enforcement substantially increases effectiveness and cost.
Rationing	++	++	++	Moderate	Effects greater on heavy drinkers.
Government monopoly of retail sales	++	+++	++	Low	Effective way to limit alcohol consumption and harm. Public health and public order goals increase beneficial effects.
Hours and days of sale restrictions	++	++	+++	Low	Effective where changes in trading hours meaningfully reduce alcohol availability or where problems such as late night violence are specifically related to hours of sale.
Restrictions on density of outlets	++	+++	++	Low	Evidence for both consumption and problems. Changes to outlet numbers affect availability most in areas with low prior availability, but bunching of outlets into high-density entertainment districts may cause problems with public order and violence.
Different availability by alcohol strength	++	++	+	Low	Mostly tested for strengths of beer.
Modifying the Drinking Environment					**Generally evaluated in terms of how staff training, enforcement, and legal liability affect alcohol-related violence and other harms.**
Staff training and house policies relating to responsible beverage service (RBS)	0/+	+++	++	Moderate	Not all studies have found a significant effect of RBS training and house policies; needs to be backed by enforcement for sustained effects.

continued

TABLE I-1 Continued

Strategy or Intervention	Effectiveness	Breadth of Research Support	Cross-National Testing	Cost to Implement or Sustain	Comments
Staff and management training to better manage aggression	++	+	++	Moderate	Evidence currently limited to one randomized control study and supportive results from multi-component programs.
Enhanced enforcement of on-premises laws and legal requirements	++	++	++	Moderate	Sustained effects depend on making enhanced enforcement part of ongoing police practices.
Server liability	++	++	+	Low	Effect stronger where efforts made to publicise liability. Research limited to the United States and Canada.
Community action projects	++	++	++	Moderate to high	Need commitment to long time frame; uncertain which components are responsible for effects.
Voluntary codes of bar practice	O	++	++	Moderate	Ineffective when strictly voluntary but may contribute to effects as part of community action projects.
Late-night lockouts of licensed premises	O	+	+	Low to moderate	Limited research and no studies have identified effective approaches.
Drink-Driving Countermeasures					**Most research has focused on intervention effects on traffic accidents and recidivism after criminal sanctions.**
Sobriety checkpoints	++	+++	+++	Moderate	Effects of police campaigns typically short-term. Effectiveness as a deterrent is proportional to frequency of implementation and high visibility.
Random breath testing	+++	++	+	Moderate	Effectiveness depends on number of drivers directly affected and the extent of consistent and high-profile enforcement.
Lowered BAC Limits	+++	+++	++	Low	The lower the BAC legal limit, the more effective the policy. Very low BAC levels ("zero tolerance") are effective for youth, and can be effective for adult drivers but BAC limits lower than 0.02 are difficult to enforce.

Administrative license suspension	++	++	++	Moderate	When punishment is swift, effectiveness is increased. Effective in countries where it is applied consistently. Target population: high-risk drinkers.
Low BAC for young drivers ("zero tolerance")	+++	++	+	Low	Clear evidence of effectiveness for those below the legal drinking or alcohol purchase age.
Graduated licensing for novice drivers	++	++	++	Low	Can be used to incorporate lower BAC limits and licensing restrictions within one strategy. Some studies note that "zero tolerance" provisions are responsible for this effect.
Designated drivers and ride services	O	+	+	Moderate	Effective in getting impaired drinkers not to drive but do not affect alcohol-related accidents, perhaps because these services account for a relatively small percent of drivers.
Severity of punishment	0/+	++	++	Moderate	Mixed evidence concerning mandatory or tougher sanctions for drink-driving convictions. Effects decay over time unless accompanied by renewed enforcement or media publicity.
Restrictions on Marketing					**Better quality studies evaluate impact in terms of youth drinking and attitudes. Impact also studied in terms of ability to limit youth exposure to marketing campaigns.**
Legal restrictions on exposure	+/++	+++	++	Low	Strong evidence of dose-response effect of exposure on young peoples' drinking, but mixed evidence from ecological on per capita consumption; advertising bans or restrictions may shift marketing activities into less regulated media (e.g., Internet).
Legal restrictions on content	?	O	O	Low	Evidence that advertising content affects consumption but no evidence of the impact of content restrictions as embodied in industry self-regulation codes.
Alcohol industry's voluntary self-regulation codes	O	++	++	Low	Industry voluntary self-regulation codes of practice are ineffective in limiting exposure of young persons to alcohol marketing, nor do they prevent objectionable content from being aired.

continued

TABLE I-1 Continued

Strategy or Intervention	Effectiveness	Breadth of Research Support	Cross-National Testing	Cost to Implement or Sustain	Comments
Education and Persuasion					**Impact generally evaluated in terms of knowledge and attitudes; effect on onset of drinking and drinking problems is equivocal or minimal. Target population is young drinkers unless otherwise noted.**
Classroom education	0	+++	++	Moderate	May increase knowledge and change attitudes but has no long-term effect on drinking.
College student education — universal	0	+	+	Moderate	May increase knowledge and change attitudes but has no effect on drinking.
Brief interventions with high-risk students	+	+	+	High	Brief motivational interventions can impact drinking behaviour.
Mass media campaigns, including drink-driving campaigns	0	+++	++	Moderate	No evidence of impact of messages to the drinker about limiting drinking; messages to strengthen policy support untested.
Warning labels and signs	0	+	+	Low	Raise public awareness, but do not change drinking behaviour.
Social marketing	0	++	+	Moderate to high	Raises public awareness but alcohol specific campaigns do not change behaviour.
Treatment and Early Intervention					**Usually evaluated in terms of days or months of abstinence, reduced intensity and volume of drinking, and improvements in health and life functioning. Target population is harmful and dependent drinkers, unless otherwise noted.**
Brief intervention with at-risk drinkers	+++	+++	+++	Moderate	Can be effective but most primary care practitioners lack training and time to conduct screening and brief interventions.

Mutual help/self-help attendance	++	++	++	Low	A feasible, cost-effective complement or alternative to formal treatment in many countries.
Mandatory treatment of drink-driving repeat offenders	+	++	+	Moderate	Punitive and coercive approaches have time-limited effects, and sometimes distract attention from more effective interventions.
Medical and social detoxification	0	++	++	High	Safe and effective for treating withdrawal syndrome but have little effect on long-term alcohol consumption unless combined with other therapies.
Talk therapies	++	+++	++	Moderate	A variety of theoretically-based therapies to treat persons with alcohol dependence in outpatient and residential settings. Population reach is low because most countries have limited treatment facilities.
Pharmaceutical therapies	+	++	++	Moderate	Consistent evidence for a modest improvement over talk therapies and clinical management only for naltrexone.

The following rating scale was used to evaluate effectiveness

- 0 Evidence indicates a lack of effectiveness
- + Evidence for limited effectiveness
- ++ Evidence for moderate effectiveness
- +++ Evidence of a high degree of effectiveness
- ? No controlled studies have been undertaken or there is insufficient evidence upon which to make a judgment

SOURCE: Reprinted from Babor, T. F., R. Caetano, S. Casswell, G. Edwards, N. Giesbrecht, K. Graham, J. Grube, L. Hill, H. Holder, R. Homel, M. Livingston, E. Osterberg, J. Rehm, R. Room, and I. Rossow. 2010. *Alcohol: No ordinary commodity: Research and public policy.* Oxford, UK: Oxford University Press.

Appendix J

Biosketches of Committee Members and Staff

Charles P. O'Brien, M.D., Ph.D. (*Chair*), is Kenneth E. Appel professor and vice chair of psychiatry at the University of Pennsylvania and director of the Center for Studies of Addiction. Dr. O'Brien's work involves the discovery of central nervous system changes involved in relapse, new medications for addiction, behavioral treatments, and instruments for measuring the severity of addictive disorders. He led the discovery of the effects of alcohol on the endogenous opioid system and developed a completely new treatment for alcoholism. Many of his discoveries are now utilized in common practice for the treatment of addictive disorders throughout the world. Dr. O'Brien was elected to the Institute of Medicine (IOM) of the National Academies in 1991 and has received numerous national research awards, as well as an honorary doctorate from the University of Bordeaux in 1994. He received the Nathan B. Eddy award for research on addiction from the College on Problems of Drug Dependence in 2003, the American Psychological Association (APA) Research Award for 2000, the 2010 Gold Medal for Research from the Society on Biological Psychiatry, the 2010 Sarnat Award from the Institute of Medicine for Mental Health Research, and the 2012 Jellinek award for research on alcoholism. He has been an adviser on drug policy to local and national governments since the 1970s and has chaired or served as a member of numerous IOM committees dealing with the science and policy of abused drugs. He is currently chair of the substance use disorders committee for the *Diagnostic and Statistical Manual of Mental Disorders*, Fifth Edition (DSM-5). Dr. O'Brien is past president of the American College of Neuropsychopharmacology and the Association for Research in Nervous and Mental Disease. He earned his M.D. and Ph.D.

degrees from Tulane University. He received residency training at Harvard, Tulane, the University of London, and the University of Pennsylvania in internal medicine, neurology, and psychiatry and is board certified in both neurology and psychiatry.

Hortensia D. Amaro, Ph.D., is associate vice provost for community research initiatives and dean's professor of social work and preventive medicine at the University of Southern California. For the past 10 years, she served as associate dean and distinguished professor of health sciences and of counseling psychology in the Bouve College of Health Sciences, and director of the Institute on Urban Health Research at Northeastern University. Her research has focused on alcohol and drug use and addiction among adolescents and adults, the development and testing of behavioral interventions for HIV/AIDS prevention, substance abuse and mental health treatment for Latinos and African Americans, alcohol and drug use among college populations, behavioral interventions for adherence to HIV medications, and integration of behavioral health care into the pediatric medical home. She has authored more than 135 publications on these topics. Dr. Amaro has served on the editorial boards of the *American Psychologist, American Journal of Public Health, Cultural Diversity and Ethnic Minority Psychology*, and other leading publications. She was elected to the IOM of the National Academies in 2011 and has received numerous awards from professional, government and community organizations and honorary degrees from Simmons College and the Massachusetts School of Professional Psychology. Additionally, she has served on review and advisory committees for the National Institutes of Health (NIH), the U.S. Department of Health and Human Services, the Substance Abuse and Mental Health Services Administration, and the Centers for Disease Control and Prevention. Dr. Amaro founded five substance abuse treatment programs for women in Boston and served on the board of the Boston Public Health Commission for 14 years. She received her B.A., M.A., and Ph.D. degrees in psychology from the University of California, Los Angeles.

Rhonda Robinson Beale, M.D., is chief medical officer for OptumHealth Behavioral Solutions, a leading provider of solutions for mental health and substance use disorders in California. Dr. Robinson Beale develops quality initiatives and clinical systems for OptumHealth Behavioral Solutions. She has more than 20 years of experience in behavioral health and quality management and is an active member of the behavioral health community. Dr. Robinson Beale has been involved with the National Committee for Quality Assurance as a surveyor; a member of the Review Oversite Committee, which makes accreditation decisions; and a member of advisory panels that developed the managed behavioral health care organization

(MBHO) and disease management standards. She has also been a member of the board of directors for the IOM's Neuroscience and Behavioral Health and Health Care Services Boards and has served on several IOM committees. Dr. Robinson Beale participated on the National Quality Forum's board of directors as co-chair for the Evidence-Based Practices to Treat Substance Use Disorders Steering Committee. Before joining OptumHealth Behavioral Solutions, she was chief medical officer for PacifiCare Behavioral Health. She also served as senior vice president and chief medical officer for CIGNA Behavioral Health, national medical director for Blue Cross Blue Shield, executive medical director of medical and care management clinical programs for Blue Cross Blue Shield of Michigan, and senior medical director for behavioral medicine for Health Alliance Plan. Dr. Robinson Beale received her medical degree from Wayne State University and her psychiatric training at Detroit Psychiatric Institute. She is certified in psychiatry by the American Board of Psychiatry and Neurology.

Robert M. Bray, Ph.D., a fellow of the APA, is a senior research psychologist and director of the Substance Abuse Epidemiology and Military Behavioral Health Program at RTI International. His research interests focus on the epidemiology of substance use and other health behaviors in military and civilian populations, with an emphasis on understanding the prevalence, causes, correlates, and consequences of these behaviors. He has directed nine comprehensive worldwide Department of Defense health behavior surveys of active duty military personnel that have furnished the most widely cited data on substance use and health behaviors in the military and is preparing a book summarizing findings from these studies. He has directed and supported other studies in the military assessing health-related behaviors among the reserve component, risk and protective factors for initiation of tobacco and alcohol use, mental fitness and resilience among Army basic trainees, and a Web-based intervention to reduce heavy alcohol use. He is currently leading the RTI component of a large multi-institutional clinical trial to optimize usual primary care for soldiers with posttraumatic stress disorder and depression. Dr. Bray is principal editor of *Drug Use in Metropolitan America*, which integrates findings from a large-scale study of drug use among diverse populations in the Washington, DC, metropolitan area. He has published and presented widely in the area of substance use– and health-related behaviors. Dr. Bray previously served on an IOM committee examining drug use in the workplace. He received his Ph.D. in social psychology from the University of Illinois and his M.S. and A.B. degrees in psychology from Brigham Young University.

Raul Caetano, M.D., Ph.D., is regional dean and professor of epidemiology at the Dallas Regional Campus of the University of Texas School of Public

Health. He also is dean and professor of health care sciences and psychiatry at the School of Health Professions, University of Texas Southwestern Medical Center, in Dallas. His area of expertise is the epidemiology of substance use by minorities, including studies of the association between intimate partner violence and substance use. He is well published in this area and also serves on the editorial boards of many substance abuse journals. Dr. Caetano also serves on the advisory boards for several substance abuse agencies in his community. Before coming to the University of Texas system in 1998, he was a senior scientist and director of the California-based Alcohol Research Group, a National Alcohol Research Center funded by the National Institute on Alcohol Abuse and Alcoholism. He previously served on an IOM committee that examined coverage for substance abuse treatment. Dr. Caetano earned his M.D. in psychiatry from the State University of Rio de Janeiro in Brazil. From 1973 to 1974 he was at the London School of Hygiene and Tropical Medicine, and from 1973 to 1976 he was a research psychiatrist at the Institute of Psychiatry of the University of London in England. He also earned an M.P.H. in behavioral sciences and a Ph.D. in epidemiology, both from the School of Public Health, University of California, Berkeley.

Mathea Falco, J.D., is president of Drug Strategies, a nonprofit research institute in Washington, DC, established in 1992, that promotes more effective approaches to the nation's drug problems. She is a visiting scholar at the Harvard Law School Center for International Criminal Justice and was a fellow at Harvard's Weatherhead Center for International Affairs, as well as associate professor of public health, Weill Medical College/Cornell University, in New York City. The author of *The Making of a Drug Free America: Programs That Work* (Times Books, 1994), as well as numerous articles, Ms. Falco comments frequently on drug policy in the media and in public speeches across the country. Until 1993, she was director of health policy, Department of Public Health, Cornell University Medical College, in New York City. From 1977 to 1981, Ms. Falco was assistant secretary of state for International Narcotics Matters. Earlier, she served as chief counsel and staff director for the U.S. Senate Judiciary Committee's Juvenile Delinquency Subcommittee, special assistant to the president of the Drug Abuse Council, and senior associate of the Carnegie Endowment for International Peace. Ms. Falco received her B.A. from Radcliffe College and her J.D. from Yale Law School.

Joyce M. Johnson, D.O., M.A., is vice president of health sciences and chief medical officer in Battelle's Health and Life Sciences Global Business, located in Arlington, Virginia. She joined Battelle in December 2003 upon her retirement from the U.S. Public Health Service (Rear Admiral, Upper

Half). She had been assigned to the U.S. Coast Guard, Department of Homeland Security, as chief medical officer/director, health and safety, and functioned as the Coast Guard's surgeon general. Her other government assignments included senior scientific and management positions with the Food and Drug Administration and the Substance Abuse and Mental Health Services Administration. She has held clinical positions at the National Institute of Mental Health and the VA. At the Centers for Disease Control and Prevention, she was an Epidemiologic Intelligence Service officer and staff epidemiologist in the Center for Infectious Disease. Dr. Johnson is a physician board certified in three specialties—public health and preventive medicine, clinical pharmacology, and psychiatry. In addition to her medical degree, she earned a master's degree in hospital and health administration and has received five honorary doctoral degrees. She is a certified addiction specialist and certified food service executive. Dr. Johnson earned her bachelor's degree from Luther College, her master's degree in hospital and health administration from the University of Iowa, and her medical degree from Michigan State University.

Thomas Kosten, M.D., is the J.H. Waggoner chair and professor of psychiatry, pharmacology, and neuroscience, Baylor College of Medicine, and former professor and chief of psychiatry at Yale University and the VA in Connecticut. He is research director of the VA National Substance Use Disorders Quality Enhancement Research Initiative, based in Houston, Texas. Dr. Kosten is founder of the Division of Substance Abuse at Baylor and Yale and directs their NIH Medications Development Center for substance abuse. He has been supported by a Research Scientist Award from NIH since 1987 and has served on national and international review groups for medications development in substance abuse. Dr. Kosten has been a congressional fellow in the House of Representatives and a visiting professor in Canada, China, Germany, Greece, and Spain. He is founding vice chair for Added Qualifications in Addiction Psychiatry of the American Board of Psychiatry and Neurology, a distinguished fellow in the APA, a fellow of the American College of Neuropsychopharmacology, and past president of both the American Academy of Addiction Psychiatry and the College on Problems of Drug Dependence. Dr. Kosten received his B.S. from the Rensselaer Polytechnic Institute, his M.A. from Yale, and his M.D. from Cornell University Medical College.

Mary Jo Larson, Ph.D., is senior scientist at the Institute for Behavioral Health, Schneider Institutes for Health Policy, Heller School for Social Policy and Management, Brandeis University. She is a health services researcher specializing in access to and quality and cost of care delivered in mental health and substance abuse service delivery systems. She also has expertise in the military health care system and the impact of the Operation Iraqi Freedom and Operation Enduring Freedom conflicts on military families. With funding from the National Institute on Drug Abuse, she is conducting a study on recent combat veterans using longitudinal military health care data. Dr. Larson has conducted primary data collection studies on the outcomes of care in community-based detoxification programs and outpatient addiction programs within managed care and public systems, outcomes of integrated services for comorbid disorders for women with trauma and posttraumatic stress disorder, and other studies of service delivery systems for populations that are disenfranchised or experiencing chronic homelessness or incarceration. She has conducted secondary data analysis projects (Medicaid, Medicare, National Endangered Species Act Reform Coalition [NESARC]), including studies that merged large public-sector databases. Dr. Larson received her Ph.D. from The Heller School at Brandeis University, her M.P.A. from the John F. Kennedy School of Government at Harvard University, and her B.A. in psychology from the University of Minnesota.

David C. Lewis, M.D., is professor emeritus of community health and medicine and Donald G. Millar emeritus distinguished professor of alcohol and addiction studies at Brown University. In 1982 he founded and for 18 years he directed the Brown University Center for Alcohol and Addiction Studies. Dr. Lewis is a graduate of Brown University and Harvard Medical School. Trained in internal medicine, he is a fellow of the American College of Physicians. He has been a member of several boards of directors, including those of the National Council on Alcoholism and Drug Dependence (where he was chairman of the board), the American Society of Addiction Medicine, the Drug Policy Alliance, the Veterans Healing Initiative and the Association for Medical Education and Research in Substance Abuse. He is the founder of Physician Leadership on National Drug Policy (PLNDP) and now serves on the board of directors of the new PLNDP—Physicians and Lawyers for National Drug Policy. Dr. Lewis has an international reputation for his work on substance abuse treatment, medical education, and public policy.

Dennis McCarty, Ph.D., is professor in the Department of Public Health and Preventive Medicine at Oregon Health & Science University in Portland, Oregon, and co–principal investigator for the Western States Node of the National Drug Abuse Treatment Clinical Trials Network. Dr. McCarty collaborates with policy makers in state and federal government and with community-based programs to conduct studies that examine the organization, financing, and delivery of substance abuse treatment services. Between 1989 and 1995, Dr. McCarty served as director of the Massachusetts

Bureau of Substance Abuse Services for the Massachusetts Department of Public Health. He currently serves on Oregon's Alcohol and Drug Policy Commission. Dr. McCarty served on two prior IOM committees and was a co-editor for both committee reports: *Managing Managed Care: Quality Improvement in Behavioral Health Care* and *Bridging the Gap Between Practice and Research: Forging Partnerships with Community-Based Drug and Alcohol Treatment*. He received his B.A. degree in psychology and his M.A. and Ph.D. degrees in social psychology from the University of Kentucky. In 2007, he was named a fellow in the APA. He is a member of the editorial boards for the *Journal of Substance Abuse Treatment* and the *Journal of Behavioral Health Services and Research*.

Mary Ann Pentz, Ph.D., is professor of preventive medicine and director of the Institute for Health Promotion and Disease Prevention Research at the University of Southern California. Her research focuses on community and policy approaches to tobacco, alcohol, and drug abuse prevention in youth. She is widely published in psychology, public health, and medical journals on the use of multicomponent approaches to community-based prevention that include mass media. The findings from her longitudinal prevention trials contributed to the formulation of a U.S. Senate bill, as well as the use of evidence-based criteria for appropriating funds for prevention under the Safe and Drug Free Schools Act, for which she provided U.S. congressional testimony sponsored by Senator Kennedy. Dr. Pentz has chaired the National Institute on Drug Abuse Epidemiology and Prevention study section. She has served on the evaluation advisory boards for the Center for Substance Abuse Prevention's Community Partnership grants program and the Robert Wood Johnson Foundation's Fighting Back Initiative; on the Office of National Drug Control Policy's Campaign Design expert panel, tasked to design the new anti-drug abuse media campaigns; on the U.S.A. Horn General's Methamphetamine Task Force (under Janet Reno); and as a member of the NIH Peer Review Oversight Group (under the Clinton administration). Dr. Pentz received her B.A. in psychology from Hamilton College and her Ph.D. in psychology from Syracuse University.

Tracy Stecker, Ph.D., is assistant professor at the Psychiatric Research Center, Department of Community and Family Medicine, at Dartmouth Medical School and a health services researcher at the White River Junction VA. Dr. Stecker is a psychologist and mental health services researcher who focuses on help-seeking behavior in individuals with mental illness. She has received funding from the National Institute of Mental Health to develop and test cognitive-behavioral interventions designed to increase mental health treatment seeking among veterans returning from the wars in Iraq and Afghanistan, with a focus on those with symptoms of PTSD and suicidality. She has also received funding through the National Institute on Alcohol Abuse and Alcoholism to assess whether these interventions increase attendance at addiction treatment among individuals with alcohol use disorders. Dr. Stecker received her Ph.D. degree from the University of North Dakota, her M.A. degree from Austin Peay State University, and her B.A. degree from Clemson University.

Constance Weisner, Dr.P.H., M.S.W., is associate director for health services research at the Division of Research, Kaiser Permanente Medical Care Program, Northern California, and professor in the Department of Psychiatry at the University of California, San Francisco. She directs the Drug and Alcohol Research Team, a large program of substance use research in Kaiser Permanente. Dr. Weisner is a member of the World Health Organization's International Expert Advisory Council on Drug Dependence and Alcohol Problems, and a former member of the National Advisory Council of the National Institute on Drug Abuse and of the National Advisory Council of the Center for Substance Abuse Treatment, Substance Abuse and Mental Health Services Administration. Her research has been funded by the National Institute on Alcohol Abuse and Alcoholism, the National Institute on Drug Abuse, and the Robert Wood Johnson Foundation, and includes the epidemiology of alcohol and drug problems and access to, outcomes of, and cost impacts of substance use treatment. Dr. Weisner has served on several IOM committees addressing topics related to mental health and addiction, including the recent Committee on Improving the Quality of Health Care for Mental and Substance Use Conditions. Dr. Weisner received her doctorate in public health from the University of California, Berkeley, and her M.S.W. from the University of Minnesota.

Institute of Medicine Staff

Maryjo M. Oster, Ph.D., is a program officer and study director at the IOM. Prior to holding this position, she served as director of research and evaluation at the Pennsylvania Coalition to Prevent Teen Pregnancy (PCPTP), a statewide organization providing leadership on the issue of adolescent pregnancy prevention through advocacy, education, and support for community efforts. At PCPTP, she was the lead evaluator for a Centers for Disease Control and Prevention–funded project to promote science-based approaches to teen pregnancy prevention in schools and community settings. Dr. Oster earned her Ph.D. in educational theory and policy from The Pennsylvania State University. Research for her doctoral dissertation investigated sex education policies across the state of Pennsylvania and examined the social, political, and economic factors that influence the design and adoption of these policies.

Emily C. Morden, M.S.W., is a research associate with the Board on the Health of Select Populations at the IOM. Prior to working at IOM, she interned in the U.S. Senate, researching issues ranging from international trade relations to veteran health services. Before moving to Washington, DC, Ms. Morden resided in Oregon and worked as a medical social worker for a home hospice program. She has several years of experience working as a residential counselor in both adult and adolescent mental health treatment facilities for the largest community mental health care provider in the state of Oregon. In this role, Ms. Morden gained expertise and clinical skills in supporting clients in their recovery from mental illness. Ms. Morden holds an M.S.W. degree from Portland State University and a bachelor's degree in sociology from the University of Oregon.

Jon Q. Sanders is a veteran program associate with the Board on the Health of Select Populations at the IOM. He received his B.A. in anthropology with a minor in geosciences from Trinity University and recently completed the program management certification at George Mason University. In his 10 years with the National Academies, Mr. Sanders has worked on a variety of projects on topics ranging from childhood obesity to national security. He is coauthor of *Sitting Down at the Table: Mediation and Resolution of Water Conflicts* (2001). His research interests include public health, emergency management, and environmental decision making.

Frederick (Rick) Erdtmann, M.D., M.P.H., is a graduate of Bucknell University, where he received a B.S. degree in biology. He earned an M.P.H. from the University of California, Berkeley. He attended Temple University School of Medicine in Philadelphia, where he earned his doctorate of medicine. Dr. Erdtmann is board certified in preventive medicine. He spent 30 years as a commissioned officer in the U.S. Army Medical Department with a variety of assignments, including chief of the Preventive Medicine Services at Fitzsimons Army Medical Center, Frankfurt Army Medical Center in Germany, and Madigan Army Medical Center. He also served as division surgeon for the Second Infantry Division and as chief of the Preventive Medicine Consultant's Division in the surgeon general's office. Dr. Erdtmann served as commander of Evans Army Community Hospital from 1995 to 1997. He was deputy chief of staff for clinical operations within TRICARE Region 1 prior to assuming Hospital Command at Walter Reed Army Medical Center in March 1998. He then was assigned to the Office of the Surgeon General as deputy assistant surgeon general for force development. Following military retirement in 2001, Dr. Erdtmann joined the IOM. He currently serves as director of the Board on the Health of Select Populations (formerly the Board on Military and Veterans Health).